Practic
Transo
Echocardiography

# Practical Perioperative Transoesophageal Echocardiography

Edited by:

## David Sidebotham MBChB FANZCA
Anaesthetist
Departments of Anaesthesia and Intensive Care
Green Lane Hospital
Auckland, New Zealand

## Alan Merry MBChB FANZCA FFPMANZCA
Professor of Anaesthesiology
Department of Anaesthesia
University of Auckland
Auckland, New Zealand

## Malcolm Legget MBChB FRACP FACC
Consultant Cardiologist
Green Lane Hospital and Auckland Heart Group
Honorary Lecturer in Cardiology, University of Auckland
Auckland, New Zealand

BUTTERWORTH
HEINEMANN

Edinburgh • London • New York • Oxford • Philadelphia • St Louis • Sydney • Toronto • 2003

BUTTERWORTH-HEINEMANN
An imprint of Elsevier Limited

First published 2003
  Reprinted 2003, 2004

ISBN 0 7506 5496 1

**British Library Cataloguing in Publication Data**
A catalogue record for this book is available from the British Library.

**Library of Congress Cataloging in Publication Data**
A catalog record for this book is available from the Library of Congress.

**Notice**
Medical knowledge is constantly changing. Standard safety precautions must be followed, but as new research and clinical experience broaden our knowledge, changes in treatment and drug therapy may become necessary or appropriate. Readers are advised to check the most current product information provided by the manufacturer of each drug to be administered to verify the recommended dose, the method and duration of administration, and contraindications. It is the responsibility of the practitioner, relying on experience and knowledge of the patient, to determine dosages and the best treatment for each individual patient. Neither the Publisher nor the editors/contributors assume any liability for any injury and/or damage to persons or property arising from this publication.
The Publisher

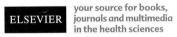
ELSEVIER
your source for books,
journals and multimedia
in the health sciences

**www.elsevierhealth.com**

The
publisher's
policy is to use
paper manufactured
from sustainable forests

Commissioning Editor: *Paul Fam*
Project Development Manager: *Belinda Henry*
Project Manager: *Mick Ruddy*
Designer: *Andy Chapman*
Illustrator: *Lily Ng*

Printed in China
C/03

To Jane Ferguson, Sally Merry and Carrie Hobson

# Contents

**CD-ROM** developed by David Sidebotham, John Faris, Alan Merry, Andrew Kerr

# Contributors

**Gerard Bashein** MD PhD
Professor of Anesthesiology
and Adjunct Professor of
Bioengineering
Department of Anesthesiology
University of Washington
School of Medicine
Seattle, Washington, USA

**Paul R Detmer** PhD
Principal Engineer
Ultrasound Engineering
Philips Medical Systems –
Ultrasound
Bothell, Washington, USA

**John Faris** MBChB DAvMed
FAFOM FANZCA BA
Fellow in Cardiac Anaesthesia
Department of Anaesthesia
Green Lane Hospital
Auckland, New Zealand

**Thomas Gentles** MB ChB
DCH FRACP
Paediatric Cardiologist
Department of Paediatric
Cardiology
Green Lane Hospital
Auckland, New Zealand

**Roger Hall** MBChB FANZCA
Consultant Cardiothoracic
Anaesthetist
Anaesthetic Department
Papworth Hospital
Cambridge, UK

**Marian Hussey** MBBCh
DA(SA) FCA(SA) FANZCA
Deputy Clinical Director and
Specialist Anaesthetist
Department of Anaesthsia
Green Lane Hospital
Auckland, New Zealand

**Mario Kalpokas** MBBS
FANZCA
Senior Visiting Anaesthetist
Department of Anaesthesia
St Vincent's Hospital
Melbourne, Australia

**Andrew Kerr** MA MBChB
FRACP
Head of Cardiology Department
Middlemore Hospital
Senior Clinical Lecturer
University of Auckland
Auckland, New Zealand

**Roman Kluger** MBBS
FANZCA Dip EpidBiostat
Senior Staff Anaesthetist
Department of Anaesthesia
St Vincent's Hospital
Melbourne, Australia

**Malcolm Legget** MBChB
FRACP FACC
Consultant Cardiologist
Green Lane Hospital and
Auckland Heart Group
Honorary Lecturer in Cardiology
University of Auckland
Auckland, New Zealand

**Andrew McKee** MBChB
FANZCA FFICANCA
Cardiothoracic Anaesthetist and
Intensivist
Department of Anaesthesia
Green Lane Hospital
Auckland, New Zealand

**Alan Merry** MBChB
FANZCA FFPMANZCA
Professor of Anaesthesiology
Department of Anaesthesia
University of Auckland
Auckland, New Zealand

**Colin Royse** MBBS MD
FANZCA
Consultant Cardiac Anaesthetist
Department of Anaesthesia and
Pain Management
Royal Melbourne Hospital
Melbourne, Australia

**David A Scott** MBBS
FANZCA
Deputy Director of Anaesthesia
Department of Anaesthesia
St Vincent's Hospital
Melbourne, Australia

**David Sidebotham**
MBChB FANZCA
Anaesthetist
Departments of Anaesthesia
and Intensive Care
Green Lane Hospital
Auckland, New Zealand

**Murali Sivarajan** MBBS
Professor of Anesthesiology
Department of Anesthesiology
Yale University
School of Medicine
New Haven, Connecticut, USA

**Damon C Sutton** MBBS
FANZCA
Senior Visiting Anaesthetist
Department of Anaesthesia
Monash Medical Centre
Melbourne, Australia

**Selwyn Wong** MBChB
FRACP
Consultant Cardiologist
Department of Medicine
Middlemore Hospital
Auckland, New Zealand

# Foreword

Transoesophageal echocardiography (TOE) has rapidly become the most powerful monitoring technique and diagnostic tool for the management of cardiac surgical patients. The explosive growth of this technology has been accompanied by widespread efforts to educate clinicians in its proper use through review courses, cardiac ultrasound textbooks, and electronic educational media. What has been needed, however, is a multimedia text that is focused specifically on the needs of the cardiac anaesthetist and intensivist. Fortunately, the publication of *Practical Perioperative Transoesophageal Echocardiography* now fills this void.

There are a number of features that distinguish this work. First and foremost, TOE is an image-based diagnostic technique and is best learned through the review of clear video loops that demonstrate the relevant pathology and its often subtle features. The CD-ROM portion of this work does an admirable job supplying this information in a clearly annotated form. While those beginning to learn TOE would want to use the CD in conjunction with the book, which provides much more complete information, the more advanced reader will find the CD to be a wonderful stand-alone review of a topic or a useful tool for a quick check of the important diagnostic features of a cardiac condition.

A second unique strength of this work is its attention to descriptive clarity, pertinent detail, and perioperative focus, accomplished largely through the editorial efforts of Drs Sidebotham, Merry and Legget. It is rare to find a multi-authored text with such consistent style from chapter to chapter, particularly since the chapter authors hail from no fewer than eight major cardiovascular units in New Zealand, Australia, the United Kingdom and the United States. The reader benefits in several ways. Nomenclature used to describe images and scan planes is consistent throughout and highlighted with wonderful line drawings that have striking explanatory power and visual appeal. There is little, if any, redundancy, and related topics are clearly linked through cross-referencing in the text and CD. Finally, perioperative echocardiographers will find just what they need to know in this work, without wading through an exhaustive discussion of echocardiography that is more relevant to the general practice of cardiac ultrasound. A perfect example of this was highlighted in my own practice recently when caring for a patient who had an unusually high, 5-m/sec peak velocity measured across a mechanical aortic valve following cardiopulmonary bypass. Critical clinical pearls relevant to this case were rapidly found in this book, including the effect of anaemia on pressure gradients, the distal pressure recovery phenomenon, the importance of using the reduced and not the simplified Bernoulli Equation when the proximal velocity is elevated, the relationship between flow and pressure gradient, and the flow independence of the continuity equation for estimating valve area.

*Practical Perioperative Transoesophageal Echocardiography* will appeal to an international readership, owing to the recognised expertise and experience of the authors and editors and their commitment to a consistent practice of perioperative echocardiography around the world. Indeed, I have had the privilege of working closely with many of these outstanding clinician-echocardiographers.

Perusal of the recently updated National Board of Echocardiography Perioperative Transesophageal Echocardiography Examination Content Outline reveals just how well this multimedia textbook covers the field of perioperative TOE. Sidebotham, Merry, Legget and their co-authors are to be applauded for producing a work that should be on the bookshelves of all perioperative echocardiographers, whether their primary fields are anaesthesia, intensive care medicine, cardiovascular surgery, or cardiology.

**Jonathan B. Mark, MD**
Professor and Vice Chairman
Department of Anesthesiology
Duke University Medical Center

Chief, Anesthesiology Service
Veterans Affairs Medical Center
Durham, North Carolina

January 2003

# Preface

Over the last decade transoesophageal echocardiography (TOE) has become integral to cardiac anaesthesia. It is now being used increasingly during non-cardiac surgery and in the intensive care unit. In consequence, large numbers of anaesthetists, intensivists, and cardiac surgeons have undertaken, or are considering undertaking, training in TOE. While establishing a perioperative TOE service in our own institution (Green Lane Hospital), it became apparent to us that a practical, up to date textbook on perioperative TOE, aimed at anaesthetists, intensivists and cardiac surgeons was not available; hence *Practical Perioperative Transoesophageal Echocardiography*.

This book does not attempt to provide a comprehensive review of TOE – instead the focus is on what really matters in the operating room and intensive care unit. Thus, there is extensive discussion of topics such as the examination of the mitral valve, common pitfalls in diagnosis and the assessment of haemodynamic instability, but very little information on issues not directly related to perioperative care (e.g. the differential diagnosis of restrictive cardiomyopathy).

This book is designed for use in the operating room or at the bedside in intensive care, as a practical reference. Numerous line drawings are included to facilitate an understanding of the important echocardiographic-anatomic relationships, with clear descriptions of probe manipulations and pitfalls in diagnosis. However, practical skills must be underpinned by a sound theoretical knowledge and we have sought to support the elements of a didactic manual with sufficient information and explanation to meet the needs of day-to-day practice. In doing this, we have attempted to cover the syllabus of the National Board of Echocardiography examination in perioperative TOE and to use the recommendations of the American Society of Echocardiography/Society of Cardiovascular Anesthesiologists regarding nomenclature, standard views and the conduct of a systematic examination. We hope, therefore, that in addition to its value in clinical practice, the book will prove very useful for candidates preparing for this formal examination.

All the authors are practising anaesthetists, cardiologists or intensivists (except Paul Detmer who is an ultrasound engineer). They come from several countries, with a wide range of expertise and experience between them. However, this book is not just a series of loosely related chapters by different authors. As editors we have worked hard with the authors to achieve a uniform style, avoid unnecessary duplication, provide appropriate cross-referencing between chapters and cover the overall subject of perioperative TOE in a coherent and logical fashion.

The book begins with five general chapters that introduce the role of TOE, the physics that underpins this modality, a description of normal views and how to obtain them, and a discussion of common pitfalls. Chapters 6 to 15 cover specific clinical topics ranging from the assessment of hypotension to the evaluation of the common congenital abnormalities encountered in adult practice. Because the calculations involved in elementary quantitative echocardiography share a common theoretical basis, we have dealt with this in one place (Chapter 16), with references to the relevant chapters for details of practical application.

The essence of echocardiography is the interpretation of abnormalities within and around a beating heart. As these appearances cannot be conveyed fully with text and still images alone, we have included a CD-ROM which contains over 400 short video clips illustrating a range of cardiovascular pathology. Each movie clip is accompanied by a short description of its contents and (in most cases) an annotated still frame. Virtually all of the topics discussed in the book have examples provided on the CD. In addition, one or two topics are covered on the CD which are not dealt with in the book (e.g. Ebstein's anomaly).

Together, we hope these two resources will prove useful and interesting to a wide range of practitioners and will benefit patients by promoting a higher standard of perioperative echocardiography.

David Sidebotham
Alan Merry
Malcolm Legget

Auckland

January 2003

# Acknowledgements

If we had known how much work would be involved in this book, we might not have started to write it. Fortunately, we have received an enormous amount of help from a great many individuals. We would like to thank them.

Lily Ng provided extensive assistance with the graphics; Diana Emmons and Jo Shepperson maintained and checked our database of references; David Linker (University of Washington Medical Center) provided advice on Chapter 9; Catherine Otto (University of Washington Medical Center) clarified a difficult point in relation to Chapter 3; and Jorry Lee and Charles Cruikshank (Philips Ultrasound) gave advice on cleaning and disinfecting the probe. Michael Harrison, Henry Connell, Neil Middleton, Jeremy Cooper, Bruce Anderson, Shay McGuinness, Jon Skinner, Ian Chapman, David Bain, Jane Ferguson, Mark Edwards and Geeta Sangamneker assisted with proof reading the manuscript and providing critical commentary on it. In addition, some chapter authors assisted with proofing other parts of the book and CD, including Selwyn Wong, Roger Hall, Andrew McKee, Marian Hussey and John Faris. We are very grateful to all these people.

The CD was a substantial project in its own right. Matthew Rowe of Webhead Ltd designed it. Additional video clips and images were identified and provided by Paul Forrest (Royal Prince Alfred Hospital, Sydney), James Lai and Lenore George (Westmead Hospital, Sydney), Cornelius Kruger (University of Washington Medical Center, Seattle), Neena Raizeda, Jon Skinner, the staff of the echocardiography lab at Green Lane Hospital (particularly Sally Greaves), and by the echocardiography lab at Middlemore Hospital. Several chapter authors also provided images and video clips, notably Selwyn Wong, Colin Royse and Roman Kluger. Jane Ferguson provided substantial help with editing the clips and John McDougall spent many hours checking them. Again, we are very grateful.

A grant from the Green Lane Research and Education Trust covered a number of incidental costs in the development of this book, and was very much appreciated. We would like to pay tribute to the ongoing value of this trust to many worthwhile activities in our hospital.

Working on a project of this type takes a great deal of time away from the normal duties and interactions of family life and on occasion also places an extra burden on colleagues at work. We acknowledge this and thank our families for their support. We would also like to thank all the members of the Department of Anaesthesia at Green Lane Hospital, including Sonia Botica and Louise Larsen, for their enthusiastic support for this undertaking.

# Abbreviations

The following abbreviations are used throughout the book.

2-D .... Two-dimensional
ASA .... American Society of Anesthesiologists
ASD .... Atrial septal defect
ASE .... American Society of Echocardiography
AV ..... Aortic valve
CW .... Continuous wave (Doppler)
EDA .... End diastolic area
EDV .... End diastolic volume
ECG .... Electrocardiograph
ECMO .. Extracorporeal membrane oxygenation
EF ..... Ejection fraction
ERO .... Effective regurgitant orifice
ESA .... End systolic area
ESPVR .. End systolic pressure–volume relationship
ESV .... End systolic volume
FAC .... Fractional area change
FFT .... Fast Fourier transform
HOCM .. Hypertrophic obstructive cardiomyopathy
ICU .... Intensive care unit
IVC ..... Inferior vena cava
IVRT .... Isovolumetric relaxation time
LA ..... Left atrium, left atrial
LV ..... Left ventricle, left ventricular
LVAD ... Left ventricular assist device
LVOT ... Left ventricular outflow tract
MV ..... Mitral valve
NL ..... Nyquist limit
OPCAB . Off-pump coronary artery bypass
PA ..... Pulmonary artery
PAC .... Pulmonary artery catheter
PAWP ... Pulmonary artery wedge pressure
PDA .... Posterior descending artery
PEEP ... Positive end-expiratory pressure
PFO .... Patent foramen ovale
PISA .... Proximal isovelocity surface area
PRF .... Pulse repetition frequency
PV ..... Pulmonary valve
PW ..... Pulse wave (Doppler)
RA ..... Right atrium, right atrial
RV ..... Right ventricle, right ventricular
RVOT ... Right ventricular outflow tract
SPTA ... Spatial peak temporal average
SAM .... Systolic anterior motion
SCA .... Society of Cardiovascular Anesthesiologists
SVC .... Superior vena cava
SWMA .. Segmental wall motion anomalies
TGC .... Time gain compensation
TOE .... Transoesophageal echocardiography, transoesophageal echocardiographic
TV ..... Tricuspid valve
VSD .... Ventricular septal defect

# The Role of Perioperative Transoesophageal Echocardiography

*David Scott*
*David Sidebotham*
*Alan Merry*

Transoesophageal echocardiography (TOE) has revolutionised cardiac anaesthesia, and has become increasingly important in the management of patients in the ICU and during certain non-cardiac surgical procedures. It provides the capacity to obtain detailed information about the structure and function of the heart and great vessels. Decisions guided by this information have the potential to substantially improve surgical, anaesthetic and intensive care management of patients during the perioperative period. However, TOE will improve patient outcome only if used competently and appropriately.

Many anaesthetists have adopted TOE without formal training.[1] This book is aimed at those who wish to undertake such training, and need a concise source of the essential information. Before considering *how* to use TOE competently it is important to know *when* to use it. It is also important to be familiar with matters (such as training, credentialling and quality assurance) that are critical to the setting up and running of a safe and effective perioperative TOE service.

## IMPACT OF PERIOPERATIVE TOE

It is very difficult to demonstrate that *any* monitoring device improves patient outcome; for instance, the value of pulse oximetry is almost universally accepted, yet a systematic review in the Cochrane library, which includes data from a randomised outcome trial in over 20 000 patients,[2,3] concludes by saying

> The results of the studies, despite an intense, methodical collection of data from a large population, indicate that perioperative monitoring with pulse oximetry does not improve reliable outcomes, effectiveness and efficiency.[4]

It also makes clear, however, that pulse oximetry enables the detection and treatment of hypoxaemia and promotes changes in patient care. Pulse oximetry is used in anaesthesia and intensive care for precisely this reason – it informs clinical decision making by providing objective information about the patient's status that otherwise could only be inferred from clinical signs, which often manifest late and unreliably. In the same way TOE provides a wealth of timely information about the filling status, systolic and diastolic function, the function of the intracardiac valves, the presence and effect of fluid in the pericardial cavity, and the state of the great vessels (amongst other things). A number of studies have demonstrated that TOE has a significant influence on surgical and medical decision making in anaesthesia and in intensive care.[5–15] In many instances these decisions lead to changes in therapy, in which the benefit to the individual patient is obvious. In some cases the advantage of TOE lies in the timeliness and confidence with which a decision is reached – in the treatment of postoperative pericardial tamponade, for example. In others the advantage may be more absolute; a therapeutic option is made possible because critical information is obtained during the operative period – reanastomosing an inadequately functioning coronary artery graft for example, or revising the strategy of aortic cannulation to take account of atheroma.

Similar comments apply to the cost–benefit analysis of intraoperative TOE.[16,17] Financial savings have been identified for the repair of valvular or congenital heart lesions, and appear likely for coronary artery bypass graft surgery or valve replacement. However, many questions remain unanswered. In particular, it is not clear whether such benefits apply to the routine, in contrast to the targeted, use of TOE.

## INDICATIONS FOR PERIOPERATIVE TOE

In 1996 the American Society of Anesthesiologists (ASA) and the Society of Cardiovascular Anesthesiologists (SCA) published the results of a task force on TOE entitled *Practice Guidelines for Perioperative Transesophageal Echocardiography*.[18] The task force divided indications into three categories (I–III) on the basis of the strength of evidence or expert opinion supporting a clinical benefit (Table 1.1).

- Category I indications are supported by the strongest evidence or expert opinion: TOE is *frequently useful* in improving outcome.

- Category II indications are supported by weaker evidence or expert consensus; TOE *may be useful* in improving outcome.

- Category III indications have little current scientific or expert support: TOE is *infrequently useful* in improving clinical outcome.

During the years since the guidelines were published new evidence has emerged in relation to the indications for TOE, and surgical practice has undergone certain changes. Some indications have become less important (e.g. the surgical correction of hypertrophic obstructive cardiomyopathy is now rare owing to advances in percutaneous alcohol injection techniques); other indications are now supported by new data

| **Table 1.1** Indications for TOE (modified from the ASA/SCA practice guidelines) |
| --- |
| **Category I:** supported by the strongest evidence or expert opinion; TOE is frequently useful in improving clinical outcome |
| Evaluation of acute, persistent and life-threatening haemodynamic instability in the operating room or ICU, in which ventricular function and its determinants are uncertain and have not responded to treatment |
| Intraoperative use in valve repair |
| Intraoperative use in congenital heart surgery for most lesions requiring cardiopulmonary bypass |
| Intraoperative use during repair of hypertrophic obstructive cardiomyopathy |
| Intraoperative use for endocarditis when preoperative testing was inadequate or extension of infection to perivalvular tissue is suspected |
| Preoperative use in unstable patients with suspected thoracic aortic aneurysms, dissections or disruptions who need to be evaluated quickly |
| Intraoperative assessment of aortic valve function in repair of aortic dissections |
| Intraoperative evaluation of pericardial window procedures |

| **Table 1.1** Continued |
|---|
| **Category II:** supported by weaker evidence or expert opinion; TOE may be useful in improving clinical outcome |
| Perioperative use in patients at increased risk of myocardial ischaemia or infarction |
| Perioperative use in patients at increased risk of haemodynamic disturbances |
| Intraoperative assessment of valve replacement |
| Intraoperative assessment of repair of cardiac aneurysms |
| Intraoperative evaluation of removal of cardiac tumours |
| Intraoperative detection of foreign bodies |
| Intraoperative detection of air emboli during cardiotomy, heart transplant and upright neurological procedures |
| Intraoperative use during intracardiac thrombectomy or pulmonary embolectomy |
| Intraoperative use for suspected cardiac trauma |
| Preoperative assessment of patients with suspected acute thoracic aortic dissections, aneurysms or disruptions |
| Intraoperative use during repair of thoracic aortic dissections without suspected aortic valve involvement |
| Intraoperative evaluation of aortic atheromatous disease or other sources of aortic emboli |
| Intraoperative evaluation of pericardectomy, pericardial effusions or evaluation of pericardial surgery |
| Intraoperative evaluation of anastomotic sites during heart and/or lung transplantation |
| Monitoring placement and function of assist devices |
| **Category III:** little current scientific or expert support; TOE is infrequently useful in improving outcome |
| Intraoperative evaluation of myocardial perfusion, coronary artery anatomy, graft patency or cardio-plegia administration |
| Intraoperative use during cardiomyopathies other than hypertrophic obstructive cardiomyopathy |
| Intraoperative use for uncomplicated endocarditis during non-cardiac surgery |
| Intraoperative monitoring for emboli during orthopaedic procedures |
| Intraoperative assessment of repair of thoracic aortic injuries |
| Intraoperative use for uncomplicated pericarditis |
| Intraoperative evaluation of pleuropulmonary diseases |
| Monitoring placement of intra-aortic balloon pump, automatic implantable cardiac defibrillators or pulmonary artery catheters |

(e.g. the routine use of TOE during aortic valve replacement[19]) and new indications not addressed by the 1996 guidelines have emerged (e.g. thoracic aortic endoluminal stent placement[20]). Some of these more recently established indications are discussed below.

## Consolidated and emerging indications

### Assessment of ventricular function in high-risk patients

The routine use of TOE in high-risk patients undergoing coronary artery surgery has a significant impact on decision making.[15] It is likely that TOE is also of benefit in other patients who are at increased risk of important haemodynamic instability (e.g. patients with impaired left ventricle (LV) function undergoing valve replacement or aortic surgery). A benefit has also been demonstrated in patients with coronary artery disease or ventricular dysfunction undergoing non-cardiac surgery in general[13] and major vascular surgery in particular.[14]

### TOE as a substitute for the pulmonary artery catheter

Advantages have been demonstrated for TOE over the use of a pulmonary artery catheter (PAC) for monitoring global and regional systolic LV function, and for guiding fluid administration.[5,6–11] In particular, in the setting of reduced LV compliance, TOE provides information on preload reserve (p.90) not available from a PAC.[21–23]

In many situations, rapid assessment with TOE may rule out significant ventricular dysfunction or tamponade and negate the need to place a PAC. In emergencies, TOE provides a more immediate source of information about cardiac function than a PAC because the probe can be inserted within seconds, whereas it may take some time to set up and place a PAC.

Although TOE has almost certainly reduced the requirement for pulmonary artery catheterisation, it is unlikely to replace it entirely. Some diagnoses are more easily made with a PAC (e.g. low systemic vascular resistance; p.91) and, while LA pressure can be estimated from TOE (p.126), in most circumstances this information is more accurately obtained from a PAC. In some situations each of these monitors contributes information important in making the diagnosis (e.g. in reduced LV compliance; p.90). Furthermore, the PAC is more suitable for ongoing monitoring in the ICU.

### Assessment of atheroma

Dislodgement of aortic atheroma is a leading cause of stroke and neurocognitive dysfunction following cardiac surgery. The likelihood that clinically important atheroma will be present is strongly associated with increasing age. Assessment of aortic atheroma with a combination of TOE and epiaortic scanning should be considered a routine part of the assessment of all cardiac surgical patients over 70 years of age (pp.173–176).

### Assessment of the risk of gas embolism

Gas retention within the heart or pulmonary veins is well recognised during open heart procedures such as valvular surgery, but is also seen following coronary artery bypass grafting – particularly if a venting device is used. This retained gas may embolise into the systemic circulation on restoration of cardiac output and cause harm to the brain and other organs.

The time required to de-gas the heart varies considerably from patient to patient, even if carbon dioxide flooding of the pericardium has been performed. TOE provides a means of identifying patients in whom de-airing has been inadequate and in whom additional steps, such as prolonged venting, may be required to ensure complete wash-out of gas before weaning from cardiopulmonary bypass.

In patients at risk of venous air embolism during neurosurgery TOE may identify the presence of a patent foramen ovale or atrial septal defect that might contraindicate a head-up position.

## Use during placement of left ventricular assist device

TOE provides information on the presence of atrial shunting, aortic regurgitation, intra-cardiac thrombus and right ventricle (RV) function relevant to patients undergoing LV assist device placement (pp.217–219).[24] TOE is also useful in the assessment of ventricular function during weaning from temporary LV assistance or extracorporeal membrane oxygenation (ECMO).

## Positioning of cannulae

In patients undergoing standard bicaval cannulation TOE is useful for visualisation of the relationship between the venous cannula, the inferior vena cava (IVC) and the hepatic veins. For patients undergoing femoral venous cannulation (e.g. aortic aneurysm surgery or ECMO), TOE facilitates correct placement of the cannula tip in the right atrium (RA). TOE may also identify abnormalities of the coronary sinus and facilitate the correct placement of a coronary sinus cannula.

## Deployment of intravascular devices and minimally invasive surgery

TOE is helpful in a number of techniques involving percutaneous intravascular device placement, such as endoluminal stenting of thoracic aortic aneurysms[20] and transcatheter closure of atrial septal defects (p.223).

There is growing interest in minimally invasive approaches to coronary revascularisation and valve repair or replacement. In such procedures surgical inspection of the heart is limited and the ability to visualise the heart with TOE is very important.

## Off-pump coronary artery bypass graft surgery

The benefit of TOE in off-pump coronary surgery has not yet been demonstrated. However, TOE provides important information on global and regional LV function, RV function, the development of new mitral or tricuspid regurgitation, volume status and the presence of aortic atheroma. Furthermore, it may provide early warning of impending cardiovascular collapse (pp.114–115).

## Assessment of myocardial perfusion

Contrast echocardiography, an evolving technique that is not widely available, has the potential to allow assessment of myocardial perfusion in real time (p.9).

## Differential diagnosis of pulmonary oedema in the ICU

Up to 50% of patients with acute pulmonary oedema have normal systolic function (p.127). TOE is useful in differentiating between systolic and diastolic dysfunction and in ruling out other causes of pulmonary oedema, such as mitral regurgitation.

## Valve replacement surgery

Further evidence supporting the use of TOE in valve replacement surgery has been published since 1996 (p.183).

## Echocardiography in the ICU

Echocardiography has a number of indications in the ICU (Table 1.2). In the ICU, unlike the operating room, patients can readily be examined with transthoracic echocardiography. Transthoracic imaging is less invasive than TOE, and is more reliable for the visualisation of the LV apex and the ventricular aspect of a prosthetic mitral valve (MV). Furthermore, it can more easily be performed in non-ventilated patients. However,

| Table 1.2 Indications for TOE in a mixed ICU environment[25] | |
|---|---|
| **Indication** | **No. (%) (total patients 113)** |
| Suspected endocarditis | 33 (29%) |
| Aortic dissection | 25 (22%) |
| Source of emboli | 19 (17%) |
| Haemodynamic instability | 15 (13%) |
| Miscellaneous | 21 (19%) |
|     Prosthetic valve assessment | 8 |
|     Suspected shunt in hypoxic patients | 3 |
|     Limited transthoracic echocardiogram | 3 |
|     Follow up of endocarditis | 3 |
|     Suspected pulmonary embolus | 2 |
|     Suspected mediastinal mass | 1 |
|     Mitral regurgitation following aortic valve replacement | 1 |

image quality in ventilated patients in the ICU is usually much better with TOE; for example, in a study of hypotensive, ventilated ICU patients, transthoracic imaging produced inadequate views in 64% of cases (compared with 3% of cases studied using TOE).[10] Factors that predispose to poor image quality with transthoracic echocardiography include mechanical ventilation, recent sternotomy, obesity and chronic obstructive respiratory disease. In some situations it may be necessary to use both imaging modalities (e.g. the assessment of prosthetic AV function).

## SAFETY AND CONTRAINDICATIONS

TOE is minimally invasive and complications are infrequent (Table 1.3), provided care is exercised and contraindications are respected (Table 1.4). In two large series involving over 17 000 surgical[26] and cardiological patients,[27] only one death directly related to TOE was reported. Gastrointestinal haemorrhage and oesophageal perforation are rare, but potentially fatal. Furthermore, in the anaesthetised patient, their diagnosis may be delayed. Preoperative assessment should include questions regarding dental status, swallowing difficulties, the presence of a hiatus hernia and prior gastric or oesophageal surgery. To minimise the potential for pharyngeal or oesophageal damage it is important that if significant resistance is met the probe is not advanced. In such situations, if simple manipulations to advance the probe are unsuccessful (p.45) it is preferable to abandon the procedure rather than risk injury to the patient.

The probe should not be left in a fixed, flexed position in the oesophagus for prolonged periods of time, because its pressure may cause damage. It may also become hot, relative to the patient (especially during cardiopulmonary bypass), so ultrasound output should be suspended (by turning the power output down or freezing the image) while the probe is not in use.

| Table 1.3 Complications associated with the use of intraoperative TOE[26] | |
|---|---|
| **Complication** | **Incidence (%)** |
| Odynophagia | 0.10 |
|    Swallowing abnormality | 0.01 |
|    Oesophageal abrasions | 0.06 |
|    No associated pathology | 0.03 |
| Upper gastrointestinal haemorrhage | 0.03 |
| Oesophageal perforation | 0.01 |
| Dental injury | 0.03 |
| Endotracheal tube malposition | 0.03 |
| Total | 0.20 |

| Table 1.4 Contraindications to perioperative TOE[28] | |
|---|---|
| **Absolute** | **Relative** |
| Perforated viscus | Atlantoaxial joint disease |
| Oesophageal stricture | Prior irradiation to the chest |
| Active upper gastrointestinal bleeding | Hiatal hernia |
| Oesophageal tumours | |
| Oesophageal diverticula | |
| Oesophageal scleroderma | |
| Recent upper gastrointestinal surgery | |
| Oesophageal varices | |

Misinterpretation of data is an obvious risk of TOE. The consequences of this may range from the inappropriate administration of fluid to an incorrect decision to replace a valve or to leave a non-functioning coronary graft. A rigorous programme of education, credentialling and quality assurance is strongly recommended to minimise this risk (see below).

## THE REQUIREMENTS OF A PERIOPERATIVE TOE SERVICE

The cardiac anaesthesia community has adopted perioperative TOE with enthusiasm. As early as 1992, 91% of anaesthesia training programmes in the USA used intraoperative TOE, with the anaesthetist being primarily responsible for interpretation in 54% of cases.[29] Current figures are not available but it is likely that the anaesthetist is now the primary echocardiographer for the great majority of perioperative TOE services. This new role as cardiac diagnostician has created exciting opportunities for improved patient care and enhanced cooperation between anaesthetists, cardiologists and cardiac surgeons. However, with this new role has come additional responsibility.

Ideally these responsibilities should be formalised within the framework of a perioperative TOE service. This will typically consist of a number of credentialled physicians under the guidance of a director of perioperative TOE. The director should develop practice guidelines, a credentialling process and a quality assurance programme. Proper procedures for the cleaning and maintenance of equipment should be established (see Appendix 1). A close working relationship with on-site echocardiologists will enhance any perioperative TOE service; advantages include assistance with training and quality assurance, advice with difficult cases and cooperation with research.

## Training and credentialling

Given the potential for harm to patients of the misinterpretation of findings with TOE, it is absolutely essential that TOE is undertaken by appropriately trained and skilled practitioners who understand its indications, contraindications, limitations and risks – and who appreciate their own limitations. Knowing when to ask for a second opinion from a more experienced practitioner is very important. The ASA/SCA guidelines[18] identify two levels of training: basic and advanced.

Practitioners with basic training are considered able to use TOE for indications that lie within the customary practice of anaesthesia (e.g. assessment of ventricular function and gross valvular pathology).

Practitioners with advanced training are considered able to use the full diagnostic potential of TOE (e.g. to assess valvular pathology using the techniques of quantitative Doppler).

In the USA certification in perioperative TOE is administered by the National Board of Echocardiography (NBE: http://www.echoboards.org/) and involves passing an examination (syllabus published by the NBE at http://www.echoboards.org/pte/outline.html) and completing specified training. The requirements for training, established by a working party of the SCA/ASE,[30] involve:

- Basic training – 150 TOE examinations, of which at least 50 must be personally performed, interpreted and reported by the trainee.

- Advanced training – 300 TOE examinations, of which at least 150 must be personally performed, interpreted and reported by the trainee.

The NBE examination is available to people from all countries. As yet, no other organisation has established an international process of certification.

Credentialling is a hospital-specific process by which physicians are granted privileges to practise perioperative TOE. Credentialling may or may not utilise NBE certification, and needs to take into account the resources and needs of the particular institution. Credentialling should be formalised and explicit. Furthermore, to reduce the risk of incorrect or missed diagnoses, all trainees should work under the direct supervision of a credentialled physician until they have completed their training.

There is a strong argument against the use of TOE by occasional, non-credentialled, practitioners who have undergone no formal training.[1]

## Reporting, archiving and quality assurance

Every TOE examination should be recorded on archivable media. These studies should be reviewed at regular quality assurance meetings. Off-line review is limited in a significant proportion of cases by poor quality of the recorded images,[31] so attention should be paid to ensuring that the recorded studies are suitable for review by independent echocardiographers. In addition, a written report should be provided and archived by the service, and a copy included in the patient's notes. A model report is available from the SCA website (http://www.scahq.org/sca3/teereport.shtml).

## Should TOE be used routinely in all cardiac surgical patients?

The routine use of TOE in all patients undergoing cardiac surgery has become the norm in many units. This approach promotes the acquisition and maintenance of skill on the part of practitioners, facilitates the teaching of novices and results in important changes in surgical and anaesthetic management in some patients in whom TOE might not otherwise have been used. However, it is more costly, in terms of equipment and staffing, to use TOE routinely rather than selectively. The need to cover cases outside normal working hours, and the need to avoid compromising anaesthetic vigilance, should also be considered.[32] The resolution of these issues will to a large part depend on the resources of each particular institution.

## Informed consent

In a cardiac surgical unit in which TOE has become an integral part of anaesthetic monitoring, it can be argued that explicit informed consent (over and above that obtained for anaesthesia) is unnecessary. However, the position of the courts in this matter varies from jurisdiction to jurisdiction. In many countries the landmark Australian case of *Rogers v. Whittaker* ((1992) 67 ALJR 47) has been influential. In this case the judges held that the information to be disclosed was not that thought reasonable by other doctors, but rather that which a reasonable patient in the circumstances of the particular patient might wish to know. Unfortunately this is somewhat unpredictable.[33] It would therefore seem prudent to discuss with patients the serious risks associated with all aspects of their anaesthetic management, including the use of TOE. In circumstances in which TOE is not routine in a particular institution, or its risk is unusually high (e.g. in the presence of oesophageal varices), it would be wise to obtain explicit consent.

## Future directions

Progress in computer technology, and the development of more compact and capable transducers, will bring developments from the research setting into standard clinical practice.

Three-dimensional image reconstruction is already possible, but depends on the acquisition of suitable images and requires significant computer processing power. Considerable expertise may be required to interpret these images.

Real-time continuous assessment of LV function is a goal that is close to realisation. Newer techniques for improved image definition, such as first- and second-order harmonic detection, are being used to enhance existing automated endocardial border detection technologies (p.104). Tissue Doppler imaging permits the quantitative assessment of muscle contraction and relaxation and has already had a major impact in the diagnosis of diastolic dysfunction (p.126). Defining the epicardial border presents more of a challenge, but will allow better assessment of wall motion abnormalities.

The distribution of blood flow and cardioplegia can be identified with contrast echocardiography.[34] Ultrasonic contrast media (sonicated albumin, micelles, saccharides) for facilitation of cavity detection are already available. The routine verification of graft function and assessment of myocardial perfusion should become possible using improved probes with these media as contrast.

TOE machines designed specifically for intraoperative use and more ergonomically suited to this working environment are becoming available, and are likely to become less expensive (and therefore more attractive for routine clinical use). The equipment is becoming smaller, and in some cases more specialised: already, devices that can perform simple two-dimensional imaging from compact probes are available for the measurement of cardiac output.[35,36]

The rapid uptake and development of TOE, which has occurred over the last 15 years, is likely to continue as the indications for its use become clearer, the equipment becomes less expensive and formal training programmes are developed. The use of TOE is likely to increase, particularly in the critical care setting and in high-risk patients undergoing non-cardiac surgery and minimally invasive cardiac surgical procedures.

# REFERENCES

1. Jacka MJ, Cohen MM, To T, et al. The use of and preferences for the transesophageal echocardiogram and pulmonary artery catheter among cardiovascular anesthesiologists. *Anesthesia and Analgesia* 2002;94:1065–1071.
2. Moller JT, Pedersen T, Rasmussen LS, et al. Randomized evaluation of pulse oximetry in 20,802 patients: I. Design, demography, pulse oximetry failure rate, and overall complication rate. *Anesthesiology* 1993;78:436–444.
3. Moller JT, Johannessen NW, Espersen K, et al. Randomized evaluation of pulse oximetry in 20,802 patients: II. Perioperative events and postoperative complications. *Anesthesiology* 1993;78:445–453.
4. Pedersen T, Dyrlund Pedersen B, Moller AM. Pulse oximetry for perioperative monitoring. *The Cochrane Database of Systematic Reviews* 2002.
5. Bergquist BD, Bellows WH, Leung JM. Transesophageal echocardiography in myocardial revascularization: II. Influence on intraoperative decision making. *Anesthesia and Analgesia* 1996;82:1139–1145.
6. Mishra M, Chauhan R, Sharma KK, et al. Real-time intraoperative transesophageal echocardiography – how useful? Experience of 5,016 cases. *Journal of Cardiothoracic and Vascular Anesthesia* 1998;12:625–632.
7. Couture P, Denault AY, McKenty S, et al. Impact of routine use of intraoperative transesophageal echocardiography during cardiac surgery. *Canadian Journal of Anesthesia* 2000;47:20–26.
8. Sutton DC, Kluger R. Intraoperative transoesophageal echocardiography: impact on adult cardiac surgery. *Anaesthesia and Intensive Care* 1998;26:287–293.
9. Michel-Cherqui M, Ceddaha A, Liu N, et al. Assessment of systematic use of intraoperative transesophageal echocardiography during cardiac surgery in adults: a prospective study of 203 patients. *Journal of Cardiothoracic and Vascular Anesthesia* 2000;14:45–50.
10. Heidenreich PA, Stainback RF, Redberg RF, et al. Transesophageal echocardiography predicts mortality in critically ill patients with unexplained hypotension. *Journal of the American College of Cardiology* 1995;26:152–158.
11. Benjamin E, Griffin K, Leibowitz AB, et al. Goal-directed transesophageal echocardiography performed by intensivists to assess left ventricular function: comparison with pulmonary artery catheterization. *Journal of Cardiothoracic and Vascular Anesthesia* 1998;12:10–15.
12. Poelaert JI, Trouerbach J, De Buyzere M, et al. Evaluation of transesophageal echocardiography as a diagnostic and therapeutic aid in a critical care setting. *Chest* 1995;107:774–779.
13. Kolev N, Ihra G, Swanevelder J, et al. Biplane transoesophageal echocardiographic detection of myocardial ischaemia in patients with coronary artery disease undergoing non-cardiac surgery: segmental wall motion vs. electrocardiography and haemodynamic performance. *European Journal of Anaesthesiology* 1997;14:412–420.
14. Gillespie DL, Connelly GP, Arkoff HM, et al. Left ventricular dysfunction during infrarenal abdominal aortic aneurysm repair. *American Journal of Surgery* 1994;168:144–147.
15. Savage RM, Lytle BW, Aronson S, et al. Intraoperative echocardiography is indicated in high-risk coronary artery bypass grafting. *Annals of Thoracic Surgery* 1997;64:368–374.
16. Benson MJ, Cahalan MK. Cost-benefit analysis of transesophageal echocardiography in cardiac surgery. *Echocardiography* 1995;12:171–183.
17. Ionescu AA, West RR, Proudman C, et al. Prospective study of routine perioperative transesophageal echocardiography for elective valve replacement: clinical impact and cost-saving implications. *Journal of the American Society of Echocardiography* 2001;14:659–667.
18. American Society of Anesthesiologists and the Society of Cardiovascular Anesthesiologists Task Force on Transesophageal Echocardiography. Practice guidelines for perioperative transesophageal echocardiography. *Anesthesiology* 1996;84:986–1006.
19. Nowrangi SK, Connolly HM, Freeman WK, et al. Impact of intraoperative transesophageal echocardiography among patients undergoing aortic valve replacement for aortic stenosis. *Journal of the American Society of Echocardiography* 2001;14:863–866.
20. Rapezzi C, Rocchi G, Fattori R, et al. Usefulness of transesophageal echocardiographic monitoring to improve the outcome of stent-graft treatment of thoracic aortic aneurysms. *American Journal of Cardiology* 2001;87:315–319.
21. Çiçek S, Demirkiliç U, Kuralay E, et al. Prediction of intraoperative hypovolemia in patients with left ventricular hypertrophy: comparison of transesophageal echocardiography and Swan–Ganz monitoring. *Echocardiography* 1997;14:257–260.
22. Cheung AT, Savino JS, Weiss SJ, et al. Echocardiographic and hemodynamic indexes of left ventricular preload in patients with normal and abnormal ventricular function. *Anesthesiology* 1994;81:376–387.

23. Swenson JD, Bull D, Stringham J. Subjective assessment of left ventricular preload using transesophageal echocardiography: corresponding pulmonary artery occlusion pressures. *Journal of Cardiothoracic and Vascular Anesthesia* 2001;15:580–583.

24. Savage RM, Scalia G, Smidera N, et al. Intraoperative echocardiography is indicated in implantable left ventricular assist device placement [abstract]. *Journal of the American Society of Echocardiography* 1996;9:375.

25. Chenzbraun A, Pinto FJ, Schnittger I. Transesophageal echocardiography in the intensive care unit: impact on diagnosis and decision-making. *Clinical Cardiology* 1994;17:438–444.

26. Kallmeyer IJ, Collard CD, Fox JA, et al. The safety of intraoperative transesophageal echocardiography: a case series of 7200 cardiac surgical patients. *Anesthesia and Analgesia* 2001;92:1126–1130.

27. Daniel WG, Erbel R, Kasper W, et al. Safety of transesophageal echocardiography: a multicenter survey of 10,419 examinations. *Circulation* 1991;83:817–821.

28. Kallmeyer I, Morse DS, Body SC, et al. Case 2–2000. Transesophageal echocardiography-associated gastrointestinal trauma. *Journal of Cardiothoracic and Vascular Anesthesia* 2000;14:212–216.

29. Poterack KA. Who uses transesophageal echocardiography in the operating room? *Anesthesia and Analgesia* 1995;80:454–458.

30. Cahalan MK, Abel M, Goldman M, et al. American Society of Echocardiography and Society of Cardiovascular Anesthesiologists task force guidelines for training in perioperative echocardiography. *Anesthesia and Analgesia* 2002;94:1384–1388.

31. Rafferty T, LaMantia KR, Davis E, et al. Quality assurance for intraoperative transesophageal echocardiography monitoring: a report of 846 procedures. *Anesthesia and Analgesia* 1993;76:228–232.

32. Weinger MB, Herndon OW, Gaba DM. The effect of electronic record keeping and transesophageal echocardiography on task distribution, workload, and vigilance during cardiac anesthesia. *Anesthesiology* 1997;87:144–155.

33. Garden AL, Merry AF, Holland RL, et al. Anaesthesia information – what patients want to know. *Anaesthesia and Intensive Care* 1996;24:594–598.

34. Kaul S. Myocardial contrast echocardiography: 15 years of research and development. *Circulation* 1997;96:3745–3760.

35. Marik PE. Pulmonary artery catheterization and esophageal Doppler monitoring in the ICU. *Chest* 1999;116:1085–1091.

36. Madan AK, UyBarreta VV, Aliabadi-Wahle S, et al. Esophageal Doppler ultrasound monitor versus pulmonary artery catheter in the hemodynamic management of critically ill surgical patients. *Journal of Trauma* 1999;46:607–611

# 2

# Physical Principles, Ultrasonic Image Formation and Artifacts

*Gerard Bashein*
*Paul R. Detmer*

At first glance, two-dimensional (2-D) ultrasound images have much the same appearance as images made by two other common medical imaging modalities: X-ray computed tomography and magnetic resonance. However, ultrasonic images are formed by the reflection of pulses of energy from tissues, rather than by absorption of energy (as with X-ray images) or secondary emission of energy (as with magnetic resonance images). Thus, the principles of ultrasonic imaging bear more similarity to those of sonar or radar imaging than they do to other forms of medical imaging. Ultrasonic imaging has different advantages, limitations and artifacts from other medical imaging modalities. These must be understood by the practitioner in order to use the technique effectively.

The purpose of this chapter is to provide an introduction to the physical principles, design considerations and sources of artifacts in ultrasonic imaging systems. Readers seeking to study this material in more depth are referred to the text by Kremkau,[1] the chapter on echocardiography physics and instrumentation by Geiser in *Marcus Cardiac Imaging*[2] and the comprehensive textbook of echocardiography by Weyman.[3]

## PRINCIPLES OF ULTRASOUND

**Sound** is defined as vibrations transmitted through an elastic medium that are capable of being detected by the human organs of hearing. Vibratory waves alternately cause **compression** and **rarefaction** (i.e. positive and negative changes in pressure within the medium through which they pass; Figure 2.1). The compression and rarefaction vary periodically over time at any fixed position in the medium and also vary periodically in space for any fixed time during passage of the sound wave.

The number of cycles of a sound wave per unit time is called its **frequency**, which is measured in cycles per second or Hertz (abbreviated Hz and named after Heinrich Rudolf Hertz, a 19th century German physicist). The frequency $f$ is the reciprocal of the **period** $T$, which is the time between successive pressure peaks or troughs (or other specific reference points) on the wave when measured at a fixed observation position, i.e.

$$f = \frac{1}{T}$$
(Equation 2.1)

Frequencies within the range of human hearing (about 20–20 000 Hz) are referred to as **audio frequencies,** while those above this range are referred to as **ultrasonic frequencies.** Echocardiography machines commonly operate in the frequency range of 2–10 million cycles per second (2–10 MHz). Some specialised ultrasound instruments (e.g. those made for intracoronary imaging) may operate at frequencies as high as 30 MHz.

At any fixed time the distance between corresponding reference points on adjacent cycles of a sound wave is called the **wavelength** ($\lambda$). Frequency and wavelength are related by the equation

$$c = f\lambda$$
(Equation 2.2)

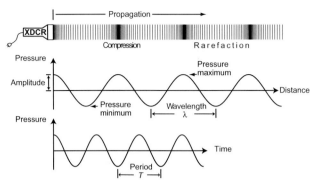

**Figure 2.1** Diagram of the compression and rarefaction of a medium in which a continuous pure tone generated by a transducer (XDCR) is travelling from left to right. Below is shown the corresponding graph of the sinusoidal pressure wave versus distance at some instant in time, drawn on the same distance scale as the diagram above. The wavelength is indicated between successive pressure minima. Below that is shown the corresponding graph, also sinusoidal, of pressure versus time at some fixed point within the medium. The distance and time scales of the graphs are related by the equation $\lambda = cT$ (from Equations 2.1 and 2.2), where $c$ is the speed of propagation in the particular medium.

where $c$ is the speed of propagation in the medium. This relationship between frequency and wavelength requires specification of the medium through which the wave is travelling, because the speed of propagation of sound varies with the medium. The average propagation speed in soft tissues and blood is about 1540 m/s (1.54 mm/μs), the speed for which most medical ultrasound instruments are calibrated.

Among different media, the speed of sound propagation varies inversely with density (mass per unit volume) and directly with stiffness (tendency to resist compression). Paradoxically, sound usually travels faster in higher density materials because they also tend to be stiffer and because stiffness differences among materials are usually larger than density differences. In general, the propagation speed of sound is low in gases, higher in liquids and highest in solids. It is much faster in any tissue than in air (approximately 330 m/s).

The acoustic waves emitted by typical TOE transducers have a centre frequency of 5 MHz, giving a wavelength of 0.308 mm in tissue (by Equation 2.2). Wavelength is important to image quality, because physical principles limit the **spatial resolution** of an ultrasonic image to approximately 1 wavelength (p.26). Thus shorter wavelengths, obtained with higher frequencies, produce better resolution. When the imaging frequency is selectable, the operator has to make a choice that balances the improved image quality with the reduced penetration obtained with higher frequencies. Accordingly, higher frequencies are used when imaging paediatric patients or shallow structures in adults.

As an acoustic wave passes from one medium into another, its frequency does not change. However, if the speed of propagation $c$ differs between adjacent media, the wavelength of the sound will change upon passage from one medium to the other (by Equation 2.2).

Once the medium has been specified, a sound wave that is a pure tone is completely characterised by its frequency and its **amplitude**. The amplitude of a wave is defined as the distance from the baseline to the peak of the waveform. In the case of sound it is measured in units of pressure (Figure 2.1). The **power** (rate of energy delivery) of a sound wave is proportional to the pressure amplitude squared, and is measured in watts.

Because the biological effect of a sound wave is determined by the concentration of the power within the tissues, the output of ultrasound instruments is specified as **intensity** or power per unit area (usually watts/cm²).

For introductory purposes, we have considered sound waves that are generated for an indefinite time period, called **continuous wave** (CW) sound. However, CW signals are used in echocardiography only for purposes of some Doppler measurements (Chapter 3). The use of **pulsed wave** (PW), rather than continuous wave, ultrasound is necessary in order to construct images from the returned echoes. Pulses are brief bursts of sound (typically only a few cycles) transmitted into the medium, followed by a relatively long period of silence, during which the receiver in the ultrasound instrument awaits returned echoes (Figure 2.2). In addition to the underlying frequency and amplitude of the pulses, a pulsed ultrasound signal is described by the **pulse duration** (in microseconds) and the **pulse repetition frequency** (PRF, in Hz), which is the reciprocal of the **pulse repetition period**. For any given speed of propagation, setting the pulse duration also determines the **pulse length** in the medium. The pulse length is critical in that it limits the longitudinal or axial resolution of an ultrasound image (pp.26–27).

Because the average propagation speed of sound in tissue is 1.54 mm/µs, a pulse will travel 1 cm (10 mm) in 6.5 µs. Twice this time (13 µs) is required for each centimetre of round-trip travel from the transducer to a reflector and back. In order to display all objects uniquely within a typical 10 cm viewing window and avoid **range ambiguity**, there must be only a single ultrasonic pulse present within 10 cm of the transducer at any given time. This implies that the minimum time between transmitted pulses is $10 \times 13$ or 130 µs, or equivalently, that the PRF must be no more than 1 s/130 µs $\approx$ 7700 Hz = 7.7 kHz (see Figure 2.2).

Together, the pulse duration and PRF determine the **duty cycle**, or fraction of time that the pulse is "on." The duty cycle and amplitude, in turn, determine the average power output by an ultrasound system, which determines the biological effect on the tissues (p.31).

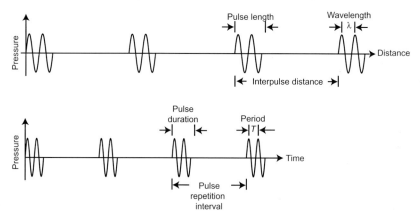

**Figure 2.2** Graphs of pressure versus distance (upper) and pressure versus time (lower) for a hypothetical train of ultrasonic pulses. The period $T$ is the reciprocal of the underlying frequency (e.g. 0.2 µs, with a 5 MHz probe) and bears the same relation to the wavelength ($\lambda = cT$) as in Figure 2.1. The pulse itself is usually 2–3 cycles of the underlying wave, making the pulse duration (or pulse length) 2–3 times the pulse period (or pulse wavelength). Typical values for pulse duration are about 0.5 µs and for pulse length about 0.8 mm. In order to avoid range ambiguity in imaging, the interpulse distance must be at least twice the depth setting of the echocardiography machine (e.g. 20 cm for a 10 cm imaging window, corresponding to a pulse repetition period of about 130 µs). Thus, an actual transmitted ultrasonic pulse train would have pulses much more widely spaced than those shown here, and the pulses themselves would look more like damped sine waves.

**Table 2.1** Examples of power ratios and their decibel equivalents

| Power ratio | dB |
|---|---|
| 2:1 | 3 |
| 10:1 | 10 |
| 20:1 | 13 |
| 40:1 | 16 |
| 100:1 | 20 |
| 1000:1 | 30 |
| 100 000:1 | 50 |
| 10 000 000:1 | 70 |

Relative power may often be obtained by the simple manipulation of logarithms for which the value is known. For example, a power level of 200 W relative to a reference power level of 1000 W is given by Relative Power (dB) = $10 \log_{10}(200/1000) = 10 \log_{10}(0.2)$, but it can also be estimated as $10(\log_{10} 2 - \log_{10} 10) = 10(0.3-1) = -7$.

Because useful ultrasonic power levels vary greatly, power is usually expressed on a relative logarithmic scale called the decibel (dB, after Alexander Graham Bell), expressed as

$$\text{Relative Power (dB)} = 10 \log_{10}\left(\frac{P}{R}\right) \qquad \text{(Equation 2.3)}$$

where $P$ is the power of the signal and $R$ is the reference power level. For example, the control adjusting the transmitted power of an ultrasound instrument may be calibrated in dB relative to the maximum possible transmitted power.

Because $\log_{10}(2) \approx 0.3$, a doubling of power corresponds to a 3 dB increase, while a halving corresponds to a −3 dB change. Overall, the strength of useful returned echoes in ultrasound imaging may be as small as $10^{-10}$ of the transmitted signal strength, corresponding to a power reduction of $10 \log_{10} 0.0000000001$ or −100 dB. Other examples of power ratios and decibels are given in Table 2.1.

## INTERACTION OF ULTRASOUND WAVES WITH TISSUES

The formation of an ultrasonic image is dependent upon wave reflections occurring at the interfaces between different media. The strength of the reflection at an interface depends upon the difference in **acoustic impedance** between the two media. Acoustic impedance is the product of the media density and the propagation speed of sound within that medium, but, because propagation speed varies only slightly between soft biological tissues, differences in impedance depend primarily upon the differences in their density. For example, a blood–fat interface produces a stronger reflection than a blood–muscle interface, because there is a greater difference in density between blood and fat than between blood and muscle. A very large **acoustic impedance mismatch** occurs between tissue and air, preventing imaging within the lung. Another large mismatch occurs between the transducer material that generates the ultrasound wave and the tissue. The transducer manufacturers place an impedance matching layer of an intermediate material on the surface of the transducer; otherwise this mismatch would prevent transfer of most of the energy from the transducer into the patient (see Figure 2.6).

Relatively smooth boundaries between tissues having lateral dimensions much larger than a wavelength produce **specular** or mirror-like reflections, in which the incident and reflected beams make the same angle with respect to a line perpendicular to the boundary (the angle of incidence is equal to the angle of reflection). Thus, reflected energy returns to the receiver only when the boundary is perpendicular to the beam (Figure 2.3a,b). With a rough surface, the bulk of the reflected energy follows the same path as it would with a true specular reflector, but a portion will be returned in other directions (Figure 2.3c,d). The strength of received echoes from a rough surface is maximal when the interface is perpendicular to the beam, and it diminishes to zero as the angle of intersection approaches 0°. The tissue interfaces can thus be viewed from a range of angles, but are best imaged when the ultrasound beam intersects them nearly perpendicularly (e.g. the mitral leaflets in closure as seen from a retroatrial transoesophageal view). At the other extreme, the endocardial and epicardial borders are poorly imaged (a phenomenon called **dropout**) around the 10 and 2 o'clock positions on short axis transoesophageal views because the beam intersects the surfaces nearly tangentially. Rougher surfaces (e.g. the endocardium) give reflections that are less angle-dependent than smoother surfaces (e.g. the epicardium or large vessel walls).

Non-homogeneous tissues (e.g. muscle) generate echoes internally due to **scattering** that give the image texture, while homogeneous substances (e.g. blood or fluid) appear echo-lucent (black) on 2-D images. However, very weak ultrasonic back-scattering does occur from blood cells (Figure 2.3e), and it is the back-scattered signal that is used in Doppler echocardiography (see Chapter 3). In either case, the portion of the incident

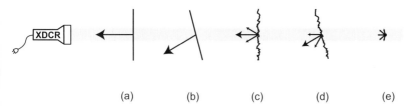

|  |  |  |  |  |
|---|---|---|---|---|
| (a) | (b) | (c) | (d) | (e) |

**Figure 2.3** Schematic diagram of an ultrasound beam impinging upon a series of interfaces. The strength of the returned echoes is indicated by the length of the arrows. (a) A perfectly specular reflector oriented perpendicularly to the incident beam, giving a very strong reflection directly back to the transducer. (b) An identical reflector oriented obliquely to the beam, causing all of the reflected energy to be directed away from the source. In practice, steel needles behave as nearly perfect specular reflectors and are therefore very difficult to visualise on ultrasonic examinations. (c) A rough surface, more typical of tissue interfaces, oriented perpendicularly to the beam. While most of the reflected energy returns to the source, a portion is back-scattered in other directions. When a rough surface is oriented obliquely to the beam, as in (d), there is some loss of returned signal strength, but the target would probably be visible unless the intercept angle were very acute. A target smaller than a wavelength of the ultrasound (e) scatters only tiny amounts of energy over a wide range of angles. For purposes of illustration, attenuation in the tissues, refraction and the reduction in transmitted signal strength due to each successive reflector have been ignored.

acoustic energy that is not reflected or back-scattered is transmitted onward, where it may generate another echo upon contacting a third medium, and so on (see Figure 2.5).

If an incident beam obliquely encounters an interface between tissues having different velocities of propagation, the transmitted beam will undergo bending or **refraction**, behaviour similar to that of light (Snell's law). The direction and degree of bending depend on the relative speeds of propagation in the two media (Figure 2.4). Bending does not occur when the incident beam encounters the interface perpendicularly. **Refraction artifact** can cause errors in making dimensional measurements of deep structures (e.g. in obstetric ultrasonography) but is usually of little importance in TOE.

As an ultrasound beam propagates through a single tissue it progressively diminishes in amplitude (power) owing to internal frictional heating, reflection and scattering from inhomogeneities within the tissue. This phenomenon is called **attenuation**. For a given frequency in a given tissue, the **attenuation coefficient** (in dB/cm) is the attenuation for each centimetre of sound travel. Attenuation in soft solid tissue (muscle, organs, etc.) increases linearly with frequency, with a typical value of 0.5 dB/cm per MHz of frequency. Thus, lower frequency ultrasound waves have better tissue penetration, allowing imaging at greater depths, albeit with a sacrifice in resolution due to their increased wavelength. Liquids (blood, body fluid collections, water) cause much less attenuation than soft tissues. Solid tissues (bone, cartilage) and air produce very high attenuation.

The returned signal strength from any given tissue interface will vary with the amount of overlying tissue and resultant signal attenuation. In order to make tissue interfaces of the same reflectivity have the same appearance anywhere in the image, **time-gain compensation** (TGC) is employed, wherein the receiver gain progressively increases when "listening" for echoes from deeper and deeper tissues (Figure 2.5). The standard TGC assumes an average attenuation of the overlying tissues. Superimposed upon the standard TGC are slider-type controls to allow the operator to adjust the TGC at any particular depth of interest. Some ultrasound instruments also incorporate **lateral gain compensation** to compensate for image dropout where the ultrasound beam strikes the endocardial borders tangentially.

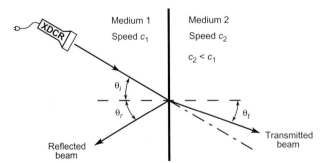

**Figure 2.4** An ultrasonic beam directed obliquely to a specular reflector. The angles of the incident beam ($\theta_i$) and the reflected beam ($\theta_r$), with respect to the perpendicular to the interface are equal. Whenever the propagation speeds in the two media differ, following Snell's law, the transmitted beam will be angled with respect to the incident beam. When $c_2 < c_1$, the transmitted beam angle $\theta_t$ will be less than the incident beam angle $\theta_i$, and vice versa. Mathematically,

$$\frac{\sin(\theta_t)}{\sin(\theta_i)} = \frac{c_2}{c_1} .$$

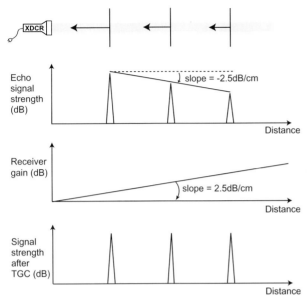

**Figure 2.5** The reflection and transmission of an ultrasound beam directed perpendicularly to interfaces between tissues of differing acoustic impedance. The intensity of each echo is represented by the length of its arrow. Below is plotted the returned signal amplitude versus distance (i.e. an A-mode image). For purposes of illustration, the strength of the successive returned echoes are assumed to diminish by 2.5 dB/cm of depth. The middle graph shows the receiver gain, or number of decibels of signal strength added to the returned echoes, as a function of depth. In this case, the time gain compensation (TGC) is uniformly increasing and exactly compensates for the loss of signal strength in succeeding echoes, as shown in the bottom graph. Most real-world situations are more complex and require a hand-tailored gain-versus-depth curve to produce the desired image.

## ULTRASONIC TRANSDUCERS

A **transducer** is a device that converts energy from one form into another. Ultrasonic transducers exhibit a reciprocal property: when transmitting, they convert electrical energy from the ultrasound instrument into acoustic energy, and when receiving they convert the acoustic energy reflected from the tissues into electrical energy used by the instrument in forming an image. Ultrasonic transducers work by the **piezoelectric effect** (from the Greek *piezein*, to press tight or squeeze), whereby certain crystals or ceramics will deform slightly when strong electric fields are imposed upon them and, reciprocally, will generate a voltage when deformed mechanically.

When an ultrasonic crystal gets a pulse of electrical energy it oscillates, much as a bell does, at a specific frequency called its **resonant frequency**. Piezoelectric crystals made of quartz are used to regulate the frequency of oscillations in digital wristwatches and computer clocks. The resonant frequency of a piezoelectric crystal depends upon its mechanical properties and *varies inversely with its thickness*. These properties determine the type of crystal that is selected for each specific application. The simplest ultrasonic transducer consists of a single discoid crystal, usually made of lead-zirconate-titanate, having a sound-absorbing (**damping**) material on its back, an impedance matching layer, and possibly an acoustic lens, on its face (Figure 2.6). The longitudinal or **axial resolution** of an imaging system will be improved if the tendency of the transducer crystal to

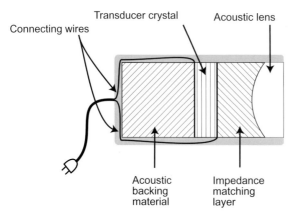

**Figure 2.6** A single crystal ultrasonic transducer with its lens, matching layer and backing materials. The electrical wires are connected to a conductive coating on the faces of the transducer. The lens can either be a separate material as shown, or may be produced by shaping the ultrasonic crystal itself. Up to half of the acoustic energy generated by the transducer can be absorbed and lost as heat in the matching layers and backing material, a price that must be paid in order to produce a short, clean pulse. This may also be the factor that limits a transducer's acoustic output.

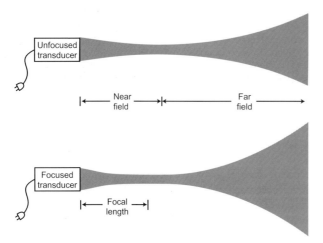

**Figure 2.7** The main beam produced by an unfocused single-element discoid transducer (top) and a focused transducer (bottom). The beam from a focused transducer is narrower at its focal depth than that of an unfocused transducer, at the expense of somewhat more rapid divergence in the far field. Side lobes are not shown here, but may generate clinically important artifacts.

continue to ring after being pulsed is limited by a damping material that keeps the pulse duration short.

In the absence of a lens, the radiation pattern of the main beam emitted by a discoid transducer is essentially cylindrical up to a certain distance from the face, known as the **near field length**. This near field length is inversely proportional to the square of the transducer diameter (**aperture**) and inversely proportional to the wavelength. Beyond the near field length the beam diverges into a conical pattern (**far field**), with an angle determined by the ratio of the wavelength to the transducer diameter (Figure 2.7). The addition of a lens, whether separate or as part of the transducer material itself, will constrict the near field beam in the region of the focal length, at the expense of more rapid divergence in the far field.

As the edge of a sound beam is not perfectly abrupt, the **beam width** is customarily defined as the lateral distance between the points where the beam intensity diminishes by 3 dB (i.e. 50% power) from that at the centre of the beam. The beam width determines the **lateral resolution** of an ultrasound system (i.e. the minimum separation, measured perpendicular to the beam, that is necessary for a pair of point reflectors, located the same distance from the transducer, to produce separate echoes when the beam is scanned).

In addition to the main beam, all transducers emit secondary beams, known as **side lobes**, that are angled obliquely to the centre of the main beam. Side lobes are generally much weaker (by 50 dB or so, at about 1/100 000 of the main lobe's power intensity), but when they encounter strong reflectors they can generate false targets (**side-lobe artifacts**), which appear in the image to be located along the centre of the main beam. Alternatively, they may produce multiple images from a single target.

## SCANNING TRANSDUCERS

A single-element transducer, like the discoid transducer discussed above, can be used to make 2-D images only if its beam is swept systematically over a region of interest within the tissues. A transducer with a mechanism to sweep the ultrasound beam automatically in a fan-like fashion is called a **mechanical sector scanner** (Figure 2.8a). Although mechanical sector scanners are mostly made for transcutaneous imaging, at least one manufacturer has offered a mechanically scanned probe for transoesophageal imaging.

More commonly the ultrasonic beam is formed and steered by firing an array of small, closely spaced transducer elements in a sequence controlled by the ultrasound instrument. In a **phased array** all elements, typically numbering 64 in a transoesophageal probe, are fired to form each beam. When their firing is simultaneous, the resulting beam is oriented perpendicular to the face of the array and has a pattern similar to that from a single, long and thin, rectangular element. However, by delaying the firing of successive elements slightly, in proportion to their distance along the array, the resulting beam will appear as though it came from a virtual, single rectangular element angulated with respect to the true array (Figure 2.8b). The summation wavefront coming from a segmented (phased or linear) array has undulations that are not present in the wavefront from a single-element transducer. These undulations introduce additional side lobes to the beam, known as **grating lobes**, which may produce artifacts in the same way as the side lobes mentioned above.

By changing the delay pattern each time the phased array is pulsed, the ultrasonic beam can be swept over a region defined by a sector of a circle, in a manner similar to the mechanical sector scanner. The **sector angle** achieved with transoesophageal probes can be as much as approximately 90°, but it may be desirable to reduce it (and the number of scan lines) under special circumstances (pp.25 and 42).

In **linear array** scanning, firing small subsets of adjacent elements simultaneously forms beams perpendicular to the array face, and a sequence of these perpendicular beams sweeps a rectangular region of tissue (Figure 2.8c). Linear arrays are able to image a relatively wide region of tissue close to the transducer, and are used primarily for

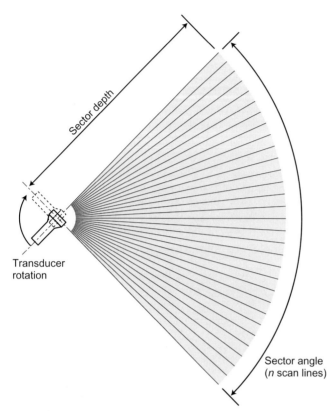

**Figure 2.8a** Scanning with a mechanical sector scanner. A single-crystal transducer is rotated through approximately 90° and the returned echo brightness is plotted along a succession (typically 128) of radial lines.

transcutaneous vascular imaging. A **curvilinear array** is simply a curved or arched version of a linear array.

A phased array or linear array beam can be focused electronically, within the imaging plane, by altering the firing delays of the elements to achieve a lens-like curvature to the summation wavefront. This **electronic focusing** can be done independently for transmission (by adjusting the timing of firing of the elements) and for reception (by changing the delays applied to the received signals from each of the array elements as they are combined). Indeed, the focus on reception can be adjusted over the receive cycle to be optimal for each expected depth of echo return, a technique known as **dynamic focusing**. The electronic focusing depth on transmission is adjustable by a panel control on most echocardiography machines. Because the beam widens rapidly beyond the focal depth, the operator should set the focus control to a depth at, or slightly deep to, the object of greatest interest in the image.

Electronic focusing can also be accomplished in *mechanical* sector scanners by using a target-shaped set of transducer elements, known as an **annular array**, in place of a single-crystal transducer. In this case, the electronic focusing will be equally effective in all radial directions around the centre of the beam, giving mechanical scanners with annular arrays better image resolution than can be achieved with phased array transducers, although at the cost of greater size, complexity and fragility of the scan head.

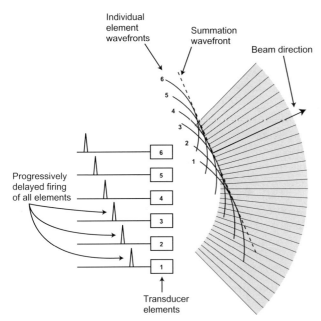

**Figure 2.8b** Scanning with a phased array. A sector is swept electronically by suitably timing the firing of all the elements generating each scan line. In this close-up view, the beam along an upwardly directed scan line is generated by firing the elements, in order, from bottom to top. The wavefronts from the individual elements form arcs, which are numbered to correspond to their source elements. The summation wavefront, shown by the dashed line, appears much as though it were coming from a virtual single-element transducer oriented perpendicular to the beam. Because the summation wavefront is not truly planar, additional side lobes, called grating lobes, are generated by phased arrays and linear arrays.

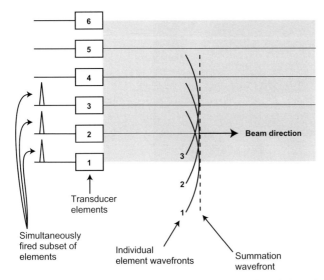

**Figure 2.8c** Scanning with a linear array. A rectangular region of tissue is scanned by simultaneously firing a subset of adjacent elements to generate a sequence of beams oriented perpendicular to the array. In this simplified illustration elements numbered 1, 2 and 3 are fired to generate the bottom line in the scanned region. Subsequent scan lines would then be generated by firing elements 2, 3 and 4, followed by elements 3, 4 and 5, etc.

## ECHO IMAGE FORMATION

The simplest type of echocardiographic image is a plot of the received signal amplitude versus time, called an **A-mode** or amplitude mode image. In such a display, each peak is likely to represent an interface between two dissimilar tissues. If the horizontal scale is calibrated in distance units for the ultrasound pulse to make a round trip (i.e. $2 \times 1.54 = 3.08$ mm/µs), the distances between tissue interfaces can be readily and accurately measured, provided they are relatively immobile (e.g. the walls of a blood vessel). This is shown diagrammatically in Figure 2.5. The A-mode image is of limited clinical usefulness, because it provides only a single-dimensional or "ice pick" view of the tissues, and it is difficult to interpret when motion is present.

Another ice-pick type of view is the **M-mode** or motion mode image (Figure 2.9). In M-mode imaging the amplitude of returning echoes is plotted as the brightness along vertical lines drawn for each transmitted echo pulse. The echo pulses are repeated at rates of thousands per second, and a raster of vertical lines, scanned along the same path, is drawn from left to right at speeds comparable to ECG recordings (25–100 mm/s). The electrocardiogram is usually recorded on the same scale to provide a timing reference. Motion of tissue interfaces can readily be discerned and distances and time intervals readily measured in M-mode imaging. It is the method of choice for measuring distances along the direction of the ultrasound beam. It is also better for observing rapidly moving structures (e.g. fluttering valve leaflets) than 2-D imaging because, without the need to scan the ultrasound beam, the pulse repetition frequency can be 100 or more times faster than in 2-D imaging.

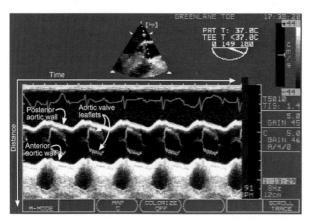

**Figure 2.9** A transoesophageal M-mode image taken across the aortic root. Each ultrasonic scan line is plotted vertically downward from the transducer (located at the top of the raster) as a column of grey pixels, with the brightness of each individual pixel representing the strength of the returned echo at that particular depth. Successive scan lines over time are plotted from left to right, with the synchronised ECG superimposed. The depth scale (12 cm) with 1 cm tick marks is shown on the right-hand side. The structures shown (in order, from top to bottom) are the posterior wall of the aorta, the aortic valve leaflets, the anterior wall of the aorta, and myocardium surrounding the right ventricular outflow tract. The rapid opening and closing of the aortic leaflets is easily appreciated. The aortic walls appear very similar and move almost synchronously, indicating that motion, but very little expansion and contraction, of the aorta occurs over the cardiac cycle. The small inset above shows the orientation of the M-line overlaid on a 2-D image for reference.

The familiar tomographic 2-D ultrasound image (also known as **B-mode** or brightness mode) is formed by scanning the ultrasound beam (mechanically, or electronically with a linear array or phased array) and using the strength of the returned echoes to modulate the brightness of points in the image corresponding to the positions of expected echo returns from the tissues. In the case of a phased-array or mechanical-sector scanner, the beam is steered along a series of lines emanating radially from the face of the transducer. Typically 128 lines are scanned to cover a 90° sector (see Figure 2.8a).

Each complete scan of the sector forms one **frame** of the image. For clinical purposes it is assumed that all parts of a 2-D image are acquired at exactly the same time. The minimum **time to generate one frame** of an image is determined by the time $t$ for a pulse of ultrasound to make the required number of round trips:

$$t = \frac{2nd}{c}$$ (Equation 2.4)

where $n$ is the number of scan lines in a frame, $d$ is the maximum depth of the sector, and $c$ is the speed of propagation in the tissue (see Figure 2.8a). For example, imaging with 128 scan lines to a depth of 10 cm (100 mm) requires $2 \times 128 \times 100/1.54$ µs, or about 17 ms. Thus, if frames were acquired repeatedly, a maximal **frame rate** of about 60 per second could be achieved. High frame rates are desirable when trying to observe fast-moving objects such as valvular vegetations. If the frame rate is insufficient for the clinical application, it becomes necessary to adjust the echo instrument to reduce the scanning depth or the number of scan lines (i.e. reduce the sector angle) to achieve the desired frame rate. The highest frame rate can be achieved with M-mode imaging, because scanning is done along only a single line ($n = 1$ in Equation 2.4).

Modern, digitally based, echocardiography machines do not display the individual 2-D scan lines directly on the video screen. Rather, they display the brightness values in a grid of tiny rectangular elements called **pixels** (short for picture elements) that typically assume one of 256 grey values. The process of transforming the brightness values along each scan line into a pixelated image is known as **scan conversion**. Electronic signal processing of the image before scan conversion (e.g. time-gain compensation) is known as **preprocessing** and that done afterward (e.g. contrast adjustment) is known as **postprocessing**.

Regardless of the frame rate, an acquired image can be stored on videotape only at a frame rate of 30 per second (in the North American NTSC system) or 25 per second (in the PAL system used in most of the rest of the world). Faster frame rates can be viewed on the live screen, captured and reviewed using a digital loop memory, or written to removable digital storage media, a feature becoming common on newer echocardiography machines.

## RESOLUTION

The **resolution** of an ultrasound system is a measure of its ability to distinguish echoes from different sources that are close to each other in space, time or returned signal strength (known as **spatial**, **temporal** and **contrast resolution**, respectively). Spatial resolution lends detail to an image and has three components, conventionally named axial, elevational and lateral because they are measured relative to the direction of the beam (Figure 2.10).

The two components of resolution perpendicular to the beam are determined by the beam width, because two targets at the same distance from the transducer cannot be distinguished if they both lie within the same beam. Beam width decreases with increasing

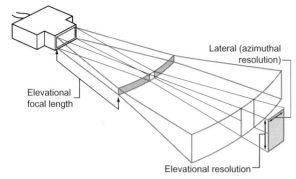

**Figure 2.10** The ultrasonic sector ("fan") emitted by a phased-array transducer and a single scan line within it. The (fixed) transducer design and acoustic lens determine the thickness of the fan, i.e. the system's elevational resolution and elevational focal length. Transducer design and electronic focusing both determine the lateral or azimuthal resolution, which is generally better than the elevational resolution and is adjustable in focal depth by the operator. The best resolution occurs along the direction of the beam (axial resolution; not shown) and is determined by the transmitted pulse duration (or length), not by the geometry of the transducer itself.

transducer aperture size or increasing frequency, for a given aperture size. Beam width can also be decreased by focusing with an acoustical lens in the elevational direction and by electronic means in the lateral direction. The component of beam-width resolution that lies in the plane of the sector scan is called **lateral** or **azimuthal resolution**, while the component perpendicular to the sector plane is called **elevational resolution** (i.e. image thickness).

In phased-array systems the elevational resolution is the poorest of the three spatial components. The face of a phased array is considerably longer than it is wide, so that the beam thickness (which varies inversely with the transducer's aperture size) will be greater in its dimension perpendicular to the imaging plane than it is in the plane (see Figure 2.10). Because of the considerable beam thickness normal to the imaging plane, it would be more realistic for the operator to imagine the ultrasonic fan as imaging a thin wedge of tissue, rather than a planar slice. Lateral resolution is somewhat better than elevational resolution, because the phased array has a larger effective aperture in that direction, and because electronic focusing is possible. Limitations in elevational and lateral resolution can produce **beam width artifacts**, which arise from strong reflectors in the beam's edge that are represented as targets located at its centre. The variation of beam width with depth can also lead to inaccurate representation of an object's size.

By far the most accurate component of resolution of the ultrasound system is the **axial resolution** (also known as **range resolution**), which is measured along the direction of the beam and is determined by the pulse length. As shown in Figure 2.11, the receiver cannot distinguish targets located closer together than half the spatial pulse length. Since pulse length is practically limited to about 2 wavelengths, the best achievable range resolution is about 1 wavelength, or 0.3 mm for the typical 5 MHz transoesophageal probe. To obtain the best resolution the operator should select ultrasonic views to image the surface of interest as nearly perpendicular to the beam as possible.

The effect of pulse length should also be considered when tracing outlines or making measurements of the distance between two surfaces, e.g. the endocardium on the near and far sides of the ventricular cavity. Because of finite pulse length, the near interface will appear (artifactually) slightly deeper than it actually is (Figure 2.12). Accordingly, with 2-D and M-mode imaging, the true dimensions of a structure are obtained

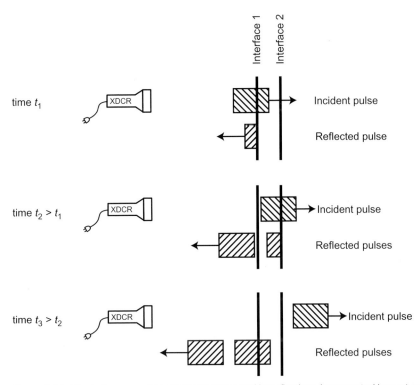

**Figure 2.11** Block diagrams of an ultrasonic pulse and its reflections (represented by rectangles), shown at three snapshots in time. The incident pulse travels from left to right and impinges on two closely spaced interfaces. For clarity, the resulting reflected pulses are shown separately below and with opposite cross-hatching to the incident pulse. At time $t_1$ (top diagram), about one-third of the incident pulse has passed through the first interface and is approaching the second interface, while the partially formed reflected pulse from the first interface is travelling back towards the transducer. At time $t_2 > t_1$ (middle diagram), the incident pulse has passed through the first interface and partially through the second interface. The reflection from the first interface is thus complete and the incomplete reflection from the second interface is headed back towards, but has not yet reached, the first interface. At time $t_3 > t_2$ (bottom diagram), the incident pulse has passed the second interface and the fully formed pair of reflected pulses is returning to the source. If the distance between interfaces were less than half of the pulse length, the trailing edge of the reflected pulse from the first interface would overlap the leading edge of the reflection from the second interface, and two reflected pulses would merge, making the two targets indistinguishable in the image.

when measurements are made from points where the leading edge of the ultrasonic pulse intersects each interface, the so-called **"leading-to-leading edge"** method. However, because the distance between the leading and trailing edges of the pulses is small, many clinicians make measurements between the inner edges of structures.

## IMAGING ARTIFACTS

Several of the artifacts that can confound the interpretation of echocardiographic images have already been mentioned in the context of the physical phenomena from which they arise. Some additional artifacts are described below.

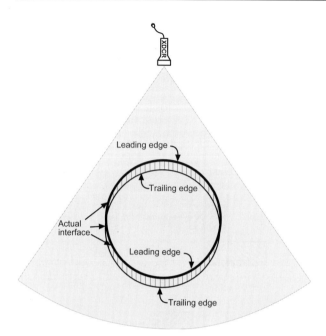

**Figure 2.12** A thin circular reflecting interface (e.g. LV endocardium) shown as a solid bold line. The cross-hatched region represents the 2-D image that would be generated by a transducer located at the top of the figure and transmitting a pulse of finite length. The leading edge of the reflection corresponds with the true border. The trailing edge lies in the far field to it. Thus, measurements or tracings of the outline of the structure should be made along leading edges at both the near and the far sides of the outline.

As a general principle, the operator of a TOE instrument should attempt to reduce the chances for artifacts to cause misinterpretation by examining each feature of interest from different viewpoints and depth settings. Image features that then appear consistently are less likely to be artifactual. Limiting the transmitted power will also help to eliminate artifacts due to strong reflectors, beam width and side lobes.

One artifact caused by unusually strong reflection is **multi-reverberation**, which occurs when a sound wave ricochets back and forth between two surfaces (commonly the transducer face and a structure near it, or occasionally two tissue interfaces) and creates image features that are not real (see Figure 11.1). Reverberation artifacts occur along the straight line of the ultrasound beam and are often multiple and equally spaced, giving a ladder-like appearance. Superposition of multiple reverberation artifacts near the transducer face is known as **near-field clutter** or **ring-down artifact** and generally renders imaging impossible very close to the transducer. For example, it prevents imaging of the anterior wall of the ascending aorta from an ordinary transducer placed upon it by a cardiac surgeon (special transducers having a layer of standoff material can be used for epiaortic imaging).

In 2-D and pulsed Doppler imaging (Chapter 3), the ultrasound machine automatically sets the PRF to display each target within its depth setting uniquely to avoid **range ambiguity**. However, when a very strong reflector lies deep to the range setting of an instrument (i.e. below the bottom of the image), the resulting echo may return to the receiver during the time when the echoes from the succeeding transmitted pulse are expected, causing the system to display the echo within the image sector as though it had occurred within the set range. Whether in a 2–D or pulsed Doppler image, changing the depth setting of the machine or using a different acoustic window will alter or eliminate the artifact.

A **mirror-image artifact** may occur when a strong reflector redirects the path of a portion of the beam and a subsequent reflection from a more distal structure travels back to the transducer along a path identical to that taken on its outward journey. The underlying assumption in image formation, that sound travels in a straight line, will then be violated, and the structure will be incorrectly located within the image. Mirroring can also give rise to duplication of image features.

When an unusually strong proximal reflection occurs (e.g. at the blood–metal interface of a prosthetic cardiac valve) or the beam passes through a highly attenuating medium, little ultrasonic energy remains to image tissues deeper to the transducer, a phenomenon called **shadowing**. Severe shadowing is usually obvious because the image appears black directly beyond the reflecting or attenuating barrier (see Figure 12.5). However, subtle shadowing (e.g. due to calcification of valve leaflets or annulus) may obscure an important diagnostic feature without casting a particularly noticeable shadow (see Figure 12.10). Shadowing may also occur as the result of refraction at the edge of a circular structure and is sometimes called an **edge shadow**.

## INSTRUMENT CONTROLS FOR IMAGING

It is critical to fine-tune the controls of the echocardiography machine in order to obtain optimal images for diagnosis. Unless indicated otherwise, the controls listed below perform preprocessing functions and can act only on the live image data as it is acquired. It is therefore incumbent upon the operator to set these controls carefully because corrections cannot be made afterwards. On the other hand, the operator can adjust postprocessing functions on both live images and those stored in the ultrasound system. Postprocessing controls are also available in offline echocardiography workstations. The main imaging controls on most echocardiography machines include:

### Transmit power
This control adjusts the amount of acoustic energy delivered to the tissues. The setting should be kept as low as possible, consistent with good image quality, in order to reduce patient exposure and to diminish some types of artifacts (e.g. multiple reverberations and beam-width artifacts).

### Receiver gain
This control adjusts the overall sensitivity of the system to the received echoes. In order to utilise the transmitted ultrasonic signal maximally, this control should be set as high as possible, without displaying more than a trace of electronic noise on echo-free portions of the image.

### Time-gain compensation (TGC)
Each of the several slider-type controls adjusts the relative sensitivity of the system to received echoes from a particular band of depths (p.18). These controls act in conjunction with the receiver gain and should be readjusted frequently to optimise the appearance of each individual image. Some systems also provide lateral-gain compensation to adjust receiver sensitivity across the image and compensate for lateral changes in attenuation or reflectivity.

## Image depth

Setting the maximum depth of the acquired image also determines the frame rate and how long the system listens for echoes along each beam. To obtain the best frame rate and image clarity, this control should be set at the smallest value that will show all of the structures of interest.

## Compression (or reject or dynamic range)

This control determines the spread of weaker echoes relative to stronger echoes within the digital storage (grey-scale range) of the system. It can be set to use the available range to display the subtle variations across weaker echoes (e.g. a thrombus amongst myocardial trabeculae) while de-emphasising variations in strong echoes, or vice versa. Because this preprocessing control acts early along the signal path it can have a more pronounced effect on image quality than similar postprocessing controls such as contrast or grey map adjustments (see below).

## Focal zone position

This control adjusts depth of optimum lateral focus in the image by setting the electronic focal point on transmission. It should be placed slightly deep to the region of interest for maximum effect.

## Sector width and sector steer

These controls adjust the sector width (angle) within the range of the normal image sector. By reducing the sector width, much higher frame rates can be obtained at the expense of field of view. The sector steer control then permits positioning of the reduced sector anywhere within normal range of the image sector without physically moving the transducer.

## Zoom

Two types of zoom function are often available. *Transmit* (or *write*) *zoom* is a preprocessing function that digitizes the image data in the selected region at a higher density than in the non-zoomed image and thus improves the displayed detail. *Receive* (or *read*) *zoom* is a postprocessing function that acts like an electronic magnifying glass: it simply enlarges the pixels within a selected region of interest. Receive zoom may enable the operator to appreciate existing image detail better, but it does not improve the spatial resolution of the image.

## Freeze

Pressing the freeze control puts the system in a standby state, stops ultrasonic transmission, and retains in digital memory a sequence of the immediately preceding image frames. The operator can then scroll through the stored frames to study evanescent phenomena, enter annotations, print selected frames, or save the sequence of frames into auxiliary storage. Advantages of reviewing digitally stored frames, rather than a videotape recording, include better spatial and temporal resolution, easier scrolling, easier selection of individual frames and an ability to apply other postprocessing manipulations to the images.

## Brightness, contrast, colourisation, grey scale

These postprocessing controls are all designed to enhance contrast resolution to enable the eye to distinguish better between nearby echoes in the image differing only slightly in their signal strength. Colourisation may be used by taking advantage of the human visual system's ability to distinguish certain colour variations better than grey levels. These controls should be adjusted to produce the most pleasing and diagnostically useful image, but they do not have the range of effects that the (preprocessing) compression control affords.

## Dosimetry and safety

Although diagnostic ultrasound has no known adverse biological effects, the prudent clinician should limit the ultrasonic power levels and time of exposure to the minimum necessary to obtain the desired information. Intraoperatively, acoustic transmission should be turned on *only* when the operator is actually viewing the image. The main effect of concern is localised heating, which depends upon the power output, frequency and focus of the transducer, tissue properties and perfusion. Freezing the image display is a simple way to halt transmission.

The American Institute of Ultrasound in Medicine has issued guidelines that suggest limiting the ultrasonic exposure to produce at most a 1°C rise in local tissue temperature. The recommended maximum power levels are expressed as spatial peak, temporal average (SPTA), which take into account that in a pulsed system the duty cycle is much less than 100%. The SPTA power recommended for unfocused beams is less than 1 W/cm$^2$ and that for focused beams 100 mW/cm$^2$. Most echocardiography machines can generate power levels that exceed these recommendations, particularly in one of the Doppler modes. The clinician should become familiar with the particulars of the instrument used and limit the use of Doppler to necessary measurements.

Heating of the face of the transducer may cause an oesophageal burn. Although transoesophageal probes have built-in thermometers that activate a safety shutoff in the echocardiography machine when the transducer temperature reaches about 40°C, burns can occur at lower temperatures than this when the patient is hypothermic. Leaving the mechanical controls in an unlocked neutral position when not actually performing an examination will reduce the risk of pressure necrosis to the oesophageal or gastric mucosa.

The electrical insulation of a transoesophageal probe can become damaged by repeated use and sterilisation, and electrical shock or electrocautery burns can occur to the oesophagus. Probes should be inspected and tested for electrical leakage regularly according to the manufacturer's recommendations (Appendix 1).

## REFERENCES

1. Kremkau FW. *Diagnostic Ultrasound: Principles and Instruments*, 6th Edition. Philadelphia: WB Saunders, 2002.
2. Geiser EA. Echocardiography: physics and instrumentation. In: Skorton DJ, Schelbert HR, Wolf GL, Brundage BH (eds) *Marcus Cardiac Imaging: A Companion to Braunwald's Heart Disease*, 2nd Edition. Philadelphia: WB Saunders, 1996:273–291.
3. Weyman AE. (ed.) *Principles and Practice of Echocardiography*, 2nd Edition. Philadelphia: Lea & Febiger, 1994.

# Principles of Doppler Ultrasound

*Gerard Bashein*
*Paul R. Detmer*

This chapter provides a brief introduction to the physics and operating principles of instruments which use the Doppler effect in cardiovascular diagnostics. Readers seeking more detail should consult Kremkau's textbook,[1] Hatle and Angelsen's classic monograph[2] and Weyman's comprehensive textbook.[3]

Most Doppler signals of interest come from blood flow. Recent advances in Doppler tracking of tissue motion will be covered only very briefly here, although the basic principles are the same. Because blood cells are much smaller than the wavelength of the ultrasound used, returned signals are generated only by scattering, and accordingly are of the order of 100-fold (–20 dB) weaker than the signals from specular reflectors. Strong signals from specular reflectors within the beam can occasionally be of diagnostic help (e.g. valve "clicks" that give important timing information), but are usually a nuisance to be eliminated by filtering (pp.36 and 37). Because the Doppler processing path in ultrasound machines must measure tiny frequency changes in extremely weak signals, Doppler measurements are particularly sensitive to environmental electrical noise. Fortunately, electrocautery and other noises are usually obvious on the Doppler display and are unlikely to lead to misdiagnoses.

To obtain sufficient signal strength and penetration for a good Doppler signal, higher ultrasonic intensity levels and lower frequencies are used than for 2-D imaging. Because the patient receives a much higher ultrasound dose during a Doppler examination, its duration should be limited to that necessary to obtain the desired information.

## DOPPLER EFFECT

The **Doppler effect** is defined as the apparent change in the frequency of waves (e.g. sound or light) occurring when the source and observer are in motion relative to each other, with the frequency increasing when the source and observer approach each other and decreasing when they move apart. It is named after Christian Johann Doppler, an Austrian physicist who first described the effect (for light) in 1842. To understand the Doppler effect imagine the distance between successive sound wave fronts becoming squeezed when the source and receiver are coming closer together, resulting in a foreshortening of the wavelength or, equivalently, an increase in the frequency. Conversely, an elongation of the wavelength of a sound wave when the source and receiver move apart results in a decrease in frequency (Figure 3.1).

Another way to understand the Doppler effect is to imagine a boat travelling through ocean waves. When the boat moves in a direction opposite to the wave motion, it encounters wave peaks more often (i.e. at a higher frequency) than if it were stationary. Conversely, when the boat moves in the same direction as the wave propagation it encounters wave peaks less frequently. The change in frequency depends on the boat speed and the original frequency and speed of the waves in the water.

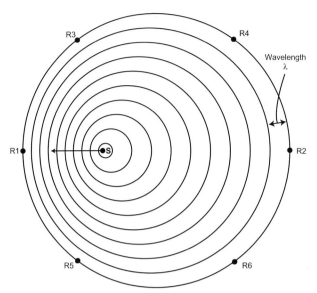

**Figure 3.1** A series of wavefronts emanating from a sound source, S, which is moving from right to left. A receiver positioned at R1 will observe the highest frequency (shortest wavelength) sound, while a receiver at R2 will observe the lowest frequency (longest wavelength). Receivers positioned at R3 and R5 will observe an identical sound frequency, which will be higher than the source frequency and lower than the frequency observed at R1; receivers positioned at R4 and R6 will observe an identical frequency, which will be lower than the source frequency but higher than the frequency observed at R2. The degree of shift and distortion of the wavefronts due to motion has been greatly exaggerated for purposes of illustration.

By combining electrical signals representing the transmitted and received acoustic frequencies, another signal can be obtained with a frequency equal to the difference of the two frequencies, the so-called **Doppler shift**. The frequency of the Doppler-shifted signal when a reflector or scatterer moves directly towards or away from the transmitter is given by the **Doppler equation**, which may be derived from the change in wavelength due to motion:

$$f_D = f_0 \left( \frac{2v}{c - v} \right)$$

(Equation 3.1)

where $f_D$ is the Doppler frequency, $f_0$ is the transmitted frequency, $v$ is the velocity directed towards the transducer from the scatterer, and $c$ is the speed of propagation in the medium. The factor of 2 appears above because the shift occurs twice, once due to the reflector's motion when it receives the signal from the source, and a second time when it becomes the source and sends the already Doppler-shifted wave back to the transmitter. When the speed of the scatterer (in the heart, typically in the range of 1 m/s) is much lower than the speed of propagation in tissue, the $v$ term in the denominator of Equation 3.1 can be neglected (i.e. $c - v \cong c$), giving the approximate form shown in most textbooks:

$$f_D = \frac{2f_0 v}{c}$$

(Equation 3.2)

For example, when a 2.5 MHz transmitted signal encounters scatterers moving at 1 m/s, the Doppler frequency is 3247 Hz, i.e. within the range of human hearing. Echocardiography machines use lower frequencies for Doppler measurements than for imaging, typically in the lower third of the useful bandwidth of the scan head. The lower frequency increases the beam penetration, resulting in a larger reflected signal strength from weak scatterers, such as blood cells. Using a lower transmitted frequency also reduces the Doppler shift frequency proportionately. Because Doppler shifts encountered clinically lie within the audible range, Doppler instruments usually provide output to a loudspeaker, which can give important diagnostic clues to the operator. More advanced machines separate the Doppler shifts of scatterers moving towards the scan head from those moving away from the scan head and present the directionally distinct signals in separate channels of a stereo loudspeaker output.

Equations 3.1 and 3.2 are based upon the assumption that the scatterer is moving directly towards or away from the transducer. When the motion is oblique to the path between the transducer and scatterer, only the component of velocity along the line connecting them will cause a Doppler shift. A term with the cosine of the **crossing angle θ** between the velocity vector and the beam path must then be included in the Doppler equation, which is rearranged to solve for the quantity of clinical interest, namely velocity:

$$v = \frac{f_D c}{2 f_0 \cos\theta} \qquad \text{(Equation 3.3)}$$

When the crossing angle θ is zero, the cosine term becomes unity, so there is no correction. Most echocardiography machines provide a steering control for the operator to indicate the assumed crossing angle, in which case the machine automatically makes the correction. However, as a practical matter, when the crossing angle is less than about 20°, the error caused by ignoring the correction is negligible (less than 6%), so most operators will choose views to minimise the crossing angle, not use the steering control, and ignore the correction. Because the cosine term can cause only underestimation of the velocity, and because the true direction of the flow generating a Doppler signal is usually not known in three dimensions, the prudent operator will take a Doppler measurement from as many viewpoints as possible and accept the largest value as the assumed true value. For example, the jet of tricuspid regurgitation may be eccentric and Doppler measurements should be evaluated from all of the available transoesophageal windows.

## DOPPLER SPECTRAL ANALYSIS AND DISPLAY

A formidable amount of electronic processing must be undertaken to extract velocity signals from the echoes returned from moving targets. Modern echocardiography machines employ a technique known as the Fourier transform (after Jean Baptiste Joseph Fourier, a 19th-century French mathematician). This process, implemented algorithmically as the **fast Fourier transform** (FFT) on a silicon chip called a **spectrum analyser**, takes the returned echo signals over a short interval of time and transforms them into a **spectrum** of signal strength versus frequency (or velocity by Equation 3.3). A spectrum is necessary to represent a range of velocities because the returned echoes come not from a point but from a **sample volume** of blood or tissue, within which the velocity is usually not uniform.

The evolution of the spectra over time is displayed in a manner similar to that of an M-mode image, with time on the horizontal axis and velocity on the vertical axis. By convention, motion towards the transducer is positive and motion away from the transducer

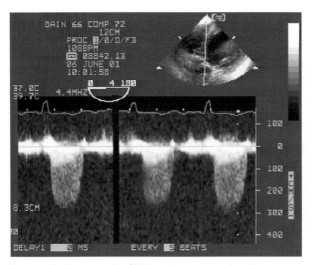

**Figure 3.2** Example of a CW Doppler display taken from a deep transgastric long axis view, with the beam nearly aligned with the centre of the ascending aorta. Each Doppler velocity spectrum is plotted vertically as a column of grey pixels, with the brightness of each individual pixel representing the strength of the returned echo at that particular velocity. Successive spectra over time are drawn from left to right, with the synchronised ECG superimposed. The velocity scale ranges from +100 cm/s (motion towards the transducer) to –400 cm/s (motion away from the transducer). Note the filled-in appearance of the spectra. The bright horizontal band around the zero velocity axis probably represents vessel walls and other strong, slow-moving specular reflectors lying within the beam. The bright band could have been reduced or eliminated by setting the wall filter appropriately. Use of CW rather than pulsed Doppler was necessary to obtain this particular measurement, because the peak velocity of about 3 m/s exceeds the maximum unambiguous velocity for pulsed Doppler (Equation 3.4) under these conditions (5 MHz probe and an AV depth of about 10 cm on the inset 2-D image). This image is taken from a patient with moderate aortic stenosis.

is negative (Figure 3.2). In the display, each vertical line of pixels represents a single spectrum, acquired over about 10 ms (depending on frequency and depth settings). The brightness (or **grey-scale value**) of each pixel along the line is assigned to represent the strength of the returned echo at that particular velocity. The ECG is usually shown as an overlay to convey timing information.

Because strong signals from specular reflectors (e.g. vessel or myocardial walls) located within the beam can easily overload the spectrum analyser, an adjustable low-frequency (velocity) filter, called a **wall filter** (p.43), is commonly employed. The wall filter creates an echo-free black band around the zero velocity line in the spectral display (see Figures 3.3 and 3.5).

## CONTINUOUS WAVE DOPPLER

**Continuous wave** (CW) Doppler requires separate transducers for transmission and reception because the beam is continuously transmitted, received and processed. Dedicated CW probes, having no 2-D imaging capability, employ two single-crystal transducers, oriented so that their beam patterns overlap. General-purpose ultrasound machines use either separate non-imaging CW probes or two subsets of the elements of a phased-array probe for transmission and reception (as with TOE probes). The general-purpose machines can also

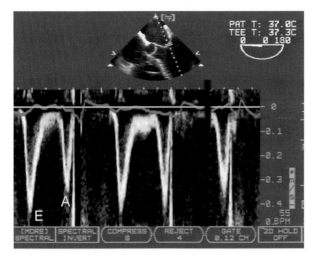

**Figure 3.3** A pulsed Doppler display of mitral inflow with the baseline set to show only negative velocities (i.e. flow directed away from the transducer, which is located behind the atrium). The Doppler sample
volume, shown on the inset 2-D image, is located near the tips of the mitral leaflets. Timing from the ECG
overlying the spectrum shows that all of the flow occurs during diastole (i.e. no mitral regurgitant flow
occurs within the selected sample volume, although it may be found elsewhere within the valve annulus).
During diastole, the negatively directed E and A waves (see Chapter 8) are clearly shown, with a peak E
velocity of about −0.45 m/s. The spectral lines themselves are quite narrow, indicating laminar flow, and
a small amount of extraneous noise can be seen within the spectra. The black band surrounding the
zero velocity axis is caused by the wall filter being set to eliminate low velocity signals. The bright vertical line following the A wave represents a closing valve "click" due to the strong reflection from the leaflet
as it enters the sample volume at the onset of systole.

overlay a 2-D image with a cursor representing the direction of the CW beam, making it
much easier for the operator to determine the source of the Doppler signals, but at the cost
of reduced Doppler and image signal quality.

The displayed spectrum represents the superimposition of the echoes returned from
*all* depths along the ultrasonic beam, so that CW spectra are filled in with speeds ranging from zero to the peak speed in each spectral sample. The operator needs experience
to determine which portion of the display contains the signal of interest.

The advantage of CW Doppler is that it can represent faster signals unambiguously.
This permits the measurement of flows of several metres per second, which can occur,
for example, in aortic stenosis (see Figure 3.2). The disadvantage of CW Doppler is that
it provides no range information about the location of source of the echoes along the
beam.

## PULSED WAVE DOPPLER

**Pulsed wave** (PW) Doppler, like 2-D imaging, employs the same transducer crystals for
both transmission and reception. It is used in conjunction with 2-D imaging (called
**duplex Doppler**) to sample velocities within a specific region of interest. Single pulses,
whose pulse lengths are typically several cycles longer than those used for 2-D imaging,
are repeatedly sent along the same beam path at the selected PRF. Echoes returned from
a selected range of depths along the selected scan line (called the **sample volume**) are

fed into the spectrum analyser and displayed in the same manner as a CW Doppler spectrum. The beam path and sample volume are displayed as overlays on the associated 2-D image, and the operator can adjust their position to interrogate the anatomical region of interest. When acquiring the Doppler signal, the 2-D image will either be frozen or updated at a very low frame rate in order to enable frequent updating of the Doppler spectrum.

PW spectra tend to have a linear, rather than a filled-in, appearance because they come from a small sample volume that usually has a limited range of velocities within it (Figure 3.3). Flow at a single constant velocity would appear as a single white horizontal line on the spectral display (and a pure tone in the audio output). In a region of disturbed (turbulent or complex) flow, the wider range of velocities produces **spectral broadening**. This appears as a much wider and changing line in the spectral display (and a harsh audio output), often filling the entire range with intermediate grey values from baseline to the peak velocity. In general, choosing a larger sample volume will also yield a greater range of velocities within it and thus a broader spectrum. The operator should select the sample volume according to the specific application. For example, a bigger sample volume is used when evaluating pulmonary vein flow because the precise location of the region of fastest flow is difficult to anticipate, whereas a smaller sample volume is used when measuring mitral inflow, in order to avoid the flow disturbed by the valve leaflets.

The major limitation of PW Doppler is that it can measure only a limited range of velocities unambiguously. Targets with velocities outside the limits of the spectral display, called the **Nyquist limit** (after Harry Nyquist, a physicist and engineer at Bell Telephone Laboratories) will "wrap around" and appear falsely elsewhere within the display (possibly with reversal of direction), a phenomenon known as **aliasing**. The Nyquist limit will be exceeded and aliasing will occur when the Doppler frequency ($f_D$ in Equation 3.1) exceeds half the PRF or when a sinusoidal Doppler signal is sampled uniformly at a rate of less than twice per cycle (Figure 3.4). Viewers of old cowboy movies may observe aliasing when the spokes of the stagecoach wheels in chase scenes appear to rotate backwards, stand still, or rotate forwards only slowly.

Much of the "art" of reading a PW Doppler spectrum lies in recognising and interpreting aliased signals. The operator wishing to display the highest possible velocities unambiguously has several means available.

1. Select the lowest possible transducer frequency in order to reduce $f_D$ (this is often done automatically by the machine).

2. Increase the PRF by adjusting the velocity scale (p.37).

3. Shift the baseline of the spectral display when the velocities observed are primarily in one direction. In Figure 3.3, unidirectional mitral inflow is shown without aliasing, because the baseline was shifted upward to expand the range of negative velocity maximally (and thereby eliminate any display of positive velocity). The same wave is shown in Figure 3.5, with the baseline set to give equal range to negative and positive velocity. The negative velocity range is thus halved relative to Figure 3.3, and aliasing results. Such baseline correction cannot be made when the underlying signal is substantially bidirectional or when the velocity of the target is several times the Nyquist limit, wrapping the signal around the baseline multiple times. Some of the latest generation ultrasound systems have built-in pattern recognition functionality to recognise the wrap-around of aliasing and adjust the baseline automatically.

The maximum flow velocity that can be measured by PW Doppler without aliasing is a function of the depth setting of the machine, because a greater depth setting will

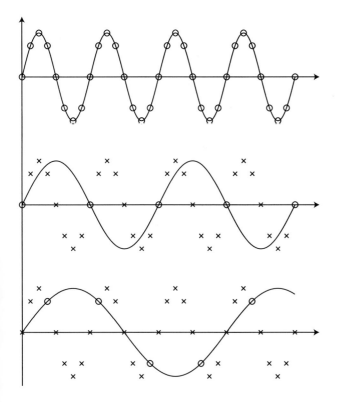

○   Active samples

×   Omitted samples

**Figure 3.4** Examples of aliasing of a sampled sine wave. The top graph shows four full cycles of a sine wave with samples, shown as small circles, occurring every eighth of a cycle. In the middle graph only one sample per cycle has been retained and the remaining seven samples (×) omitted. While the original sine wave would still pass through the retained sample points, another sine wave with a frequency half that of the original, will also fit the retained sampled points and would cause ambiguity if one were to try to reconstruct the sine wave from the sampled values. Similarly, a negative sine wave (corresponding to a negative velocity) could have been passed through the same data points. In the lower graph, only one-sixth of the original samples have been retained, resulting in a frequency one-third that of the original.

require a longer transit time, and hence a lower PRF. By combining the Nyquist criteria, the time to generate one scan (Equation 2.4) and the Doppler equation (Equation 3.3), the maximum unambiguously displayed velocity $v_{max}$ is given by:

$$v_{max} = \frac{c^2}{8f_0d} \qquad \text{(Equation 3.4)}$$

where $c$ is the speed of sound, $f_0$ is the transmitted frequency, and $d$ is the depth setting on the machine. With a 5 MHz probe, a speed of sound of 1570 m/s in blood, and $d$ measured in metres, the maximum velocity in m/s is (approximately) given by:

$$v_{max} = 0.06/d \qquad \text{(Equation 3.5)}$$

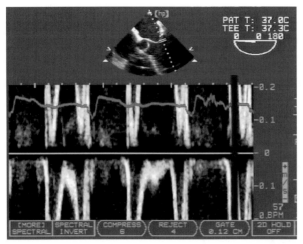

**Figure 3.5** A PW Doppler spectrum of the mitral inflow from the patient and instrument settings shown in Figure 3.3. The spectral baseline has been shifted to display equally scaled positive and negative velocities. This adjustment effectively halves the unambiguous range of negative velocities that can be displayed and introduces aliasing. Comparison with Figure 3.3 shows that the bottom halves of each E and A wave has been cut off, only to reappear as though they were "pasted in" as positive velocities above the zero-velocity baseline. Vertical lines representing both opening and closing valve clicks can be seen intermittently.

For example, when attempting to measure ascending aortic flow from a deep transgastric window at a typical depth of 10 cm (0.1 m), Equation 3.4 gives a maximum unambiguous velocity of only about 0.6 m/s without shifting the baseline (and double that value, 1.2 m/s, with maximal baseline shift). Because ascending aortic velocity can exceed 1.5 m/s, use of CW Doppler becomes necessary (see Figure 3.2).

Some ultrasound machines have an operating mode called **high-PRF Doppler**, in which two or more sample volumes occur along a scan line. This technique multiplies the base PRF (and the Nyquist velocity limit) by the number of sample volumes, at the cost of introducing range ambiguity. The 2-D display will show all the sample volumes along the beam line, and it is then up to the operator to decide which sample volume is the probable source of particular features in the Doppler spectrum. CW Doppler has, in effect, an infinite PRF, resulting in no range resolution at all.

## COLOUR FLOW DOPPLER

**Colour flow** imaging presents a real-time colourised display of blood flow information superimposed on a conventional grey-scale 2-D or M-mode image of the underlying anatomy. With 2-D images, colour is shown in an adjustable subregion of the image called the **colour box**.

Colour flow Doppler requires an enormous amount of computation. To construct the image, between 3 and 16 pulses (the **packet size** or **ensemble length**) are transmitted along each scan line, and the echoes returned from each of the transmitted pulses are recorded for some 100 or more sample volumes along each colour scan line (Figure 3.6). The line density of the colour flow image is typically one-half to one-quarter of the line density of the underlying anatomical image. Sample volumes having a velocity exceeding

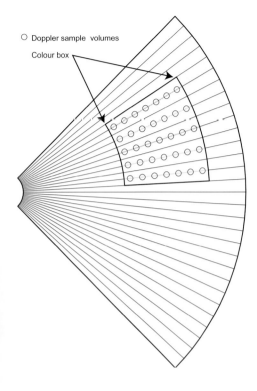

Doppler sample volumes

Colour box

**Figure 3.6** An ultrasonic sector with colour Doppler sampling. Within the colour box multiple Doppler sample volumes occur at a reduced scanning line density, and the colour is displayed overlying the 2-D image.

the wall filter value set by the operator become part of the colour image. The **echo and colour threshold** setting (or **write priority**) allows the operator to adjust the grey-scale intensity above which no colour flow signal will be displayed, preventing brightly reflecting moving wall structures from being falsely displayed as flowing blood.

The displayed colour conventionally varies over a **colour map** that can be selected from a menu by the operator. For example, the colours may range from saturated red for maximal mean velocities away from the transducer to saturated blue for maximal mean velocities towards the transducer (mnemonic: BART, blue away, red towards – this is opposite to the Doppler "red shift" observed in astronomy when a star is moving away from the Earth). Intermediate velocities are represented as colours gradually changing towards black at zero velocity. **Variance** in velocity can be set to display increasing shades of green and yellow over red and blue. Regions with high variance indicate complex or turbulent flow patterns. Activating this velocity-plus-variance option typically reduces the resolution of the velocity scale by a factor of 4 or 8.

A large number of sample volumes is present in a colour flow image. Since each pixel can display only a single colour at a time, only the **mean velocity** (and its variance, if enabled) is displayed for each sample. In contrast, PW Doppler displays the entire velocity spectrum, but only in a very small region. A simplified processing method, known as **autocorrelation**, is used to estimate these quantities in lieu of the fast Fourier transform employed in the spectrum analyser for CW and PW Doppler. For this reason, the clinician should not rely on colour flow imaging to pinpoint and measure peak velocities.

Colour flow Doppler, being a pulsed technique, is subject to the same limitations and artifacts as PW Doppler. Aliasing of the colour display occurs when the velocity in any sample volume exceeds the Nyquist limit. The wrap-around phenomenon causes individual sample volumes to change abruptly from red to blue, or vice versa, rather than transitioning through the intermediate colours. When the variance option is activated, aliased signals will sometimes assume a green–yellow hue due to the apparently high variance when the velocity crosses the Nyquist threshold. The presence of a mosaic of colour in a Doppler image can indicate either turbulent flow or flow velocity that exceeds the Nyquist threshold. As with PW Doppler, the operator can attempt to eliminate aliasing by shifting the baseline (if the flow is believed to be predominantly in one direction), increasing the PRF, or decreasing the transmitted frequency.

The major limitation of colour flow imaging is resolution, both temporal and spatial. The reduced numbers of scan lines and relatively small number of sample volumes along each line limit the spatial resolution, and the requirement for several transmitted pulses to be sent along each scan line reduces the frame rate or temporal resolution. Often the operator can increase the frame rate by narrowing the sector width to the minimum necessary to view the region of interest and adjusting the width, length and position of the colour box. Deeper colour box settings reduce frame rate by requiring the machine to wait longer for the echoes to return before sending the next pulse. A wider colour box also necessitates that more colour Doppler lines be acquired. Decreasing the depth of the sector will not only increase the frame rate but will also increase the PRF and reduce aliasing. If the maximum obtainable frame rate is inadequate to display a moving target of interest, the operator can use colour M-mode to achieve a much higher frame rate along a single scan line.

While artifacts in colour Doppler due to electrical interference are usually obvious, reflections from moving strong reflectors like valve leaflets can cause "**ghosting**" or splashes of colour that appear intermittently in otherwise colourless areas. **Reverberation** artifacts can also cause colour to appear in regions of the image where logically there should be no flow. Sometimes these are an indication of excessive signal strength and can be reduced or eliminated by reducing the colour channel gain on the machine.

The orientation of the beam with respect to the flow can also introduce colour artifacts. For example, the flow imaged in the descending aorta in a longitudinally oriented transgastric view will be red on one side of the sector and blue on the other, because the direction of flow in the vessel relative to the beam is opposite on opposite sides of the sector. On the other hand, the flow display in the centre of the sector will disappear because the Doppler angle is so extreme that the signal will drop below the wall filter threshold value. By varying the probe position or depth setting the operator can alter or eliminate these artifacts.

# DOPPLER SIGNAL PROCESSING CONTROLS

The clinician should have a thorough knowledge of the Doppler controls of the particular echocardiography machine because their misuse can easily lead to false diagnoses. Controls typically include the following:

## Doppler receiver gain

To maximise the quality of the signal, receiver gain should be set to the level that introduces very occasional splashes of noise into the spectrum or colour image. Setting the gain too high can falsely enlarge the size of a flow jet and produce spurious signals or display reverberation artifacts. Setting it too low can mean that diagnostically important flow signals are missed. There is often a separate control for colour flow and PW/CW Doppler gain.

## Wall filter

This is a high-pass filter that eliminates strong signals from slow-moving specular reflectors (e.g. ventricular or vessel walls). Its setting is a trade-off between getting strong flow signals from undesired objects and missing slow-moving blood flow. A feature called **Doppler tissue imaging**, available on some echocardiography machines, is essentially a reverse wall filter (i.e. it displays the mean velocity of slower-moving tissue structures, such as ventricular walls, to the exclusion of faster-moving structures and blood).

## Velocity scale (or range)

The scale control can expand or compress the display, within the Nyquist limits, to best show the velocity range of interest. It adjusts the PRF to match the range of velocities and determines the velocity resolution.

## Baseline shift

If the range of velocities is more in one direction than the other, the baseline can be shifted to use the available velocity range more effectively and reduce or prevent aliasing.

## Sample volume size

This control adjusts the length of the sample volume along the beam. A large sample volume allows observation of a larger region of flow at a time, but generally results in increased spectral broadening. A smaller sample volume provides a more focused view of the flow field and allows exclusion of regions of disturbed flow that may affect a measurement. However, it may take the operator more time to pinpoint and measure a region of peak flow and could lead to omission of the region of peak flow altogether.

## Colour threshold (also called echo and colour threshold or write priority)

Available on many ultrasound machines, this colour flow control sets the threshold of 2-D signal strength above which no colour information is displayed. Blood flow signals should not appear outside of vessels or chambers, whose walls produce bright echo features. Using this control and the wall filter setting the operator can adjust the amount of "bleed-through" allowed into the wall when visualising slow flow near the wall.

## Steering angle

This allows the operator to specify the angle to be used by the ultrasound machine in the cosine correction term of Equation 3.3. Although adjusting the steering angle changes the values on the velocity scale, it has no effect on the Nyquist limit or the occurrence of aliasing. It is infrequently used in cardiac diagnostics.

## Colour box size and position

These controls adjust the size and position of the region within which the colour flow information is displayed in the 2-D image and determines how much Doppler versus 2-D information will be acquired and processed. It allows the operator to trade-off the field of view for increased frame rate, higher PRF and velocity scale, and to manipulate the Doppler angle by adjusting the acquisition beam angle relative to the flow direction.

## Variance

This colour flow control activates the variance mapping. Activating it causes the instrument to use both the mean velocity and velocity variance to assign a colour within the colour sample. It reduces the resolution of displayed velocity because some of the colour display range is used to contain variance information in addition to velocity.

## Colour inversion

This control allows the operator to reverse the colour mapping, swapping red for blue and vice versa.

## Colour maps

The operator can select from different colour maps. For display purposes, this is purely a matter of aesthetics. However, different maps will reproduce more clearly on certain printers and videotape than others.

# REFERENCES

1. Kremkau FW. *Doppler Ultrasound: Principles and Instruments*, 6th Edition. Philadelphia: WB Saunders, 2002.
2. Hatle L, Angelsen B. *Doppler Ultrasound in Cardiology: Physical Principles and Clinical Applications*, 3rd Edition. Philadelphia: Lippincott Williams & Wilkins, 1994.
3. Weyman AE (ed.) *Principles and Practice of Echocardiography*, 2nd Edition. Philadelphia: Lea & Febiger, 1994.

# 4

# Image Planes and Standard Views

*David A. Scott*
*Damon C. Sutton*

To maximise the diagnostic yield from TOE it is important to have an understanding of standard imaging views and important anatomical–echocardiographic relationships. Echocardiography is a two-dimensional representation of three-dimensional structures, and it is difficult (and frequently misleading) to make functional assessments without adequate views in multiple planes. Furthermore, unanticipated pathology may easily be missed. Therefore, if time and resources permit, a comprehensive TOE examination should be performed on every patient. This should be done in a systematic way to ensure that all major structures are identified and evaluated appropriately. Performing a complete examination also increases experience, which is essential if the operator is to distinguish normal variants from pathological states. If time is limited, the primary area of interest should be examined in as much detail as possible and a restricted review of the remaining structures undertaken.

The following descriptions owe much to the significant contribution by the American Society of Echocardiography (ASE) and the Society of Cardiovascular Anesthesiologists (SCA), which appointed a task force to develop guidelines for performing a comprehensive intraoperative multiplane TOE examination.[1] With a few explicitly identified exceptions, the standard views and nomenclature recommended in the ASE/SCA guidelines are used throughout this book.

The orientation of the heart and its relationship to the TOE probe varies from patient to patient and the cardiac structures may be distorted by pathology. Therefore probe positions and angles are given as a general guide only.

Detailed assessment of specific structures, such as the MV or segmental LV wall motion, is described in the relevant chapters.

## PROBE PREPARATION, PLACEMENT AND IMAGE QUALITY

A modern adult TOE probe is a modified gastroscope suitable for use in patients weighing more than 25 kg. The probe should be chemically sterilised and free from defects (see Appendix 1).

Inserting the probe into an intubated, anaesthetised patient is usually straightforward. If teeth are present, a dental guard should be used to protect teeth and probe. The flexion control lock should be disengaged before insertion and removal. Liberal lubrication of the tip, and gentle anterior thrust of the mandible, will usually allow blind placement of the probe. A mild degree of resistance is usually experienced on passing the upper oesophageal sphincter: modest anteflexion of the tip assists passage within the mouth and slight retroflexion may facilitate entry into the oesophagus. A laryngoscope may be useful if difficulty is encountered.

Image quality with TOE is generally very good, but it is rare for every individual view to be of high quality in a particular patient. Contact of the probe with the diaphragmatic surface of the stomach is necessary for adequate transgastric imaging, but this may be impossible in patients with a diaphragmatic hernia. If image quality is poor, it may help to remove the probe, cover it well in gel, suction air from the stomach and reinsert the probe. A nasogastric feeding tube may prevent adequate contact between the probe and oesophageal wall, and so it should be removed before starting the examination. As surgical diathermy dramatically reduces image quality, it is preferable to complete the prebypass study as soon as possible after induction of anaesthesia.

Because of the orientation of the oesophagus and trachea to the cardiac structures, some regions of interest are difficult or impossible to image with TOE. In particular, the distal ascending aorta and proximal aortic arch are usually not seen at all, and complete visualisation of the LV apex is unreliable. It may be impossible to adequately align a CW Doppler signal through the AV.

## MOVEMENTS OF THE PROBE

The probe can be manipulated in a number of ways to facilitate image acquisition (Figure 4.1). The movements described below are made with reference to the echocardiographer standing at the patient's head looking towards the patient's feet.

The shaft of the probe may be **advanced** into or **withdrawn** from the oesophagus and **turned** to the right (clockwise) or to the left (anticlockwise). The tip of the probe may be **anteflexed** (anteriorly) or **retroflexed** (posteriorly) by rotating the large control wheel on the handle of the probe. Rotating the small control wheel **flexes the tip of the probe to the left** or **to the right**, although with the advent of multiplane TOE probes this manipulation is rarely necessary.

**Rotation** of the transducer refers to movement of the sector scan from 0° to 180°:

At 0° the sector scan lies in the **transverse** image plane and runs perpendicular to the shaft of the probe. At 90° the sector scan lies in the **longitudinal** or **vertical** plane and runs parallel to the shaft of the probe. At 180° the view is a mirror image of the view at 0°. At 45° the plane of the sector scan runs between the left shoulder and the right leg. At

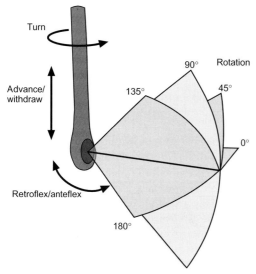

**Figure 4.1** Movements of the probe.

135° the plane of the sector scan runs between the right shoulder and the left leg. Movement of the sector scan in the direction of 0° to 180° is called **rotating forward**; movement of the sector scan in the direction of 180° to 0° is called **rotating backward**.

## THE STANDARD SECTOR DISPLAY (FIGURE 4.2)

The apex of the sector scan is shown at the top of the screen and locates the posterior cardiac structures. In the transverse image plane (0° rotation), the left of the image is towards the patient's right, and the right of the image is towards the patient's left. In the vertical image plane (90° rotation), the left side of the image is inferior and points towards the patient's feet and the right side of the image is anterior and points towards the patient's head.

## CENTRING THE IMAGE

Once a structure of interest has been **centred** within one image plane, it will remain in the centre of successive image planes as the transducer is rotated between 0° and 180°. This greatly facilitates the three-dimensional assessment of any particular structure.

To centre a structure in the transverse image plane (0° rotation), the shaft of the probe should be **turned** to the left or to the right so that the structure of interest is aligned in the middle of the display. If the probe is in the vertical image plane (90° rotation), **advancing** or **withdrawing** the probe will achieve the same result.

## STANDARD VIEWS AND SYSTEMATIC EXAMINATION

Before starting the examination, the recording media should be cued, patient details entered and the machine controls adjusted for optimal resolution. In particular, adjust:

- **2-D gain** so that the chambers are black while the tissues remain white/grey.

- **Colour gain** to a level just below that which produces background noise and speckling.

- **Sector depth** to optimise the view of the structures being assessed. This is usually between 6 and 16 cm; the aorta is usually best seen at 6 cm.

The terms **short axis** and **long axis** are used throughout the following sections. Generally speaking, short axis refers to an image plane *perpendicular* to the length of the structure of interest and long axis refers to an image plane *parallel* to the length of the

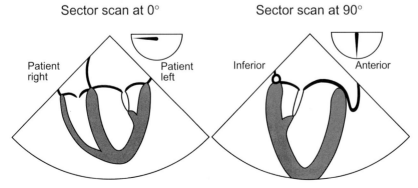

Figure 4.2 The standard sector display.

structure of interest. With respect to the LV, the term long axis has a specific meaning; it applies to any image plane in which both the aortic and mitral valves can be seen simultaneously. Because of the orientation of the heart many structures are seen in short axis in (or close to) the transverse image plane, and in long axis in (or close to) the longitudinal image plane. However this is not always the case – notably for the aortic arch.

Images are collected at four depths: **upper oesophageal** (20–30 cm), **mid oesophageal** (30–40 cm), **transgastric** (40–45 cm) and **deep transgastric** (45–50 cm). The great majority of images are obtained at the mid oesophageal and transgastric levels.

The mid oesophageal views fall into two convenient groups: the **mid oesophageal aortic views** and the **mid oesophageal ventricular views**. The aortic views are slightly higher than the ventricular views, and the **mid oesophageal five-chamber view** provides a useful link between these two levels. The ASE/SCA recommends 20 standard images for a systematic TOE examination; these are described below. Various other views are in common usage, notably the five-chamber view and the views of the coronary sinus, pulmonary and hepatic veins, and pleural spaces.

The views used in the assessment of each of the major cardiac structures are summarised in Table 4.1. Normal dimensions and velocities are given in Appendix 2.

## Mid oesophageal aortic views

The mid oesophageal aortic views are useful for assessing the AV and proximal ascending aorta. Two additional views are also obtained at this level: the mid oesophageal RV inflow–outflow view, which is used for assessing the RV and TV, and the mid oesophageal bicaval view, which is used for assessing the interatrial septum and vena cavae.

### Mid oesophageal five-chamber view (0°; Figure 4.3)

The five-chamber view is easy to obtain and serves as a convenient starting point. With the sector scan at 0° the probe is advanced into the oesophagus 35–40 cm until the AV is seen in oblique cross-section. The "five chambers" are the RA, RV, LA, LV and LVOT.

### Mid oesophageal AV short axis view (40°; Figure 4.4)

To obtain a true short axis view of the AV the probe is withdrawn slightly from the five-chamber view and the transducer rotated (to 40°) until the characteristic three leaflets of the AV are seen in short axis (the "Mercedes Benz sign"). The **non-coronary cusp** lies

| Table 4.1 Primary views for each of the major cardiac structures | |
|---|---|
| Views | Key structures and assessments |
| **The aortic valve** | |
| MO AV SAX | *En face* view of all three leaflets, CFD for AR |
| MO AV LAX | Non-coronary (or possibly left) and right cusps, root measurements, CFD for AR |
| Deep TG LAX view | CWD and PWD through AV and LVOT |
| TG LAX view | CWD and PWD through AV and LVOT |
| **Left ventricle** | |
| MO four-chamber | Septal and lateral walls (basal, mid, apical levels) |

| Table 4.1 Continued | |
|---|---|
| MO two-chamber | Inferior and anterior walls (basal, mid, apical levels) |
| MO LAX | Posterior and anteroseptal walls (basal and mid levels) |
| TG basal SAX | All segments at basal level |
| TG mid SAX | All segments at mid level, FAC, volume status |
| TG two chamber | Inferior and anterior wall (basal and mid levels) |
| **Mitral valve** | |
| MO four-chamber | A3, A2/P1 segments, LA dimension, CFD for MR |
| MO commissural | P3/A2/P1 segments, CFD for MR |
| MO two-chamber | P3/A3, A2, A1 segments, CFD for MR |
| MO LAX | P2/A2 segments, annular size, leaflet length, CFD for MR, PWD for MR |
| TG basal SAX | *En face* view of all leaflet segments with CFD |
| TG two-chamber | MV subvalvular apparatus |
| **RV, RA, tricuspid and pulmonary valves** | |
| MO four-chamber | Lateral free wall, septal and posterior tricuspid leaflets, CFD for TR |
| MO coronary sinus | Coronary sinus |
| MO RV inflow–outflow | Inferior free wall, RVOT, posterior and anterior tricuspid leaflets, CFD of PV, CWD for $TR_{max}$ |
| TG RV inflow-view | TV subvalvular apparatus |
| **Ascending aorta and pulmonary artery** | |
| MO asc aortic SAX | Proximal ascending aorta, VTI through MPA |
| MO asc aortic LAX | Proximal ascending aorta |
| MO RV inflow-outflow | Pulmonary valve |
| **Interatrial septum and vena cavae** | |
| MO four-chamber | Fossa ovalis, PFO, CFD across IAS |
| MO bicaval | Fossa ovalis, PFO, eustachian valve, CFD across IAS |
| **Descending thoracic aorta** | |
| Descending aortic SAX | Left pleural effusion |
| Descending aortic LAX | PWD flow in descending aorta |
| UO aortic arch LAX | Distal arch |
| UO aortic arch SAX | Distal arch, origin of LSA |

MO = mid oesophageal, TG = transgastric, UO = upper oesophageal, SAX = short axis, LAX = long axis, CFD = colour flow Doppler, PWD = pulsed wave Doppler, CWD = continuous wave Doppler, MPA = main pulmonary artery, MR = mitral regurgitation, TR = tricuspid regurgitation, $TR_{max}$ = maximum tricuspid regurgitant velocity, AR = aortic regurgitation, FAC = fractional area change, IAS = interatrial septum, PFO = patent foramen ovale, LSA = left subclavian artery, VTI = velocity–time integral

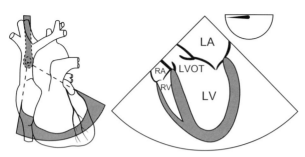

**Figure 4.3** Mid oesophageal five-chamber view.

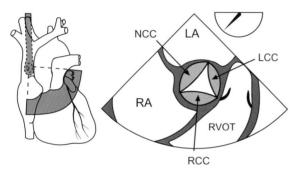

**Figure 4.4** Mid oesophageal AV short axis view. NCC = non-coronary cusp, LCC = left coronary cusp, RCC = right coronary cusp.

adjacent to the interatrial septum (on the left of the display), the **right coronary cusp** is the most anterior (lowermost on the display – recall that, during cardiac surgery, intra-aortic air usually enters the right coronary artery) and the **left coronary cusp** is seen on the right of the display.

The probe may be withdrawn slightly to visualise the origin of the **coronary arteries**.

### Mid oesophageal AV long axis view (130°; Figure 4.5)
From the short axis view of the AV the transducer is rotated (through 90°) to 130° to obtain a long axis view of the AV. The probe is turned right and left until leaflet excursion is clear. The **right coronary cusp** is the most anterior of the three cusps and is therefore seen lowermost on the display, adjacent to the **RVOT**. The cusp seen adjacent to the **anterior mitral leaflet** is either the **non-coronary** (usually) or the **left coronary cusp** (the association between the anterior mitral leaflet and the AV is very useful when trying to identify which mitral leaflet is seen in a particular view).

An echo-free structure caused by fluid in the **transverse pericardial sinus** is sometimes seen between the posterior wall of the ascending aorta and the LA. If fluid has collected behind the heart the **oblique pericardial sinus** may be seen between the posterior wall of the LA and the oesophagus (from any mid oesophageal view).

### Mid oesophageal ascending aortic short axis view (40°; Figure 4.6)
From the five-chamber view the transducer is rotated to 40° and the probe withdrawn until the short axis view of the ascending aorta is seen. This view shows the **proximal ascending aorta, main pulmonary artery, right pulmonary artery** and the **SVC**. As the

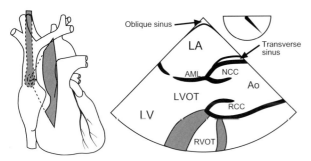

**Figure 4.5** Mid oesophageal AV long axis view. NCC = non-coronary (or left coronary) cusp, RCC = right coronary cusp, AML = anterior mitral leaflet, Ao = aorta.

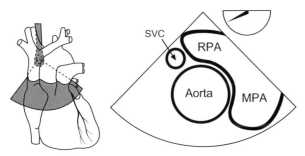

**Figure 4.6** Mid oesophageal ascending aortic short axis view. MPA = main pulmonary artery, RPA = right pulmonary artery.

probe is progressively withdrawn the main pulmonary artery, which is initially seen as a circle, becomes oval shaped as it curves posteriorly (towards the probe) before branching into the left and right pulmonary arteries. At this level the aorta is separated from the probe by the right pulmonary artery, not the LA.

## Mid oesophageal ascending aortic long axis view (130°; Figure 4.7)

From the ascending aortic short axis view the transducer is rotated to 130° to show the ascending aorta in long axis. The right pulmonary artery is now seen in short axis. Both walls of the ascending aorta can be examined by withdrawal of the probe and minor backward rotation.

In many patients the ascending aortic views are obscured by interposition of the large airways between the oesophagus and the structures of interest.[2]

## Mid oesophageal RV inflow–outflow view (80°; Figure 4.8)

From the mid oesophageal AV short axis view, the transducer is rotated to 80° and the probe turned to the *left* (anticlockwise) to show the tricuspid and pulmonary valves. The **RV inferior free wall** is seen on the left and the **RVOT** on the right of the display. If a pulmonary artery catheter is in situ, it can be seen passing through the RA, TV and RVOT as they appear to "wrap around" the AV from left to right on the display. This view usually provides good alignment between a CW Doppler signal and a jet of

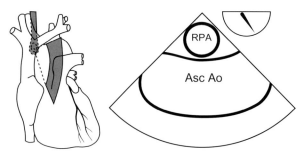

**Figure 4.7** Mid oesophageal ascending aortic long axis view. RPA = right pulmonary artery, Asc Ao = ascending aorta.

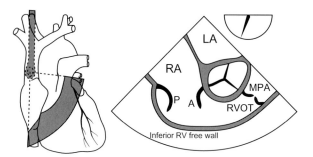

**Figure 4.8** Mid oesophageal RV inflow–outflow view. MPA = main pulmonary artery. P and A refer to the posterior and anterior leaflets of the TV.

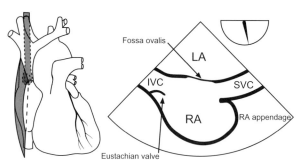

**Figure 4.9** Mid oesophageal bicaval view.

tricuspid regurgitation. The **posterior leaflet** of the TV appears on the left and the **anterior leaflet** on the right.

## Mid oesophageal bicaval view (110°; Figure 4.9)

Again starting from the AV short axis view the transducer is rotated to 110° and the probe turned to the *right* (clockwise) to show the RA and vena cavae. In this view, the **SVC** is seen on the right of the image and the **IVC** on the left. At the junction of the IVC and RA, a small flap of tissue is usually seen – the **eustachian valve**. This view is useful for assessment of the **interatrial septum**. The thin central **fossa ovalis** is usually well seen and a **patent foramen ovale** can be sought (p.222).

## The mid oesophageal ventricular views

The mid oesophageal ventricular views (four-chamber, commissural, two-chamber and long axis views) are important in the assessment of the MV and LV. Progressive rotation of the transducer from the four-chamber to the long axis view allows visualisation of all segments of the MV and a complete evaluation of LV wall motion. The LV is divided into three levels: **basal**, **mid** and **apical**.

The basal and mid levels are each divided into six segments: the **septal, inferior, posterior, lateral, anterior** and **anteroseptal** walls.

The apical level is divided into four segments: **septal, inferior, lateral** and **anterior**, giving a total of 16 segments (p.109).

In any view showing the LV, it is important to identify which segments are being observed (basal anterior wall, mid inferior wall, etc.). The mid-level segments are commonly referred to as **mid-papillary** and the apical segments are poorly visualised in many patients (the segmental anatomy of the MV is discussed in Chapter 9). The orientations of the mid oesophageal ventricular views with respect to the MV and LV are shown in Figure 4.10.

### Mid oesophageal four-chamber view (0–20°; Figure 4.11)

From the five-chamber view the probe is advanced slightly until the AV and LVOT are lost from the view to obtain the four-chamber view. It may be necessary to rotate the probe forward to 15° to avoid the AV and maximise the tricuspid annular diameter. Retroflexion of the tip of the probe may be needed to prevent foreshortening of the LV

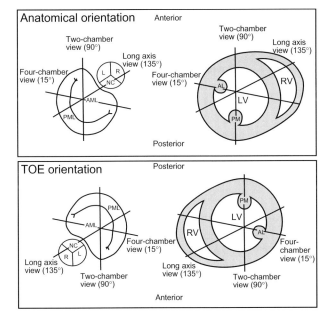

**Figure 4.10** The orientations of the mid oesophageal ventricular views with respect to the MV and the LV, shown from an anatomical and TOE orientation. The orientation of the MV shown in the lower panel corresponds to the orientation of the valve seen in the transgastric basal short axis view. PML = posterior mitral leaflet, AML = anterior mitral leaflet, AL = anterolateral papillary muscle, PM = posteromedial papillary muscle. The left, right and non-coronary leaflets of the AV are also shown.

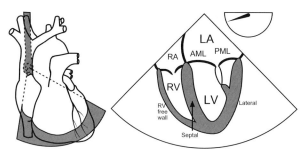

**Figure 4.11** Mid oesophageal four-chamber view. AML = anterior mitral leaflet, PML = posterior mitral leaflet.

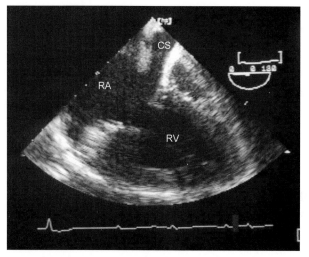

**Figure 4.12** Coronary sinus view. The coronary sinus (CS) is seen in long axis as it drains into the RA adjacent to the septal leaflet of the TV (not well seen in this frame).

(see Figure 7.4). This view is useful in the assessment of the left and right ventricles, the interatrial septum and the interventricular septum.

To start, the image should be centred on the **LV** and **MV** and the screen depth adjusted so that as much as possible of the LV apex is seen. The **septal wall** of the LV is seen on the left and the **lateral wall** of the LV on the right. The **anterolateral papillary muscle** can usually be seen arising from the lateral wall of the LV. The longer **anterior mitral leaflet** appears on the left and the shorter **posterior mitral leaflet** on the right.

Turning the probe to the right (clockwise) centres the image on the **RV** and **interatrial septum** (see Figure 13.1). The RV appears triangular in shape and normally extends two-thirds of the way to the cardiac apex. The **RV free wall** is seen with the basal segments on the left and apical segments lowermost on the display. The **posterior leaflet** of the TV is on the left and **septal leaflet** on the right.

Turning the probe to the left (anticlockwise) and withdrawing slightly allows examination of the **left upper pulmonary vein** (p.57) and **descending thoracic aorta** (p.61).

Advancing (or retroflexing) the probe slightly beyond the four-chamber view brings the coronary sinus (in long axis) into view as it runs along the posterior atrioventricular groove behind the mitral annulus (Figure 4.12) The **coronary sinus view** is particularly useful during cannulation for cardiopulmonary bypass (p.65).

## Mid oesophageal commissural view (60°; Figure 4.13)

From the four-chamber view with the image centred on the MV, the transducer is rotated to 60° until the mitral commissural view is seen. This view is specifically indicated in the assessment of MV function (p.136). A portion of the anterior mitral leaflet appears to float in the centre of the LV inflow tract, between two scallops of the posterior mitral leaflet. The appearance is explained by the fact that the image plane runs along the **intercommissural line** and cuts the posterior leaflet twice (see Figure 9.7), and should not be confused with a mitral cleft or perforation. The **posteromedial papillary** muscle is seen on the left and the **anterolateral papillary** muscle on the right.

## Mid oesophageal two-chamber view (90°; Figure 4.14)

From the commissural view the transducer is rotated to 90° until the two-chamber view is seen. This view is useful for assessment of function of the LV and MV. It is identified by the appearance of the **coronary sinus** (in short axis) on the left and the **LA appendage** on the right of the image.

In contrast to the four-chamber view, the **posterior mitral leaflet** now appears on the left and the longer **anterior mitral leaflet** on the right, adjacent to the atrial

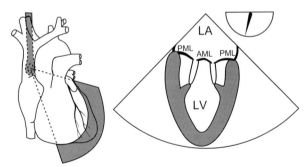

**Figure 4.13** Mid oesophageal commissural view. PML = posterior mitral leaflet, AML = anterior mitral leaflet.

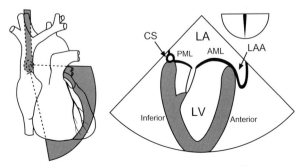

**Figure 4.14** Mid oesophageal two-chamber view. CS = coronary sinus, PML = posterior mitral leaflet, AML = anterior mitral leaflet, LAA = left atrial appendage.

appendage. The inferior wall is seen on the left of the display and the anterior wall on the right.

If the LV appears to lengthen during the rotation of the transducer, this indicates that the apex was not adequately visualised in the four-chamber view. A clue to the presence of LV foreshortening is excessive motion of the apparent apex; when the true apex is visualised, wall motion and thickening appear similar to the surrounding myocardium (see Figure 7.4) unless segmental wall motion abnormalities are present. Extension of the apex of the LV below the bottom of the screen in the two-chamber view at a depth of 15 cm indicates significant LA or LV dilatation.

The **posteromedial papillary** muscle is typically seen arising from the inferior wall of the LV.

### Mid oesophageal long axis view (130°; Figure 4.15)

From the two-chamber view the transducer is rotated to 130°. The LV long axis view is identified by simultaneously visualising the **LVOT** and the **MV**. No papillary muscles should be seen. This view is useful in the assessment of the LV and the mitral and aortic valves.

Contraction of basal and mid segments of the **posterior** and **anteroseptal walls** of the LV can be seen on the left and right of the screen respectively. In this view, the apical segments of the LV are often not visible. The cavity on the far right of the screen is the **RVOT**.

The **posterior mitral leaflet** is seen on the left and the **anterior mitral leaflet**, which forms the roof of the LVOT, on the right. (As usual, the anterior leaflet can be identified adjacent to the AV.) The image plane cuts the mid-section of the MV *perpendicularly* to the intercommissural line (see Figure 9.9). Compare this to the mid oesophageal commissural view, which is seen at 60° and cuts the valve *along* the intercommissural line. This orientation has a number of advantages in the assessment of the MV (p.137).

### Pulmonary veins

Each vein may be imaged at the mid oesophageal level with the sector scan between 0° and 90° and the probe turned to the left or right (Figure 4.16). The upper pulmonary veins are more easily seen and are better aligned with the ultrasound beam than the lower veins and are therefore more suitable for Doppler interrogation.

The **left upper pulmonary vein** (Figure 4.16b) is the easiest to visualise and lies closest to the oesophagus. It lies just lateral to the LA appendage and is best imaged from

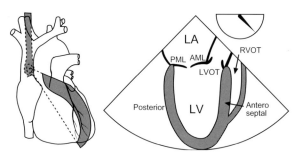

**Figure 4.15** Mid oesophageal long axis view. PML = posterior mitral leaflet, AML = anterior mitral leaflet.

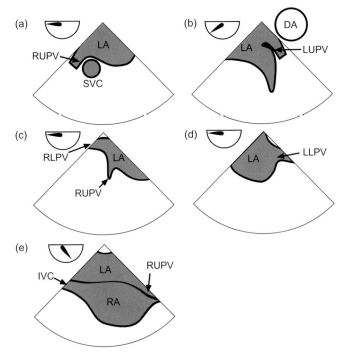

**Figure 4.16** Pulmonary veins. (a) Right upper pulmonary vein (RUPV) in transverse view. (b) Left upper pulmonary vein (LUPV). (c) Right lower pulmonary vein (RLPV). (d) Left lower pulmonary vein (LLPV). (e) Right upper pulmonary vein in longitudinal view. DA = descending aorta.

the five-chamber view after withdrawal of the probe with a slight turn to the left (anticlockwise). The sector may be rotated between 0° and 15°, or even up to 90° in some patients, to improve visualisation. It runs in an anterior–posterior direction, often nearly parallel to the direction of the ultrasound beam, and is ideally suited to Doppler interrogation.

The **left lower pulmonary vein** (Figure 4.16d) enters the LA just below the left upper vein and runs in a lateral to medial direction. It is best seen by advancing the probe slightly from the view of the left upper vein, usually coming into view as the atrial appendage disappears. It is less reliably seen than the left upper vein and is poorly aligned with the ultrasound beam.

The **right upper pulmonary vein** enters the LA in an anterior–posterior direction and lies adjacent to the SVC. In the transverse image plane (Figure 4.16a) it can be visualised by turning the probe to the right (clockwise) from the five-chamber view, and identified as it curves over the SVC. However, the right upper vein is usually better seen in a longitudinal image plane (Figure 4.16e), developed from the bicaval view either by turning the probe to the right or by rotating the transducer forward 10–20° from the standard position. The entrance of the vein into the LA usually appears on the far right of the screen as the SVC disappears from view.

The **right lower pulmonary vein** (Figure 4.16c) may be visualised by starting from the transverse view of the right upper vein and slightly advancing the probe. The vein lies adjacent to the probe but runs perpendicularly to it and is therefore very difficult to interrogate with PW Doppler.

A useful tip when trying to visualise the pulmonary veins is to use colour Doppler to identify flow in the vein. Under normal circumstances this is seen as a low velocity jet directed towards the probe.

## The transgastric views

The transgastric probe position provides a range of views useful in the assessment of the MV and left and right ventricles. In particular, the transgastric mid short axis view is commonly used in the assessment of LV function and, in conjunction with the transgastric basal short axis view, allows visualisation of 12 out of 16 LV segments. The ASE/ SCA guidelines do not describe a transgastric apical short axis view, but in practice this can often be obtained to visualise the remaining four LV apical segments.

Two views, the transgastric long axis and the deep transgastric long axis, provide the only TOE images in which there is a satisfactory alignment of a Doppler signal with the blood flow through the AV.

There is some overlap of information gained from the mid oesophageal and transgastric views but in many patients it is difficult to obtain good-quality images at both levels and the two image planes should be considered complementary.

### Transgastric basal short axis view (0°; Figure 4.17)

From the mid oesophageal four-chamber view the probe is advanced into the stomach and anteflexed until the characteristic "fish-mouth opening" of the MV is seen with all mitral segments *en face*.

Care must be taken in interpreting motion of the interventricular septum at this level: if the cut is oblique or too high the septum will seem thinned and appear to move abnormally as a result of scanning across the LVOT.

### Transgastric mid short axis view (0°; Figure 4.18)

From the basal short axis view the probe is advanced slightly and then anteflexed (to keep it apposed to the diaphragmatic surface of the stomach) to develop the transgastric mid-papillary short axis view of the LV. Gentle adjustment of flexion, with forward rotation of up to 15°, may be helpful in avoiding oblique imaging (indicated by an oval shape to the LV). The **posteromedial papillary** muscle is seen at 1 o'clock and the **anterolateral papillary** muscle at 5 o'clock.

The transgastric mid short axis view is probably the most widely employed view in perioperative TOE. It is in a stable imaging plane that can be obtained in a high proportion of

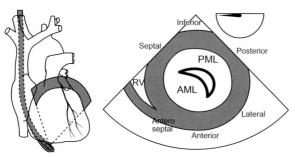

**Figure 4.17** Transgastric basal short-axis view. AML = anterior mitral leaflet, PML = posterior mitral leaflet.

patients and is useful for monitoring global LV function (**fractional area change**; p.103), regional LV function (**segmental wall motion abnormalities**; pp.109-113) and preload (**end-diastolic area**; p.90).

Appreciation of changes in function is greatly facilitated by capturing a short sequence of cardiac cycles (loops) at important stages during the procedure, and comparing these images using the dual or quad screen function of the ultrasound machine.

By turning the shaft of the probe to the right (clockwise) the image will be centred on the short axis view of the **RV** (see Figure 13.3), which has a crescent shape and more extensive trabeculae than the LV. The RV wall thickness is normally half that of the LV. Unlike that of the LV, the **RV free wall** has no formal segmental classification but the terms **basal**, **apical**, **anterior** and **inferior** are used. Note, however, that the RV is usually not cut in true short axis; this, combined with the asymmetrical shape of the RV, makes assessment of chamber size and wall thickness potentially unreliable.

## Transgastric two-chamber view (90°; Figure 4.19)

From the mid short axis view, the transducer is rotated to 90° to develop the transgastric two-chamber view. This allows evaluation of the **anterior** (at the bottom of the screen) and **inferior** (at the top of the screen) walls of the LV at the basal and mid levels. The apical segments are usually not well seen. This view usually provides the best images of the **mitral subvalvular apparatus**.

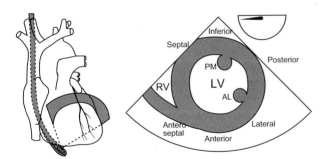

**Figure 4.18** Transgastric mid short axis view. AL = anterolateral papillary muscle, PM = posteromedial papillary muscle.

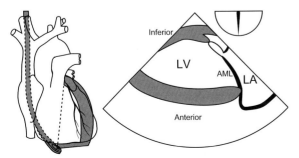

**Figure 4.19** Transgastric two-chamber view. AML = anterior mitral leaflet.

## Transgastric RV inflow view (90°; Figure 4.20)

From the transgastric two-chamber view the shaft of the probe is turned to the right (clockwise) to obtain the RV inflow view. The RV is distinguished from the LV by its diamond shape and thinner walls.

This view can be difficult to obtain. An alternative strategy is to start from the mid short axis view, centre the image on the RV and then rotate the transducer to 90°.

This view shows the RV on the left and the RA on the right of the screen, and is useful in the assessment of the **tricuspid subvalvular apparatus**.

## Deep transgastric long axis view (0°; Figure 4.21)

From the transgastric mid short axis view the probe is advanced further into the stomach and then slowly withdrawn while keeping it sharply anteflexed, until it contacts the

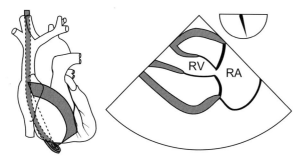

**Figure 4.20** Transgastric RV inflow view.

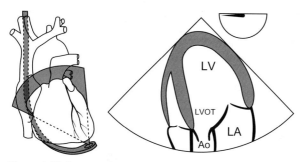

**Figure 4.21** Deep transgastric long axis view. Ao = aorta.

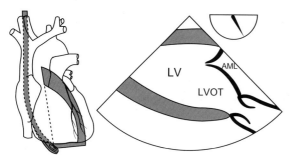

**Figure 4.22** Transgastric long axis view. AML = anterior mitral leaflet.

stomach wall. This manoeuvre is usually effective in producing the deep transgastric long axis view, which shows all four cardiac chambers, the **AV** and the **LVOT**. The tip of the probe is "wrapped around" the apex of the LV and the image is similar to an upside-down mid oesophageal five-chamber view.

Because the ultrasound beam is parallel to blood flow through the AV and outflow tract, this image is ideal for the estimation of velocity through the AV and LVOT.

### Transgastric long axis view (120°; Figure 4.22)
An alternative image, which is also suitable for Doppler evaluation of the AV and outflow tract, is the transgastric long axis view. From the mid short axis view, the transducer is rotated to 120° until the LVOT is seen at the bottom right of the screen.

The deep transgastric long axis and transgastric long axis views are often difficult to obtain.

## Descending thoracic aorta, aortic arch and pleural spaces
The **descending thoracic aorta** and **aortic arch** are each imaged in short and long axis with four standard views (Figure 4.23). Screen depth should be reduced, usually to 6 cm.

From the mid oesophageal four-chamber view, the shaft of the probe is turned to the left (anticlockwise) until the circular, short axis, cross-section of the descending thoracic aorta is centred on the screen (**descending aortic short axis view**; Figure 4.23a). The probe is then withdrawn into the upper oesophagus until the curved walls of the distal aortic arch are seen. Turning the probe slightly to the right opens out a long axis view of the distal and mid-aortic arch (**upper oesophageal aortic arch long axis view**;

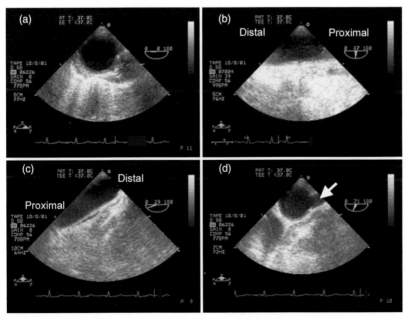

**Figure 4.23** Standard views of descending thoracic aorta. (a) Descending aortic short axis view (0°). (b) Descending aortic long axis view (90°). (c) Upper oesophageal aortic arch long axis view (0°). (d) Upper oesophageal aortic arch short axis view (90°). The arrow indicates the origin of the left subclavian artery. In both long axis views the proximal and distal orientations are shown.

Figure 4.23c). From this view the transducer is rotated to 90° until the distal arch is seen in short axis (**upper oesophageal aortic arch short axis view**; Figure 4.23d). In this view the origin of the left subclavian artery can usually be seen in the upper right of the display. The more proximal left common carotid and brachiocephalic arteries can occasionally be seen by turning the probe to the right (clockwise) to open up the view of the mid arch.

Returning to the descending aortic short axis view, the probe is advanced until the entire descending thoracic aorta has been visualised from its proximal to its distal end. The probe may need to be turned to the left or right to keep the image centred – particularly if the aorta is tortuous. The transducer is then rotated to 90° to image the aorta in long axis (**descending aortic long axis view**; Figure 4.23b).

The severity of any aortic atheroma can be assessed in all four views but it is important to note that a substantial segment of the proximal arch (and distal ascending aorta) is not seen with TOE. Epiaortic scanning is needed to rule out atheroma in this region (p.175).

Normal lung tissue is poorly visualised because of ultrasound absorption by well aerated alveoli; however, atelectatic lung tissue or pleural fluid is readily identified (Figure 4.24). In the absence of fluid or air, the pleural spaces cannot be seen. The **left pleural space** is in the far field, beyond the descending thoracic aorta in the descending aortic short axis and long axis views. In the short axis view, a left pleural effusion is seen as an echo-free space shaped like a tiger claw, which points to the *left* of the screen. The probe should be advanced and withdrawn to visualise the entire thoracic space. In contrast, the **right pleural space** has no readily identifying landmark. To search for a right pleural effusion, the shaft of the probe should be turned to the right (clockwise) from the mid oesophageal four-chamber view until the heart is just no longer visible. If present, an effusion will be identified as an echo-free space in the shape of a tiger claw pointing to the *right* of the screen. By advancing the probe from this position, the **liver** will be identified; this may be a useful landmark for the identification of a right-sided collection. In addition, identification of the liver is required for the PW Doppler evaluation of hepatic venous flow (p.211).

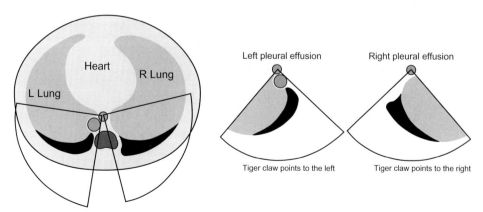

**Figure 4.24** Pleural cavities. Pleural fluid appears as a black echo-free space. Left and right effusions are distinguished by the presence of the descending aorta (left effusion) and the direction in which the effusion "points" on the screen; a left effusion points to the left and a right effusion to the right.

# SPECTRAL DOPPLER IMAGING

A comprehensive TOE examination includes spectral Doppler analysis of mitral, tricuspid, aortic, pulmonary and possibly hepatic venous flow patterns. The standard imaging of these waveforms is described below, but the clinical indications for their use are explained in the relevant chapters of the book. Normal velocities are given in Appendix 2, and the principles of Doppler analysis and display are outlined in Chapter 3.

## Transmitral Doppler (Figure 4.25)

A representative signal may be obtained from any mid oesophageal ventricular view. For the assessment of MV and diastolic function the sample volume should be placed at the level of the leaflet tips in diastole; for the calculation of stroke volume the sample volume should be placed at the level of the mitral annulus.

There is normally no flow in systole. Diastolic flow is biphasic with a large initial peak (E wave) representing early diastolic filling and a smaller peak in late diastole (A wave) representing atrial systole. This pattern changes with age (Figure 4.25). Flow is away from the probe and therefore displayed below the baseline.

A similar E and A wave pattern is seen with transtricuspid flow, but the absolute velocities are lower.

## Pulmonary venous Doppler (Figure 4.26)

The optimal views in which to visualise the pulmonary veins are described above (p.56). The left and right upper veins are usually well aligned with the Doppler signal and are therefore suited to Doppler interrogation. The sample volume should be placed centrally in the vein, 0.5–1 cm into the orifice.

Flow is towards the probe throughout most of the cardiac cycle and therefore displayed above the baseline. There are two distinct peaks, one in systole (the S wave, which itself may be biphasic; see Figure 8.1) and one in diastole (the D wave), and a brief

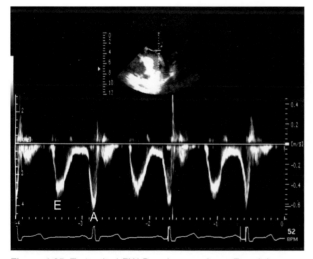

**Figure 4.25** Transmitral PW Doppler waveform. E and A waves can be seen. This image is from an elderly patient, and the A wave is greater than the E wave, which is the reverse of the pattern seen in young patients.

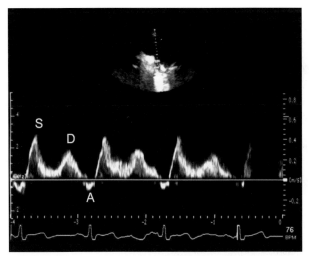

**Figure 4.26** Pulmonary venous PW Doppler waveform. S, D and reversed A waves can be seen.

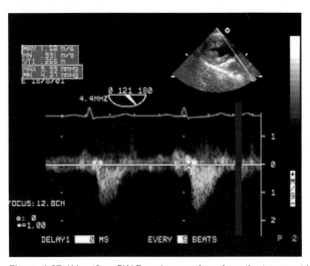

**Figure 4.27** LV outflow CW Doppler waveform from the transgastric long axis view.

reversal (A wave) in late diastole due to atrial contraction. Normally the S wave is slightly larger than the D wave.

## Left ventricular outflow Doppler (Figure 4.27)

To obtain adequate alignment of the Doppler signal and blood flow the deep transgastric and transgastric long axis views should be used. There is normally no flow in diastole. Systolic flow is away from the probe and therefore displayed below the baseline. The normal CW waveform is a smooth curve with a steep acceleration slope and a somewhat more gentle deceleration slope.

PW Doppler interrogation at the level of the LVOT is associated with two problems. Firstly, even mild AV stenosis (e.g. from a prosthetic valve) may lead to flow acceleration

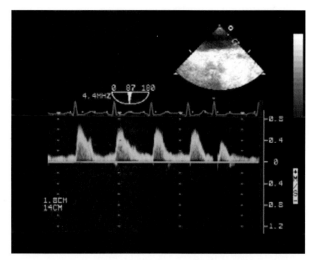

**Figure 4.28** Descending aortic PW Doppler waveform. A degree of spectral broadening is visible. A minor degree of early diastolic flow reversal is occasionally seen as a normal finding but is not apparent in this frame.

and spectral broadening; secondly, the sample depth may be too great or the velocity too high to prevent aliasing (p.38).

### Descending aortic Doppler (Figure 4.28)
With the sample volume placed proximally in the aorta (on the right of the screen) flow is towards the probe and therefore displayed above the baseline. Normally, flow is antegrade throughout the cardiac cycle, with a peak velocity in early systole that gradually tapers throughout diastole. Occasionally a brief reversal of flow is seen in early diastole.

## ECHOCARDIOGRAPHIC ASSESSMENT AND CARDIOPULMONARY BYPASS

In the context of a cardiac surgical operation there is frequently insufficient time for a complete study involving all 20 standard views during the prebypass period. Recently Miller and colleagues have published a revised basic examination with recommendations as to which views should be acquired at different stages of the surgical procedure (Table 4.2).[3] A useful approach is to acquire and record this basic set of images in every patient along with additional images relating to any specific pathology. If time allows, a complete examination of all views should be undertaken in the prebypass period.

In addition, TOE may provide specific information during cannulation and before weaning from cardiopulmonary bypass.

### During cannulation
In the mid oesophageal coronary sinus view the **coronary sinus** is seen in the posterior atrioventricular groove behind the mitral annulus entering the RA (see Figure 4.12). This is a useful view for guiding the passage of a retrograde cardioplegia cannula into the coronary sinus. If the diameter of the coronary sinus is abnormally large, this may be due to the presence of a **left SVC** (pp.81 and 224). This diagnosis is important because it

| Table 4.2 Revised basic TOE examination developed by Miller and colleagues[3] |
| --- |
| **Prebypass views** |
| Mid oesophageal AV short axis |
| Mid oesophageal AV long axis (colour flow Doppler of AV) |
| Mid oesophageal bicaval |
| Mid oesophageal RV inflow–outflow (colour flow Doppler of PV) |
| Mid oesophageal four-chamber (colour flow Doppler of mitral and tricuspid valves) |
| Mid oesophageal two-chamber |
| Transgastric mid short axis |
| Transgastric two-chamber |
| **Separation from bypass views** |
| Mid oesophageal four-chamber (colour flow Doppler of mitral and tricuspid valves) |
| Transgastric mid short axis |
| Transgastric two-chamber |
| **Post chest closure views** |
| Mid oesophageal four-chamber |
| Mid oesophageal two-chamber |
| Transgastric mid short axis |
| Transgastric two-chamber |

makes retrograde cardioplegia impossible and makes adequate emptying of the heart difficult with standard bicaval venous cannulae. The **eustachian valve** (p.69) or a **Chiari network** (p.71) may also interfere with placement of a retrograde cardioplegia cannula into the coronary sinus.

In the mid oesophageal bicaval view the IVC is seen on the left of the sector scan. By advancing the probe and turning to the right, a venous cannula can be followed as it passes through the RA into the intrahepatic portion of the IVC, where its relationship to the hepatic vein can be seen. For patients undergoing femoral venous cannulation, the bicaval view is very helpful in positioning the tip of the cannula in the RA.

During the initial administration of antegrade cardioplegia the mid oesophageal long axis view is useful when there is concern that aortic regurgitation may result in LV distension.

## Weaning from cardiopulmonary bypass

Before weaning from cardiopulmonary bypass the heart should be inspected for residual air, which may be retained in the pulmonary veins, LVOT and LA appendage, or be adherent to the walls of the LA and LV. It is important to distinguish large air collections, which appear as intensely echogenic "masses", from so-called "fireflies", which represent tiny gas particles and are likely to be benign. As the patient is weaned from bypass the transgastric mid short axis view is useful for monitoring volume status, global systolic function and the appearance of segmental wall motion abnormalities.

# REFERENCES

1. Shanewise JS, Cheung AT, Aronson S, et al. ASE/SCA guidelines for performing a comprehensive intraoperative multiplane transesophageal echocardiography examination: recommendations of the American Society of Echocardiography Council for Intraoperative Echocardiography and the Society of Cardiovascular Anesthesiologists Task Force for Certification in Perioperative Transesophageal Echocardiography *Anesthesia and Analgesia* 1999;89:870–884.

2. Royse C, Royse A, Blake D, et al. Screening the thoracic aorta for atheroma: a comparison of manual palpation, transesophageal and epiaortic ultrasonography. *Annals of Thoracic and Cardiovascular Surgery* 1998;4:347–350.

3. Miller JP, Lambert AS, Shapiro WA, et al. The adequacy of basic intraoperative transesophageal echocardiography performed by experienced anesthesiologists. *Anesthesia and Analgesia* 2001;92: 1103–1110.

# 5

# Common Diagnostic Pitfalls and Cardiac Masses

*Roman Kluger*

The appearance of many normal anatomical structures can be quite variable and may lead to pitfalls in diagnosis, unnecessary alarm and inappropriate intervention. These structures are distinct from artifacts that, although similarly misleading, are the result of an interaction between tissues and the physical properties of ultrasound (Chapters 2 and 3). When an unusual cardiac mass is seen on TOE, normal anatomical variants must be differentiated from pathological entities such as thromboses, vegetations or tumours. When an echo-free space is identified, normal structures must be differentiated from pericardial cysts, aneurysms or abscesses.

This chapter is divided into two sections: in the first section the sources of common diagnostic pitfalls are discussed, classified according to their location; in the second section pathological masses that may be identified by TOE are considered. In most instances these normal variants and pathological structures are highly characteristic, and can be positively identified. However, histological diagnoses are not provided by TOE, and the differentiation between a normal variant and a pathological mass may not be possible by TOE alone.

## COMMON DIAGNOSTIC PITFALLS

Normal structures that may cause diagnostic pitfalls with TOE are listed in Table 5.1. Readers seeking additional information are referred to the reviews by Blanchard and colleagues[1] and Seward and colleagues.[2]

### Right atrium

Embryological development of the atria gives rise to many potentially misleading anatomical structures.

#### Crista terminalis

This is a vertical ridge of muscle projecting into the cavity of the RA from the angle between the anterior SVC and the RA, and running towards the IVC. It separates the smooth from the rough walled (pectinate muscles) areas of the RA. It is best seen in the mid oesophageal bicaval view, in the region of the RA–SVC junction (Figure 5.1). During transverse imaging (at 0°) of the superior region of the RA it may appear as a bright, sometimes rounded, echo density on the lateral wall. Slight withdrawal of the probe will identify it as being in the region of the RA–SVC junction.

#### Eustachian valve

This is a commonly seen embryological remnant whose function in utero was to divert oxygenated blood flow from the IVC, through the foramen ovale, to the LA. It is seen at the junction of the IVC and RA and is best visualised in the mid oesophageal bicaval view (Figure 5.2). It is an elongated, undulating, usually membranous structure. Occasionally

| **Table 5.1** Common causes of incorrect diagnosis with TOE, classified by location | |
| --- | --- |
| **Right atrium** | |
| Crista terminalis | Right atrial appendage |
| Eustachian valve | Enlarged coronary sinus |
| Thebesian valve | Pectinate muscles |
| Chiari network | Catheters or wires |
| **Left atrium** | |
| Pectinate muscles | Inverted LA appendage |
| Warfarin (Coumadin) ridge | Accessory lobe of LA appendage |
| LA membrane | Native LA following heart transplantation |
| Stapled-off LA appendage | |
| **Interatrial septum** | |
| Double membrane fossa ovalis | Atrial septal aneurysm |
| Lipomatous hypertrophy | |
| **Right ventricle** | |
| Trabeculae | Moderator band |
| **Left ventricle** | |
| Trabeculae | Lobulated or bifid papillary muscles |
| False tendons | Spurious segmental wall motion abnormalities |
| Calcified papillary muscles and chordae | Subvalvular apparatus |
| **Valves** | |
| Valvular strands | Caseous calcification of MV annulus |
| Lipomatous hypertrophy of TV annulus | |
| **Pericardial space** | |
| Transverse sinus | Oblique sinus |
| **Extracardiac** | |
| Hiatus hernia | Aortic aneurysm |
| Pleural effusion | |
| **Great vessels** | |
| Persistent left-sided SVC | Aortic–Innominate apposition |

it may be large enough to cause obstruction of blood flow or make placement of venous bypass cannulae difficult.

## Thebesian valve[3]
This is formed by fibrous bands at the opening of the coronary sinus. Rarely, a thebesian valve may make coronary sinus catheterisation difficult.

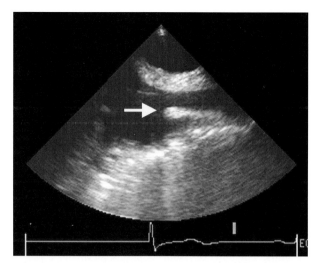

**Figure 5.1** Crista terminalis. In this mid oesophageal bicaval view, the crista terminalis (arrow) is seen as a prominent ridge at the junction of the RA and SVC.

## Chiari network[4]

This is a delicate, highly mobile, filamentous structure arising from the eustachian valve and/or the thebesian valve, and is found in 1.3–4% of normal hearts at autopsy. At surgery it presents as a fine network of delicate strands whose broad base has a variable attachment to the lateral and superior walls of the RA and the interatrial septum. It is this attachment to other parts of the RA that differentiates a Chiari network from a large eustachian valve. On TOE the motion of the filaments appears to be random and unrelated to the opening and closing of the valves.

It is sometimes difficult to differentiate a Chiari network from the leaflets of the TV. A useful technique is to attempt to visualise both structures simultaneously. This is usually

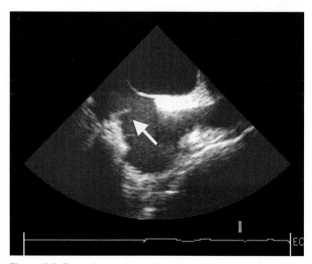

**Figure 5.2** Eustachian valve. In this mid oesophageal bicaval view, the eustachian valve (arrow) can be seen as a flap of tissue at the junction of the RA and IVC.

possible in a modified mid oesophageal RV inflow–outflow view by slowly rotating the transducer back (towards 0°) from the standard position.

The presence of a Chiari network has occasionally been associated with thrombus formation, embolus entrapment, arrhythmias and catheter entrapment. However, it is not usually considered an indication for any specific intervention.

### Right atrial appendage
The RA appendage may appear as an echo-free space anterior to the ascending aorta (i.e. in the far field, beyond the aorta) and near the RVOT in the mid oesophageal AV long axis view. It is more usually seen in the mid oesophageal bicaval view (see Figure 4.9).

### Enlarged coronary sinus[5]
The coronary sinus is considered enlarged if its diameter is greater than 1 cm. It may be confused with a cyst, a mitral annular abscess or an aneurysmal circumflex artery. Enlargement of the coronary sinus is often associated with a persistent left-sided SVC (pp.81 and 224). It can also be due to elevated RA pressure or anomalous pulmonary venous drainage into the coronary sinus. The coronary sinus is best seen in short axis in the mid oesophageal two-chamber view, and in long axis by advancing or retroflexing the probe from the mid oesophageal four-chamber view (see Figures 4.12 and 5.3).

### Pectinate muscles
These are prominent muscular ridges that give the anterior walls of the atria a roughened, irregular appearance. They are more prominent in the RA, in the atrial appendages, and within hypertrophied atria.

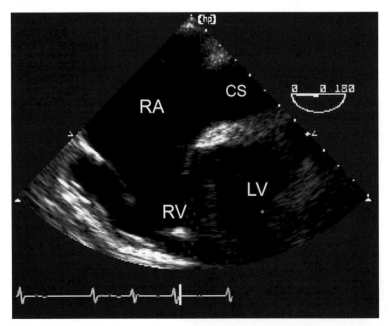

**Figure 5.3** Enlarged coronary sinus (CS). From the mid oesophageal four-chamber view, the probe is advanced (or retroflexed) and turned to the right. An enlarged coronary sinus can be seen entering the RA adjacent to the septal leaflet of the TV. The most likely reason for this finding is a left-sided SVC.

## Catheters and wires

Central venous catheters, pulmonary artery catheters and pacing wires are often seen but are usually easy to differentiate from native structures. They are imaged in the right heart views (mid oesophageal four-chamber, bicaval and RV inflow–outflow).

In the RV inflow–outflow view a pulmonary artery catheter is typically seen "wrapping around" the AV, sequentially in the RA, RVOT and pulmonary artery. It may be useful to confirm that the origin of the catheter is in the SVC by withdrawing the probe into the mid oesophageal ascending aortic short axis view. Occasionally thrombi may form on a catheter or pacing wire.

## Left atrium

### Pectinate muscles in the left atrial appendage

The normal LA appendage is lined with ridges of pectinate muscle (Figure 5.4); these must be differentiated from thrombus, which may be very difficult in the case of small thrombi (see Figure 5.16). Pectinate muscles may appear strand-like and can span the appendage; thrombus is generally rounded and may fill the appendage. Thrombus may be adherent to the wall but, unlike the pectinate muscles, it may be pedunculated and mobile (p.83). Thrombus is commonly associated with spontaneous echo contrast.

The LA appendage is usually well seen in the mid oesophageal two-chamber view but the angle at which it is best visualised varies between 0° and 90°. The clinical history may be useful; for instance thrombus is very unlikely with isolated severe mitral regurgitation but common with mitral stenosis and atrial fibrillation.

### Warfarin (Coumadin) ridge

This is a term referring to the atrial tissue between the LA appendage and the left upper pulmonary vein (Figure 5.5). This tissue may accumulate fat, creating a mass-like appearance, usually with a thin proximal part and a thicker, more bulbous, distal part.

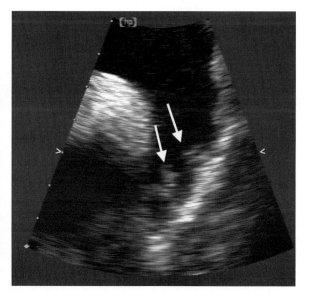

**Figure 5.4** In this view of the LA appendage, small ridges of pectinate muscle can be seen (arrows).

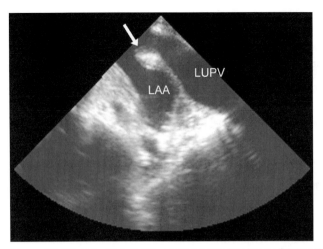

**Figure 5.5** Warfarin ridge. In this view the probe has been slightly withdrawn and turned to the left from the mid oesophageal four-chamber view to visualise the left upper pulmonary vein (LUPV) and LA appendage (LAA). The fold between these two structures may appear as a distinct atrial mass (arrow). It is commonly referred to as the warfarin ridge.

### Left atrial membrane

This is seen in partial cor triatriatum. It is a thin membrane, which extends from the common wall between the LA appendage and the left upper pulmonary vein to the superior limbus (posterior margin) of the fossa ovalis. It is usually incomplete and non-restrictive to blood flow. The first sign of this abnormality is usually the appearance of a greatly elongated warfarin ridge in the mid oesophageal two-chamber view.

### Stapled-off left atrial appendage

An incompletely stapled-off LA appendage may appear as a cavity where the appendage would normally be seen. Colour flow Doppler may demonstrate a small connection with the rest of the LA if the appendage has not been completely isolated.

### Inverted left atrial appendage[6]

Inversion of the LA appendage is a rare complication of cardiac surgery that presents as a new LA mass after cardiopulmonary bypass. The apparent mass is located just superior to the MV and inferior to the pulmonary veins. It is homogeneous, usually freely mobile, and may prolapse into the MV (usually with no haemodynamic effects). Visualisation of the appendage is no longer possible in any view.

It is important that this easily managed condition is differentiated from other masses, such as thrombi, to avoid an unnecessary reinstitution of bypass. Once alerted, the surgeon can confirm the finding by external inspection of the heart, then simply evert the appendage and ligate it. If the inverted appendage is discovered postoperatively there is controversy as to whether reoperation is indicated, because it may resolve spontaneously. However, it may also necrose, or obstruct the MV. A similar appearance has been described following heart transplantation due to invagination of redundant atrial tissue (from donor and recipient atria; Figure 5.6).[7]

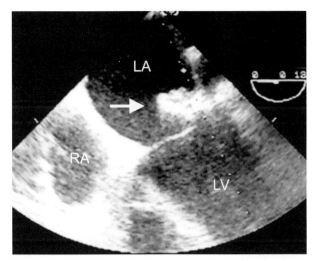

**Figure 5.6** Inverted LA appendage. This usually presents as a "new" mass in the region of the LA appendage (arrow) following cardiopulmonary bypass. In this particular case the mass developed following cardiac transplantation and may contain a combination of redundant native and donor tissue. Reprinted from reference 7 with permission of WB Saunders Co.

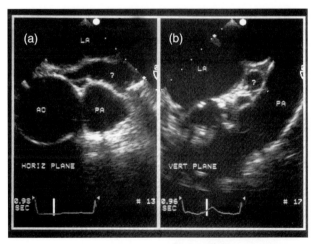

**Figure 5.7** Accessory lobe of the LA appendage within the transverse pericardial sinus. A large echo-free space (?) can be seen in the region of the transverse pericardial sinus due to an accessory lobe of the LA appendage. Reprinted from reference 8 with permission of WB Saunders Co.

## Accessory lobe of left atrial appendage[8]

The normal LA appendage may be bifid, or even trifid, and send an accessory lobe into the transverse pericardial sinus (Figure 5.7). This may appear as a confusing echo-free space in the area of the transverse sinus (p.80).

## Native left atrium following heart transplantation

In patients who have undergone heart transplantation a variable amount of native LA is left behind, creating the appearance of a fluid-filled mass behind the transplanted atrium. It is usually posterior and superior to the transplanted atrium and may show spontaneous echo contrast. In some cases the space is much larger than the transplanted LA. Close inspection usually reveals the site of connection between the native LA and the transplanted LA (see Figure 14.1).

## Interatrial septum
### Double membrane appearance of the fossa ovalis
The posterosuperior margin of the fossa ovalis membrane overlaps the superior limbus of the atrial septum; this may create the appearance of a double membrane, or even a cavity, when the interatrial septum is viewed in the mid oesophageal bicaval view.

### Lipomatous hypertrophy of the interatrial septum
Fat can accumulate in a variety of places within the heart to produce echogenic masses. When it accumulates in the interatrial septum, the peripherally thickened septum surrounds the thin fossa ovalis (which is spared fatty infiltration) and a dumbbell-shaped thickening (>1.5 cm at maximum thickness) results (Figure 5.8). When present, this hypertrophy is usually apparent in the mid oesophageal four-chamber and bicaval views. The septal fat may also involve the RA wall.

### Atrial septal aneurysm[9]
This is a localised outpouching of thin, mobile, redundant tissue in the region of the fossa ovalis (Figure 5.9). It typically prolapses predominantly into the RA, owing to the relative pressures in the atria. It is echocardiographically defined as having a basal diameter (i.e. involvement of septum) of more than 1.5 cm and an excursion between the atria greater than 1.1 cm. Atrial septal aneurysms are associated with an increased risk of cerebral ischaemic events because thrombus may form within the aneurysm and over 50% of these patients have a patent foramen ovale with the potential for paradoxical embolism.

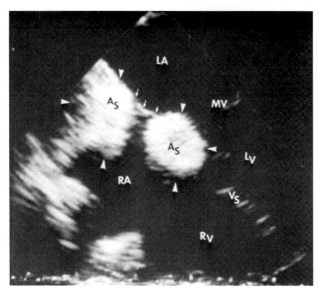

**Figure 5.8** Lipomatous hypertrophy of the interatrial septum. In this mid oesophageal four-chamber view, the thickened interatrial septum (with sparing of the fossa ovalis) can be seen. AS = atrial septum, VS = ventricular septum. Reprinted from reference 2 with permission of Mosby Inc.

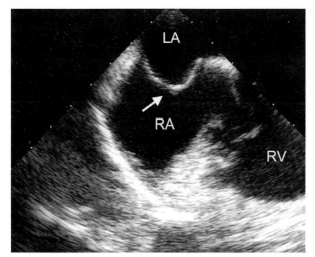

**Figure 5.9** Atrial septal aneurysm. In this modified mid oesophageal four-chamber view a bulging interatrial septum is seen (arrow). Reprinted from reference 9 with permission of WB Saunders Co.

## Right ventricle
Trabeculae
Trabeculae are a series of muscular ridges and bundles on the endocardial surface. They are characteristic of the RV and are accentuated by ventricular hypertrophy.

Moderator band
The moderator band is a prominent trabeculum, which lies in the cavity of the apical third of the RV and runs from the interventricular septum to the base of the anterior papillary muscle. It may be seen in the mid oesophageal four-chamber view with the image centred on the RV. An infundibular muscle band may also be present in the RV.

## Left ventricle
Trabeculae
These may exist but, unlike the RV, the LV usually has a smooth endocardial surface. A structure similar to a moderator band can occur but is very rarely seen on TOE.

False tendons
These are fine filamentous structures traversing the LV cavity, running from papillary muscle to papillary muscle or from papillary muscle to LV wall. They may be multiple and can be seen in any view of the LV. They are probably false chordae tendinae and are not pathologically significant.

Calcified papillary muscles and chordae tendinae[10]
These calcifications are generally mobile and may be seen anywhere in the papillary muscles (Figure 5.10) or chordae tendinae. They are of variable extent and density.

Lobulated or bifid papillary muscles
These give the appearance of small masses attached to the LV wall. They are located near to, or attached to, the papillary muscles (especially the anterolateral papillary muscle).

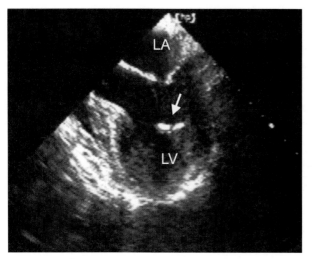

**Figure 5.10** Calcified papillary muscle. In this mid oesophageal five-chamber view, calcification of the papillary muscles can be seen (arrow) in the central part of the LV. Reprinted from reference 10 with permission of WB Saunders Co.

They may be very hard to differentiate from thrombi but the latter are usually associated with areas of abnormal wall motion. The clinical history may be helpful – notably in relation to recent myocardial infarction.

### Spurious segmental wall motion abnormalities
A number of normal and abnormal findings may be misinterpreted as segmental wall motion abnormalities (SWMA) and incorrectly attributed to myocardial ischaemia or infarction (p.112 and Table 7.2).

### Subvalvular apparatus
Ruptured papillary muscles or chordae tendinae, and spared subvalvular mitral apparatus following MV replacement, may appear as mobile masses within the LV and may be difficult to differentiate from thrombi.

## Valves
### Valvular strands (Lambl's excrescences)[11]
Valvular strands are commonly occurring, thin, mobile, thread-like structures, up to 0.1 cm thick and 1 cm long, attached to valves (Figure 5.11). They are variable in number and sometimes fusiform in shape. They occur on all native valves (particularly the aortic and mitral valves) and prosthetic valves. The strands contain a fibroelastic core covered by a single layer of endothelial tissue. It is generally difficult to see them in situ because they are usually white, or nearly transparent, but are usually obvious with TOE. Strands may be found on either side of a valve, but on a native valve usually appear near the lines of valve closure. Their incidence increases with age. It is believed that small endothelial tears initiate their formation. Valvular strands may be attached to the sewing ring, struts or hinge points of prosthetic valves. They may be differentiated from loose sutures, which appear shorter, brighter and more regularly spaced around the sewing ring.

Although they are nearly always incidental findings, valvular strands have been implicated in systemic thromboembolism and there have been reports of large valvular

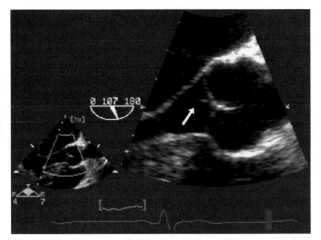

**Figure 5.11** Valvular strands. In this mid oesophageal AV long axis view, a fine filament can be seen attached to a native AV (arrow).

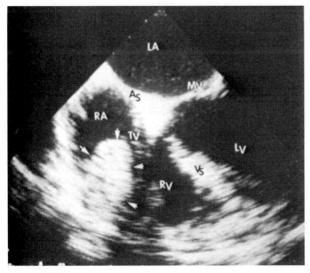

**Figure 5.12** Lipomatous hypertrophy of the TV annulus. In this modified mid oesophageal four-chamber view, a large echodensity can be seen in the region of the TV annulus in the lateral atrioventricular groove. AS = atrial septum, VS = ventricular septum. Reprinted from reference 2 with permission of Mosby Inc.

strands obstructing coronary arteries and valves. It is uncertain how they should be managed.

Valvular strands must be distinguished from papillary fibroelastomas (p.85): fibroelastomas are larger and are usually attached to the valve by a stalk or pedicle.

## Lipomatous hypertrophy of the tricuspid valve annulus
Fat may accumulate in the TV annulus and produce an echogenic mass in the groove between the RA and RV, especially laterally (Figure 5.12).

## Caseous calcification of the mitral valve annulus[12]

Fat and calcium may accumulate in the MV annulus, resulting in a large, round, echo-dense mass with smooth borders, situated in the posterior annulus. This mass produces minimal acoustic shadowing and may have central echolucencies resembling liquefaction. It seems to be benign.

### Pericardial space

### Transverse sinus

The transverse sinus is a fold of pericardium that lies between the aorta and pulmonary trunk anteriorly and the LA posteriorly. If it contains even a minimal amount of pericardial fluid it will appear as an echo-free space in the shape of a crescent or triangle. In the mid oesophageal AV long axis view, the transverse sinus is seen between the posterior wall of the aorta and the LA (see Figure 4.5). It may be misinterpreted as a cyst, aneurysm or abscess cavity, and may contain fibrinous material, which may resemble an intracardiac thrombus. Occasionally fat accumulates in the transverse sinus and may be mistaken for a mass within the LA (Figure 5.13).

The roof of the LA appendage lies within the transverse sinus and may be mistaken for thrombus if the sinus itself is erroneously assumed to be the appendage. An accessory lobe of the LA appendage may also cause confusion (p.75). The absence of colour flow in the transverse sinus on Doppler imaging is helpful in distinguishing it from the LA.

### Oblique sinus

This is a fold of pericardium between the four pulmonary veins and the posterior wall of the LA. It is a common site for blood to accumulate following cardiac surgery. This blood may appear as a space between the LA and oesophagus, which may be echo-free (if the blood is liquid) or echo-dense (if it is clotted). Fluid in the oblique sinus must be differentiated from a pericardial cyst, which may appear in the same location.

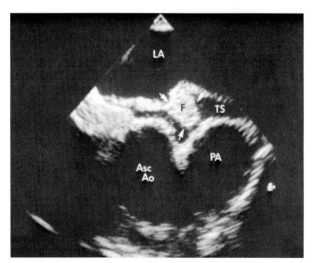

**Figure 5.13** Fat in the transverse pericardial sinus. In this mid oesophageal ascending aortic short axis view an echogenic mass can be seen in the transverse pericardial sinus (TS) due to fatty infiltration (F). Asc Ao = ascending aorta; PA = pulmonary artery. Reprinted from reference 2 with permission of Mosby Inc.

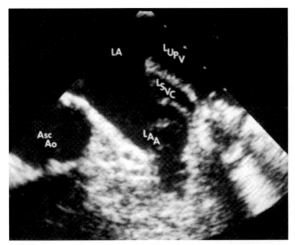

**Figure 5.14** Persistent left-sided SVC. In this view an echo-free space can be seen between the LA appendage (LAA) and left upper pulmonary vein (LUPV) due to the presence of a left-sided SVC (LSVC). Asc Ao = ascending aorta. Reprinted from reference 2 with permission of Mosby Inc.

## Vessels
### Persistent left-sided superior vena cava[5]
A persistent left-sided SVC is seen in 3–10% of patients with congenital heart disease and in 0.5% of normal people. Associations include secundum atrial septal defect and a large coronary sinus (pp.222–225). It is usually visualised (often obliquely) as an echo-free oval structure between the left upper pulmonary vein and the LA appendage (Figure 5.14). Colour flow Doppler can be used to confirm flow in the structure, which will help to differentiate it from an abscess or cyst. A simple way to confirm the diagnosis is to inject agitated saline into a left arm or left neck vein, which will result in rapid opacification of the coronary sinus.

### Aortic–innominate apposition
The left innominate vein as it courses directly anterior to the proximal aortic arch may give the appearance of an aortic dissection in imaging planes near the upper oesophageal aortic arch short axis view, particularly if the probe is turned to the right to image the more proximal arch structures (Figure 5.15). Colour flow and PW Doppler may be useful in demonstrating flow in opposite directions in the two structures.

## Extracardiac structures
A hiatus hernia, pleural effusion or descending aortic aneurysm may impinge on the heart and appear as a mass or echo-free space, adjacent to or between cardiac structures. In particular, a hiatus hernia containing fluid may appear as a thick-walled cystic mass behind the LA. A gas-filled hiatus hernia between the oesophagus and LA will substantially degrade image quality.

## CARDIAC MASSES[13]

Cardiac masses encountered perioperatively (in decreasing order of frequency) are thrombi, vegetations, abscesses, neoplasms, extracardiac masses and rarities such as foreign bodies, intramyocardial haematomas and fungal cysts.

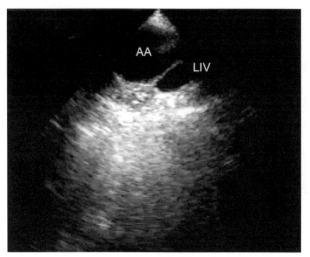

**Figure 5.15** Apposition of left innominate vein and aorta. In this upper oesophageal aortic arch short axis view, the thin tissue bridge between the proximal part of the aortic arch (AA) and the left innominate vein (LIV) may be misinterpreted as a dissection flap.

The degree of reflectance associated with these masses may assist in making a firm diagnosis; connective tissue is associated with a white appearance on ultrasound imaging (**connective tissue reflectance**), whereas soft tissue appears grey (**soft tissue reflectance**).

## Thrombi
### Left ventricular thrombi
LV thrombi occur after approximately one-third of full-thickness anterior myocardial infarctions, but are uncommon after inferior infarctions. They are usually found in the apex of the LV, which is best visualised in the mid oesophageal two-chamber view. However, apical thrombi are easily missed as they are in the far field of the image and LV foreshortening is a common problem with TOE. Using a lower probe frequency (3.7 MHz rather than 5 MHz ) may improve visualisation by increasing the depth of penetration. The apex of the heart is usually better visualised using transthoracic imaging.

Thrombi appear as masses, contiguous with the endocardium, in an area of abnormal wall motion. They are typically sessile and smooth walled, and show soft tissue reflectance. Consequently, such mural thrombi may be very difficult to differentiate from myocardium. It may also be hard to differentiate thrombi from papillary muscles, trabeculae and intracavity artifacts. Thrombi should be visible throughout the cardiac cycle, and in at least two different views. Large, irregular or mobile thrombi are easily seen, and are more likely to embolise than smaller, less easily visualised, thrombi. The centre of a LV thrombus may be relatively echo-free (suggesting liquefaction), or may have areas of calcification. Thrombi are associated with spontaneous echo contrast. A large LV thrombus can decrease the effective size of the LV cavity.

Options for management include surgical removal, a period of postoperative anticoagulation, or no treatment. If the thrombus is not removed during surgery, surgical manipulation of the area should be minimised, and the region should be carefully inspected after bypass to see whether the thrombus has changed or disappeared.

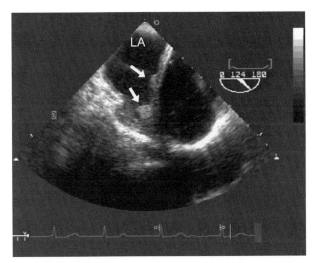

**Figure 5.16** Two thrombi in the LA appendage are identified with arrows. In this patient the LA appendage was best seen with the transducer rotated to 124°.

### Left atrial thrombi

LA thrombi are strongly associated with mitral stenosis and atrial fibrillation; they may also occur with LA enlargement secondary to LV dysfunction, but are rare with LA enlargement secondary to mitral regurgitation. The most common site of LA thrombus formation is the appendage (Figure 5.16), where it must be differentiated from pectinate muscle (p.73; Figure 5.4). An unattached freely moving clot, known as a ball thrombus, may be seen within the LA. Thrombi may be cystic but are more often homogeneous and well demarcated. They may be adherent to the MV.

### Other thrombi

Mural thrombi may occasionally develop in the RV and have features similar to those of LV thrombi. Thrombi in the RA are usually associated with chronic indwelling catheters. Occasionally thrombi in transit (i.e. in systemic venous thromboembolism) may be identified within the IVC, RA or RV.

For patients with proven severe pulmonary embolism, TOE has a high sensitivity and specificity for the detection of thrombus within the main pulmonary arteries[14] (mid oesophageal ascending aortic views).

Thrombi associated with prosthetic valves are discussed in Chapter 12.

### Vegetations[15,16]

Bacterial endocarditis most commonly involves prosthetic or abnormal heart valves. An abnormal aortic or mitral valve presents more risk of endocarditis than an abnormal PV, possibly because of higher blood velocities across the former two valves. In intravenous drug users who develop endocarditis the TV is most frequently involved.

Vegetations typically develop on the upstream, or low-pressure, side of a valve (i.e. LVOT side of AVs and LA side of MVs). Their motion is chaotic and independent of the cardiac cycle and they are commonly seen within a regurgitant pathway. Vegetations usually display soft tissue reflectance, in contrast to the connective tissue reflectance of chordae tendinae and valve leaflets. Size is variable, from 0.1 to over 1 cm in diameter. Vegetations are commonly associated with valvular regurgitation and abscess formation (particularly of the AV; see Figure 10.8).

The differential diagnosis of infective vegetations includes healed vegetations, chordal structures, degenerative valve changes, Lambl's excrescences and thrombi. All of these (except thrombi) usually display connective tissue reflectance.

Vegetations may also develop at anatomical sites other than heart valves, such as a surgically created systemic–pulmonary shunt, an uncorrected ventricular septal defect, a patent ductus arteriosus and other complex congenital heart defects. They may also develop on a chronic indwelling catheter or wire, where they may be impossible to distinguish from thrombi.

## Neoplasms[17–19]
### Secondary cardiac tumours
Secondary cardiac tumours are much more common than primary cardiac tumours. They arise from metastases (e.g. from melanoma or cancer of the colon), through direct extension of the primary lesion (e.g. carcinoma of the bronchus, oesophagus or breast) or by extension up the IVC to the right side of heart (e.g. renal cell carcinoma). These malignancies frequently infiltrate myocardial tissues without forming discrete space-occupying lesions. They are associated with pericardial effusions and patients frequently present with cardiac tamponade.

### Primary cardiac tumours: benign
#### Myxomas
Myxomas are the most common *primary* cardiac neoplasms, accounting for 50% of all primary cardiac tumours diagnosed at autopsy and 90% of those coming to surgery. The LA is the site where they are most often found (Table 5.2). Most atrial myxomas are attached by a stalk or pedicle to the interatrial septum. They should be removed because myxomas have a high embolic potential and can prolapse, causing atrioventricular valvular obstruction and/or leaflet damage. Recurrence is rare.

On TOE myxomas appear as large, polypoid, smooth-walled, gelatinous structures (Figure 5.17). Cystic echolucencies may be seen within them and they may contain dermal elements, such as bone, which give a calcified appearance. Prebypass, TOE is

| Table 5.2 Location of myxomas | |
|---|---|
| **Location** | **Incidence (%)** |
| LA | 86.5 |
| RA | 7.4 |
| Multiple locations | 2.7 |
| RV | 1.9 |
| Valvular attachment | 1.1 |
| LV | 0.3 |
| Pulmonary artery | 0.1 |

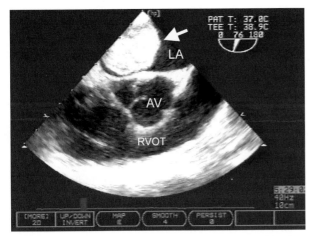

**Figure 5.17** Left atrial myxoma. In this mid oesophageal RV inflow–outflow view, a large echogenic mass (arrow) can be seen within the LA, consistent with a LA myxoma.

used to ensure that additional lesions are not present (these are rare). Postbypass, TOE is used to assess the completeness of their removal and the absence of valvular or septal damage.

## Lipomas

Lipomas may occur throughout the heart or pericardium. They are usually homogeneous, well encapsulated within the myocardium, and clinically insignificant. Lipomas are distinct from lipomatous infiltration (e.g. of the interatrial septum, TV annulus or warfarin ridge).

## Papillary fibroelastoma

These are small (usually < 1 cm in diameter), pedunculated, mobile, pompom-like masses, which may be attached to heart valves (Figure 5.18). They are more frequent on

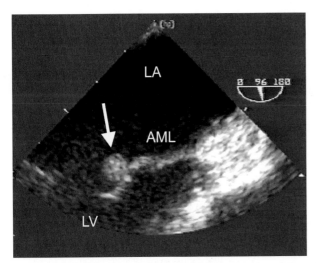

**Figure 5.18** Papillary fibroelastoma. In this close-up view of the anterior mitral leaflet (AML), a rounded mass (arrow) is attached to the distal segment of the leaflet, consistent with a papillary fibroelastoma.

left-sided valves and in older patients. Occasionally they may be attached to a ventricular wall. They display connective tissue reflectance on TOE. Fibroelastomas may provide a nidus for platelet and fibrin aggregation, leading to embolisation. If there is a history of embolic events the fibroelastomas should probably be removed; in asymptomatic patients anticoagulation should be considered.

*Miscellaneous*

Rhabdomyomas are the most common benign cardiac tumours in children and tend to involve the ventricles. LV fibromas have also been described, especially in children.

### Primary cardiac tumours: malignant

Malignant tumours are far less common than benign tumours. They include angiosarcomas, rhabdomyosarcomas, mesotheliomas, fibrosarcomas and lymphomas. Unlike benign tumours, malignancies typically disrupt, infiltrate and obscure adjacent cardiac anatomy. They are usually poorly demarcated and immobile. Additional features on TOE that suggest malignancy include the presence of fluid in the pericardium and extension of the tumour into the IVC (seen in the mid oesophageal bicaval view).

## Foreign bodies

Various foreign bodies may be seen in the heart. If metallic (e.g. a bullet), they often produce striking reverberations.

# EXTRACARDIAC MASSES

Extracardiac masses that may be detected with TOE include mediastinal tumours, pericardial tumours, cysts and haematomas.

## Pericardial cysts[20]

These benign congenital mediastinal lesions occur in approximately 1/100 000 persons. They are usually detected by routine chest radiography in adult life and do not cause symptoms unless they become very large.

The most common sites are adjacent to the RA (in the right cardiophrenic angle on chest radiograph) and adjacent to the LV (in the left cardiophrenic angle on chest radiograph). They may also occur in the posterior mediastinum adjacent to the LA, and in the anterior mediastinum adjacent to the RV and pulmonary artery. The latter two sites are more likely to result in symptoms due to compression of the heart or great vessels.

On TOE these cysts appear as echolucent, unilocular, usually spherical cavities adjacent to the pericardium. They vary widely in size (2–16 cm in diameter), and are occasionally echo-dense. They may be difficult to differentiate from other causes of juxtacardiac echolucency such as pericardial effusions (especially if loculated), pleural effusions, ascites, fluid in the oblique sinus, and aneurysms or psuedoaneurysms of the heart and great vessels.

# REFERENCES

1. Blanchard DG, Dittrich HC, Mitchell M, et al. Diagnostic pitfalls in transesophageal echocardiography. *Journal of the American Society of Echocardiography* 1992;5:525–540.
2. Seward JB, Khandheria BK, Oh JK, et al. Critical appraisal of transesophageal echocardiography: limitations, pitfalls, and complications. *Journal of the American Society of Echocardiography* 1992;5:288–305.
3. Clements F, Wright SJ, de Bruijn N. Coronary sinus catheterization made easy for port-access minimally invasive cardiac surgery. *Journal of Cardiothoracic and Vascular Anesthesia* 1998;12:96–100.
4. Schneider B, Hofmann T, Justen MH, et al. Chiari's network: normal anatomic variant or risk factor for

arterial embolic events? *Journal of the American College of Cardiology* 1995;26:203–210.

5. Hasel R, Barash PG. Dilated coronary sinus on pre-bypass transesophageal echocardiography. *Journal of Cardiothoracic and Vascular Anesthesia* 1996;10:432–435.

6. Cohen AJ, Tamir A, Yanai O, et al. Inverted left atrial appendage presenting as a left atrial mass after cardiac surgery. *Annals of Thoracic Surgery* 1999;67:1489 1491.

7. Mets B, Ahmad S, Sherman D, et al. An unusual echocardiograph after heart transplantation. *Journal of Cardiothoracic and Vascular Anesthesia* 1999;13:639–640.

8. Shanewise JS. An unusual echo-free space between the great vessels and left atrium. *Journal of Cardiothoracic and Vascular Anesthesia* 1997;11:113–114.

9. Baruch L, Goldman M. An unusual transesophageal echocardiogram. *Journal of Cardiothoracic and Vascular Anesthesia* 1993;7:243–245.

10. Suriani RJ. An unusual left ventricular transesophageal echocardiogram. *Journal of Cardiothoracic and Vascular Anesthesia* 1997;11:528–529.

11. Voros S, Nanda NC, Thakur AC, et al. Lambl's excrescences (valvular strands). *Echocardiography* 1999;16:399–414.

12. Harpaz D, Auerbach I, Vered Z, et al. Caseous calcification of the mitral annulus: a neglected, unrecognized diagnosis. *Journal of the American Society of Echocardiography* 2001;14:825–831.

13. DeRook FA, Pearlman AS. Transesophageal echocardiographic assessment of embolic sources: intracardiac and extracardiac masses and aortic degenerative disease. *Critical Care Clinics* 1996;12:273–294.

14. Wittlich N, Erbel R, Eichler A, et al. Detection of central pulmonary artery thromboemboli by transesophageal echocardiography in patients with severe pulmonary embolism. *Journal of the American Society of Echocardiography* 1992;5:515–524.

15. Schiller NB. Clinical decision making in patients with endocarditis: the role of echocardiography. In: Otto CM (ed.) *The Practice of Clinical Echocardiography.* Philadelphia: WB Saunders, 1997:389–403.

16. Ryan EW, Bolger AF. Transesophageal echocardiography (TEE) in the evaluation of infective endocarditis. *Cardiology Clinics* 2000;18:773–787.

17. Sezai Y. Tumors of the heart. Incidence and clinical importance of cardiac tumors in Japan and operative technique for large left atrial tumors. *Thoracic and Cardiovascular Surgeon* 1990;38 (special issue) 2:201–204.

18. Molina JE, Edwards JE, Ward HB. Primary cardiac tumors: experience at the University of Minnesota. *Thoracic and Cardiovascular Surgeon* 1990;38 (special issue) 2:183–191.

19. Li GY. Incidence and clinical importance of cardiac tumors in China – review of the literature. *Thoracic and Cardiovascular Surgeon* 1990;38 (special issue) 2:205–207.

20. Antonini-Canterin F, Piazza R, Ascione L, et al. Value of transesophageal echocardiography in the diagnosis of compressive, atypically located pericardial cysts. *Journal of the American Society of Echocardiography* 2002;15:192–194.

# 6

# The Evaluation of Haemodynamic Instability

*David Sidebotham*
*Andrew McKee*

Persistent or severe haemodynamic instability during the perioperative period has many causes (Table 6.1) and represents a considerable threat to the life of the patient. TOE is ideally suited to the assessment of this problem, and the evaluation of haemodynamic instability is one of the most important indications for its use in the operating room and the ICU.

In the assessment of global and regional ventricular function, and in the evaluation of volume status, TOE has clear benefits over standard haemodynamic monitoring and the pulmonary artery catheter (PAC) (p.4). Other, less common, causes of haemodynamic instability, such as mitral regurgitation and dynamic LVOT obstruction, are very difficult to diagnose by any means other than TOE during the perioperative period. Furthermore, TOE may identify coexisting pathology that contributes to the haemodynamic picture, but which is not the primary problem and would otherwise be missed (e.g. occult tamponade in a patient whose primary problem is septic shock). In some complex situations, such as the evaluation of volume status in patients with diastolic dysfunction, combined assessment with TOE and a PAC is valuable.

In this chapter the echocardiographic (and PAC) findings are discussed for a range of conditions that result in hypotension and low cardiac output. Some of these findings are summarised in Table 6.2.

## HYPOVOLAEMIA

Hypovolaemia is a well recognised cause of hypotension during the perioperative period. However, the assessment of volume status is not always straightforward as it must take into account coexisting pathology, particularly abnormal LV compliance.

| Table 6.1 Causes of hypotension or low cardiac output that may be diagnosed by TOE ||
| --- | --- |
| **Major causes** | **Minor causes** |
| LV systolic dysfunction | Dynamic LVOT obstruction |
| Low systemic vascular resistance | Other valvular pathology |
| RV systolic dysfunction | Massive pleural effusion* |
| Pericardial compression | Ventricular septal rupture |
| Hypovolaemia | Pulmonary embolus* |
| Reduced LV compliance | Traumatic myocardial contusion |
| Severe mitral regurgitation | Tension pneumothorax* |
| Rhythm disturbances* | |
| *Not the primary method of diagnosis, but TOE may help. ||

**Table 6.2** Typical echocardiographic and PAC findings in haemodynamically unstable patients

|  | TOE | | | | PAC | |
|---|---|---|---|---|---|---|
|  | Contractility | EDA | ESA | FAC | CI | PAWP |
| Hypovolaemia | Vigorous | ↓ | ↓ | ↔ | ↓ | ↓ |
| Reduced LV compliance | Vigorous | ↓ | ↓ | ↔ | ↓ | ↑ |
| Low SVR | Vigorous | ↔ | ↓ | ↑ | ↑ | ↔ |
| Systolic dysfunction | Impaired | ↑ | ↑ | ↓ | ↓ | ↑ |

CI = cardiac index, EDA = end diastolic area, ESA = end systolic area, FAC = fractional area change, PAWP = pulmonary artery wedge pressure, SVR = systemic vascular resistance.

With TOE, changes in end diastolic area (EDA) in the transgastric mid short axis view are a useful monitor of changes in preload. Within limits, fluid administration results in an increase in EDA, which is associated with an increase in stroke volume.[1,2]

## Echocardiographic findings

On 2-D imaging, hypovolaemia results in a small, vigorously contracting LV with reduced EDA and end systolic area (ESA). Reduced ESA may give the impression of systolic cavity obliteration and "kissing" papillary muscles. Even in the absence a thickened LV wall, the increased wall-to-cavity ratio can create the impression of LV hypertrophy.

On transmitral PW Doppler, hypovolaemia is associated with a reduction in the transmitral E wave and a shortened E deceleration time.

## Preload reserve volume

If LV diastolic pressure is plotted against LV diastolic volume (Figure 6.1) a curvilinear relationship is demonstrated, the slope of which (dP/dV) is an index of ventricular stiffness. For a particular pressure–volume curve, the ventricular volume at which end diastole occurs will be shifted to the right with fluid administration. The point on the curve at which further fluid administration results in a disproportionate rise in diastolic pressure, without a significant rise in diastolic volume, is known as the preload reserve volume. It represents the end diastolic volume (EDV) at which the LV is optimally filled and, from the Frank–Starling relationship, is the EDV at which stroke volume is maximal (see Figure 7.1). With TOE, EDA in the transgastric mid short axis view can be used as a surrogate for EDV to guide optimal LV filling;[3] the preload reserve volume is reached when further fluid administration is associated with a plateau in EDA.

## The effect of reduced LV compliance

Significant diastolic dysfunction is associated with reduced LV compliance (dV/dP). On Figure 6.1 this is seen as a shift of the pressure–volume curve upwards and to the left. (In contrast, conditions that lead to chronic LV volume overload, such as aortic regurgitation, shift the curve downwards and to the right.) Reduced LV compliance has important implications for the assessment of volume status. Firstly, the EDA at which the LV is optimally filled will be low; secondly, the required filling pressure will be high.

Some patients being investigated for hypotension or low cardiac output, notably those with marked LV hypertrophy (e.g. due to aortic stenosis or hypertension), have the echocardiographic appearances of hypovolaemia, but a normal, or even elevated,

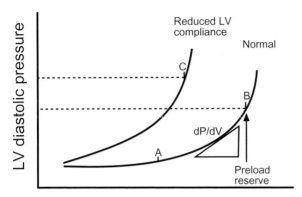

LV diastolic volume

**Figure 6.1** Ventricular stiffness and compliance. The slope of the diastolic pressure–volume curve (dP/dV) quantifies ventricular stiffness. The inverse of ventricular stiffness is ventricular compliance (dV/dP). Volume administration progressively shifts the end diastolic position along the curve A→B. Point B is at the preload reserve volume, the volume at which further volume administration results in a rapid rise in diastolic pressure with minimal change in diastolic volume. A reduction in ventricular compliance shifts the curve upwards and to the left, reducing the preload reserve volume (C).

pulmonary artery wedge pressure. In this group of patients there is evidence that fluid administration based on echocardiographic signs of hypovolaemia results in improved haemodynamics, despite the presence of a high pulmonary artery wedge pressure (>18 mmHg).[4]

In addition to reduced compliance, the EDA at which the LV is optimally filled also depends on the underlying LV systolic and RV function. For this reason there is no normal range for EDA, and most experienced echocardiographers rely on the subjective assessment of changes in EDA within an individual patient to guide fluid administration.

Hypovolaemia must also be distinguished from the related condition of low systemic vascular resistance.

## LOW SYSTEMIC VASCULAR RESISTANCE

Low systemic vascular resistance is common in patients after cardiopulmonary bypass.[5] It is also seen in sepsis, burns, anaphylaxis and as a consequence of drug therapy. It frequently coexists with hypovolaemia and has similar echocardiographic features.

### Echocardiographic and haemodynamic findings
As with hypovolaemia, the LV contracts vigorously and the ESA is reduced. However, in contrast to hypovolaemia the EDA is normal. Thus, the ventricle fills normally but empties more completely. In practice the distinction from hypovolaemia is difficult.

In cases of diagnostic uncertainty a PAC is useful. With low systemic vascular resistance, cardiac index is usually high (>3 l/min/m²). This, in combination with a low arterial pressure, results in a low calculated resistance. With pure hypovolaemia, cardiac index is low (< 2.5 l/min/m²) and the calculated resistance usually high.

# LEFT VENTRICULAR SYSTOLIC DYSFUNCTION

LV systolic dysfunction is a well recognised and important cause of perioperative haemo-dynamic instability. It may be acute or chronic. Of the two, acute (or acute on chronic) is the more troublesome problem during the perioperative period.

## Acute versus chronic left ventricular dysfunction

Chronic LV dysfunction is usually secondary to long-standing myocardial ischaemia, infarction or cardiomyopathy. The cardinal features are a reduction in global LV function and ventricular dilatation. Ventricular dilatation allows cardiac output to be maintained despite a reduction in pumping capacity, therefore chronic LV dysfunction is often well tolerated during the perioperative period. However, it does result in reduced cardio-vascular reserve, making the patient more susceptible to coexisting problems such as hypovolaemia, myocardial stunning or sepsis.

Acute systolic dysfunction is usually secondary to ischaemia, recent myocardial infarction or myocardial stunning. Ventricular dilatation has not occurred and cardiac output may be severely depressed. Such patients are at high risk of haemodynamic instability during the perioperative period – particularly following cardiopulmonary bypass.

## Echocardiographic findings

On TOE there is a reduction in the indices of global LV function (ejection fraction, frac-tional area change, etc. – see Chapter 7). Ventricular dimensions are increased to a variable extent depending on the chronicity of the problem; ESA is increased out of pro-portion to EDA. As the underlying cause is commonly myocardial ischaemia or infarction, wall motion abnormalities may be identified. The LA may be enlarged with pronounced left-to-right bowing of the interatrial septum. Significant mitral regurgita-tion may also be present.

On transmitral PW Doppler, end-stage systolic LV dysfunction is usually associated with an increased E wave, reduced A wave and a shortened E deceleration time (<140 ms) (i.e. a restrictive filling pattern – p.124).

# RIGHT VENTRICULAR DYSFUNCTION

Transient RV dysfunction occurs in most patients undergoing cardiopulmonary bypass;[6] in a small subset of patients it is associated with marked haemodynamic compromise and leads to a higher mortality rate than LV dysfunction.[7] It is a frequent (and often unexpected) finding when TOE is performed for haemodynamic instability in the ICU.[8]

Causes of RV dysfunction in cardiac surgical patients are outlined in Chapter 13, but two common clinical scenarios include:

1. pre-existing RV dysfunction in combination with poor RV myocardial protection;

2. air embolus to the anteriorly oriented right coronary artery.

## Echocardiographic and haemodynamic findings

The RV is best evaluated in the mid oesophageal four-chamber and transgastric mid short axis views. The key signs of RV dysfunction are reduced systolic wall thickening and ventricular dilatation. Associated features include RV hypertrophy, paradoxical ventricular septal motion, RA enlargement, pronounced right-to-left bowing of the interatrial septum and tricuspid regurgitation (Chapter 13).

Confirmatory haemodynamic findings include an increased RA pressure (>15 mmHg) and a reduced difference between the RA and the mean pulmonary artery pressures (<8 mmHg).

### Pulmonary embolus

In the ICU environment, the identification of new RV dysfunction should raise the possibility of pulmonary embolus (p.209). In most patients with a massive pulmonary embolus, thrombus in the pulmonary arteries can be identified with TOE.

# TAMPONADE

Pericardial tamponade is a common finding on TOE in hypotensive patients after cardiac surgery.[9] However, the clinical and echocardiographic features in this group of patients frequently differ from those with tamponade associated with medical conditions. This is because tamponade following cardiac surgery has usually developed rapidly and therefore small collections can cause marked haemodynamic compromise. Since the fluid collection is blood, it may clot and become loculated to a specific area, resulting in **regional tamponade**. In addition, in patients who are mechanically ventilated the classically described echocardiographic respiratory variations are not seen.

### Echocardiographic findings

Unclotted blood appears as a circumferential, echolucent space, and is best appreciated in the mid oesophageal four-chamber and transgastric mid short axis views. It is associated with the classical echocardiographic and haemodynamic features of tamponade and can be graded as small (<0.5 cm), moderate (0.5–2 cm) or large (>2 cm) at its maximum extent. As little as 1 cm can cause tamponade in postoperative cardiac surgical patients.[10] Small fibrinous strands may be seen within the fluid. Pericardial fat is also echolucent and has the same appearances as unclotted fluid, but is not circumferential. The ventricular cavity appears underfilled and wall thickness is increased (so-called **pseudohypertrophy**).[11] The vena cavae may appear markedly distended.

In contrast, clotted blood is echodense and has a similar echocardiographic appearance to ventricular myocardium or atelectatic lung. It is usually confined to a specific region, such as behind the LA (in the oblique pericardial sinus), posterolateral to the RV or compressing the RA free wall[12] (Figure 6.2). RA or RV regional tamponade is best appreciated in the mid oesophageal four-chamber view, with the image centred on the RV. RA compression may be sufficiently severe to produce virtual cavity obliteration; in this situation the injection of agitated saline into a central venous line can help define the atrial border. Clotted blood adjacent to the LV or RV can easily be mistaken for thickened akinetic ventricular wall – particularly anterior collections that lie in the far field. This is distinct from pseudohypertrophy, in which ventricular compression from *fluid* surrounding the heart causes the ventricle to appear thickened.

The distinction between a pericardial and pleural collection is usually straightforward. However, in the context of bleeding from the internal mammary bed with an open pleural space it can be difficult to differentiate between pleural, pericardial or combined collections. A useful landmark is the space between the LA and descending aorta, which

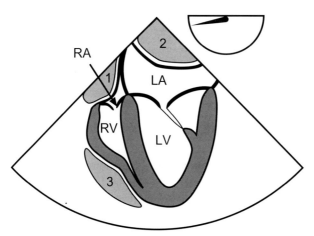

**Figure 6.2** Regional tamponade. In this mid oesophageal four-chamber view, three common sites for localised pericardial clot formation are shown: (1) overlying the RA free wall; (2) behind the LA (in the oblique pericardial sinus); (3) posterolateral to the RV.

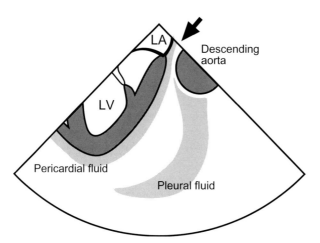

**Figure 6.3** Pleural versus pericardial fluid. In this view the probe has been turned to the left from the mid oesophageal four-chamber view to visualise the descending thoracic aorta. Fluid in the recess between the descending aorta and the LA (arrow) lies within the pericardial space. Fluid in the left pleural space appears as an echo-free space in the shape of a tiger claw which "points" to the left of the screen.

lies within the pericardium (Figure 6.3). Pericardial fluid will splay the gap between these two structures, whereas pleural fluid will not.

## Tamponade physiology

Tamponade physiology is said to exist when pericardial pressure exceeds the pressure in one or more cardiac chambers and produces a number of well defined echocardiographic findings. These include:

- RV or LV diastolic collapse (ventricular pressure is lowest during diastole).
- RA or LA systolic collapse (atrial pressure is lowest during ventricular systole).

- An *increase* in the tricuspid maximum E wave velocity with inspiration (>40%). A small *decrease* in the mitral velocity is also seen with inspiration.
- Paradoxical ventricular septal motion during inspiration (movement of septum towards RV during systole).

These signs are unreliable in the postcardiac surgical setting. Cyclical atrial and ventricular collapse are absent in most cases of postsurgical tamponade,[10] particularly in patients with a localised clot. Respiratory variations in Doppler velocities or septal motion have not been validated in patients who are mechanically ventilated. They *may* show augmented respiratory variation in a reversed pattern to that seen in spontaneously breathing patients, but in the presence of regional tamponade this may be absent.[12]

## The decision to reoperate

The decision to reoperate for suspected tamponade can be difficult and needs to take into account the clinical and echocardiographic findings. The degree to which a pericardial collection is responsible for haemodynamic instability depends not only on its size but also on the speed with which it has developed, the underlying ventricular function, vascular tone and volume status. In patients with grossly impaired ventricular function, even small collections that have accumulated rapidly may cause profound haemodynamic compromise.

# DYNAMIC LEFT VENTRICULAR OUTFLOW TRACT OBSTRUCTION

This is typically associated with three clinical situations:

- Following MV repair.
- In association with hypertrophic obstructive cardiomyopathy.
- Following AV replacement for aortic stenosis.

However, it can occur in *any* patient with marked LV (particularly septal) hypertrophy who becomes hypovolaemic or vasodilated, or receives excessive β-agonist therapy.

The mechanism of obstruction varies depending on the cause. Following MV repair the mitral coaptation line may be displaced anteriorly, pushing the anterior mitral leaflet into the LVOT. With septal hypertrophy, a reduction in the diameter of the LVOT leads to an increased velocity of blood and turbulent flow during systole. This creates a Venturi effect, which may entrain the anterior mitral leaflet. Whatever the mechanism, the end result is LVOT obstruction and (usually) a mitral coaptation defect.

## Echocardiographic findings

The following signs may be seen depending on the underlying cause:

- LV hypertrophy, particularly of the anterior septum.
- A hyperdynamic, underfilled LV.
- Systolic anterior motion of the anterior mitral leaflet and chordae (p.149).
- Mitral regurgitation.
- An elevated gradient (velocity ≥2 m/s) across the LVOT (assessed with PW Doppler in the deep transgastric long axis or transgastric long axis views).

While dynamic LVOT obstruction is relatively rare, it is extremely difficult to diagnose without echocardiography. It should always be considered in at-risk patients who fail to respond, or worsen with β-agonist or intra-aortic balloon pump therapy.

## MITRAL REGURGITATION

Severe mitral regurgitation is an important cause of haemodynamic instability and should be considered in the following situations:

- Following MV repair or replacement.
- In the setting of acute ischaemia or infarction (including papillary muscle rupture). If new mitral regurgitation is seen, a careful search for regional wall motion abnormalities should be undertaken.
- During off-pump coronary graft surgery. This may occur secondary to acute ischaemia or the mechanical effects of lifting the heart.
- In association with sepsis (due to MV endocarditis).
- In association with dynamic LVOT obstruction.

The echocardiographic features of mitral regurgitation are described in Chapter 9.

## MASSIVE LEFT PLEURAL EFFUSION

Pleural effusions do not typically cause haemodynamic instability but occasionally a massive (>1.5 l) left-sided collection can cause direct compression of the heart. This appears as a large echolucent space below the aorta. There may be associated collapse of the left lower lobe, which appears as an echodense area adjacent to the lateral LV wall.

## VENTRICULAR SEPTAL RUPTURE

Ventricular septal rupture causing shock can occur as a late complication of myocardial infarction (p.113). The septal defect is frequently difficult to see on 2-D imaging; however, on colour flow Doppler a turbulent jet on the RV side of the septum, or a region of flow acceleration on the LV side of the septum, may be identified. Associated echocardiographic findings include biventricular dysfunction and pulmonary hypertension (identified by a tricuspid regurgitation jet velocity >3 m/s). An apical defect may be missed on TOE owing to ventricular foreshortening.

## HYPOTENSION DURING SEPARATION FROM CARDIOPULMONARY BYPASS

The period immediately following separation from cardiopulmonary bypass is frequently associated with haemodynamic instability. A TOE checklist for hypotension during this period is given in Table 6.3.

## THE DIFFICULT DIAGNOSIS

Sometimes the cause of haemodynamic instability is not readily apparent from TOE: "the heart looks fine but the patient looks terrible". It is important to remember that haemodynamic instability frequently occurs in the presence of vigorous systolic function (e.g. with hypovolaemia, low systemic vascular resistance, pericardial tamponade, mitral

**Table 6.3** Haemodynamic instability during separation of the patient from bypass: a TOE checklist

**Left ventricular dysfunction**

Myocardial stunning (e.g. due to prolonged bypass, pre-existing ischaemia, inadequate myocardial protection, inadequate time for reperfusion following release of the aortic cross-clamp)

Exacerbation of pre-existing LV dysfunction by above mechanisms

Acute ischaemia involving left or right coronary systems (e.g. due to inadequate revascularisation, intracoronary air, or kinking of a coronary graft)

**Right ventricular dysfunction**

Myocardial stunning (e.g. due to prolonged bypass, poor myocardial protection associated with the use of retrograde cardioplegia)

Acute ischaemia involving the right coronary system (particularly intracoronary air)

Exacerbation of pre-existing pulmonary hypertension and RV dysfunction with the development of tricuspid regurgitation

Acute pulmonary hypertension secondary to protamine administration

RV compression during chest closure

**Hypovolaemia, reduced LV compliance and low systemic vascular resistance**

Hypovolaemia secondary to inadequate filling during separation from bypass or as a consequence of fluid loss

The effects of vasodilating and inodilating drugs (e.g. protamine or milrinone)

Vasodilation secondary to the systemic inflammatory response to bypass

Reduced LV compliance secondary to pre-existing LV hypertrophy or acute ischaemia

**Left ventricular outflow tract obstruction and SAM**

Following MV repair

Secondary to pre-existing LV hypertrophy (particularly following AV replacement) or HOCM

**Mitral regurgitation**

Secondary to failed MV repair or inadequate MV prosthesis function

Secondary to ischaemia or volume overload

Secondary to SAM

**Rhythm disturbance**

Loss of atrioventricular synchrony or atrial fibrillation (examine transmitral E and A waves if diagnosis unclear from ECG)

SAM = systolic anterior motion, HOCM = hypertrophic obstructive cardiomyopathy.

regurgitation, LVOT obstruction or a rhythm disturbance). Some diagnoses are difficult to make confidently with TOE alone (e.g. low systemic vascular resistance), and in many situations the cause of the haemodynamic instability is multifactorial. The following points should be considered when the diagnosis is not obvious on examination with TOE.

## Multifactorial causes

Hypovolaemia frequently coexists with other pathology including diastolic dysfunction, systolic dysfunction, low systemic vascular resistance and occult tamponade.

In the presence of a secondary condition (e.g. systolic LV dysfunction) small pericardial collections that would normally be benign can lead to marked haemodynamic compromise.

RV dysfunction can result in impaired filling of the LV due to the effects of ventricular interdependence and low cardiac output. Further volume administration in this situation is usually inappropriate.

Subclinical valvular lesions (e.g. mitral and aortic stenosis) may exacerbate the haemodynamic consequences of other pathology such as low systemic vascular resistance or myocardial ischaemia.

## The effect of inotropic agents

It is usual for hypotensive patients to be receiving inotropic support during the echocardiographic examination. These agents give the ventricular motion a "snappy" appearance, which can mask poor systolic function and low cardiac output. It is useful to measure fractional area change or ejection fraction formally in this setting. A "normal" heart appears hyperdynamic under the influence of inotropic agents and in the presence of sepsis.

## The effect of sepsis

Sepsis and the systemic inflammatory response (e.g. to cardiopulmonary bypass) produces a hyperdynamic dilated circulation with a cardiac index that may be as high as 4–6 l/min/m$^2$. In this setting, conditions that reduce cardiovascular reserve (e.g. chronic systolic LV dysfunction, pericardial fluid, RV dysfunction) may limit the cardiac index to less than this. On TOE the heart may look vigorous, and no abnormality may have been apparent on a presepsis examination, but the patient may be in a relatively low cardiac output state. Despite these difficulties, TOE is useful in this setting to gauge the response to further volume loading and inotropic therapy.

## The effect of rhythm disturbances

Rhythm disturbances are an important cause of haemodynamic compromise and the diagnosis is not always obvious from the ECG, particularly loss of atrioventricular synchrony or nodal rhythm. On TOE the LV may appear hyperdynamic despite low cardiac output or hypotension. A clue to the presence of a rhythm disturbance is provided by the loss of the normal E and A wave pattern on the transmitral PW Doppler waveform.

## REFERENCES

1. Greim CA, Roewer N, Apfel C, et al. Relation of echocardiographic preload indices to stroke volume in critically ill patients with normal and low cardiac index. *Intensive Care Medicine* 1997;23:411–416.
2. Thys DM, Hillel Z, Goldman ME, et al. A comparison of hemodynamic indices derived by invasive monitoring and two-dimensional echocardiography. *Anesthesiology* 1987;67:630–634.
3. Swenson JD, Bull D, Stringham J. Subjective assessment of left ventricular preload using transesophageal echocardiography: corresponding pulmonary artery occlusion pressures. *Journal of Cardiothoracic and Vascular Anesthesia* 2001;15:580–583.
4. Çiçek S, Demirkiliç U, Kuralay E, et al. Prediction of intraoperative hypovolemia in patients with left ventricular hypertrophy: comparison of transesophageal echocardiography and Swan-Ganz monitoring. *Echocardiography* 1997;14:257–260.
5. Johnson MR. Low systemic vascular resistance after cardiopulmonary bypass: are we any closer to understanding the enigma? *Critical Care Medicine* 1999;27: 1048–1050.
6. Rafferty T, Durkin M, Harris S, et al. Transesophageal two-dimensional echocardiographic analysis of right

ventricular systolic performance indices during coronary artery bypass grafting. *Journal of Cardiothoracic and Vascular Anesthesia* 1993;7:160–166.

7. Reichert CLA, Visser CA, van den Brink RBA, et al. Prognostic value of biventricular function in hypotensive patients after cardiac surgery as assessed by transesophageal echocardiography. *Journal of Cardiothoracic and Vascular Anesthesia* 1992;6:429–432.

8. Heidenreich PA, Stainback RF, Redberg RF, et al. Transesophageal echocardiography predicts mortality in critically ill patients with unexplained hypotension. *Journal of the American College of Cardiology* 1995;26:152–158.

9. Reichert CLA, Visser CA, Koolen JJ, et al. Transesophageal echocardiography in hypotensive patients after cardiac operations. *Journal of Thoracic and Cardiovascular Surgery* 1992;104:321–326.

10. Bommer WJ, Follette D, Pollock M, et al. Tamponade in patients undergoing cardiac surgery: a clinical–echocardiographic diagnosis. *American Heart Journal* 1995;130:1216–1223.

11. Feinberg MS, Popescu BA, Popescu AC, et al. Assessment of pseudohypertrophy as a measure of left-ventricular compression in patients with cardiac tamponade. *Cardiology* 2000;94:213–219.

12. Saner HE, Olson JD, Goldenberg IF, et al. Isolated right atrial tamponade after open heart surgery: role of echocardiography in diagnosis and management. *Cardiology* 1995;86:464–472.

# 7

# Systolic Left Ventricular Function

*Murali Sivarajan*

During cardiac surgery a patient's ability to separate from cardiopulmonary bypass and sustain an adequate haemodynamic state depends primarily on LV systolic function. In most patients TOE provides detailed images of the LV and is therefore ideally suited for the rapid and accurate evaluation of global and regional function and ventricular filling.

Before cardiopulmonary bypass, assessment of global systolic function with TOE can help to identify those patients at risk of difficulty in separating from bypass and in need of haemodynamic support. Following bypass TOE provides an ongoing monitor of the response to therapy. Identification of new SWMAs alerts the anaesthetist to the presence of myocardial ischaemia that may require further surgical intervention. Throughout the perioperative period TOE provides information on LV volume status that is superior to that provided by any other monitoring device. Hence, assessment of systolic LV function is a major component of, and sometimes the only indication for, perioperative TOE.

## FACTORS AFFECTING SYSTOLIC FUNCTION

The primary function of the heart is that of a pump. The force of systolic contraction provides the propulsive force for the pump. The main determinants of the force of contraction are the intrinsic contractile function of the heart (**contractility**) and loading conditions (**preload** and **afterload**).

### Loading conditions

The resting tension just before the onset of contraction represents preload and determines the end diastolic fibre length. An increase in end diastolic fibre length will, within physiological limits, increase the force of contraction (the Frank–Starling effect). In vivo, an increase in LV end diastolic volume (EDV) by distending and increasing the length of myocardial fibres will result in an increase in the force of contraction, and augment stroke volume.

Afterload is defined as the force opposing ventricular ejection, and depends on a number of factors, including systemic vascular resistance, systolic blood pressure and ventricular dimensions. An increase in systemic vascular resistance will increase afterload and decrease stroke volume.

### Ventricular function curves and pressure–volume loops

To isolate the effect of contractility from the effect of loading conditions on cardiac performance it is necessary to examine ventricular function curves and pressure–volume loops (Figure 7.1).

Ventricular function curves are constructed by plotting EDV against stroke volume. Over a physiological range of values an increase in EDV will result in an increase in stroke volume (by the Frank–Starling effect). Administration of an inotropic agent, which

Ventricular function curves

Pressure–volume loops

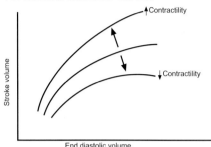
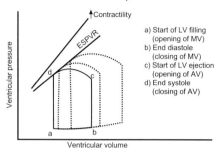

**Figure 7.1** Left panel: clinical application of the Frank–Starling relationship in which, at constant contractility, an increase in LV end diastolic volume results in an increase in LV stroke volume. An increase in contractility shifts the curve upwards and to the left, and a decrease in contractility shifts the curve downwards and to the right. Right panel: three LV pressure–volume loops under different preload conditions. The end systolic points form a straight line known as the end systolic pressure–volume relationship (ESPVR), which represents a measure of contractility that is independent of preload and largely independent of afterload. An increase in contractility shifts the line upwards and to the left.

increases contractility, will shift the curve upwards and to the left. Stated differently, an increase in contractility will result in an increase in stroke volume without an increase in EDV. A decrease in contractility will shift the curve downwards and to the right. In other words, it will decrease stroke volume without a decrease in the EDV.

A pressure–volume loop is constructed by plotting ventricular volume against pressure during a single cardiac cycle. The coordinates of pressure and volume at end systole are known as the end systolic pressure–volume relationship (ESPVR). If EDV is increased, the loop will shift to the right and stroke volume will be augmented. If a number of loops are constructed by varying preload, the coordinates at end systole form a single straight line, the slope of which is a (relatively) load-independent measure of contractility; it is steeper at higher contractility and shallower at lower contractility.

Although it is technically feasible to construct ventricular function curves and pressure–volume loops in the operating room, this is very rarely done. Instead, it is simply accepted that the indices of systolic function available for routine clinical use (pp.103–108) are influenced by both contractility and loading conditions.

## CAUSES OF SYSTOLIC DYSFUNCTION

Acute systolic dysfunction is usually due to myocardial ischaemia, infarction or stunning. Myocardial ischaemia results in SWMAs, which, when extensive, lead to a global reduction in systolic function.

A variety of conditions may result in chronic LV systolic dysfunction including coronary artery disease, aortic regurgitation and stenosis, mitral regurgitation, hypertensive heart disease and the cardiomyopathies (dilated, restrictive and obstructive). There is significant overlap between systolic LV dysfunction and the clinical syndrome of congestive cardiac failure, but not all congestive cardiac failure is due to systolic dysfunction (other causes include diastolic dysfunction, mitral stenosis and constrictive pericarditis). Furthermore, it is possible for a patient to have significant LV dysfunction and yet be asymptomatic.

# ECHOCARDIOGRAPHIC ASSESSMENT OF GLOBAL LEFT VENTRICULAR FUNCTION

A key component of the echocardiographic assessment of ventricular performance is the measurement of one or more of the indices of global LV function outlined below. In addition, a range of other signs may be apparent in patients with systolic LV dysfunction which can help assess the chronicity of the process and help distinguish between different pathologies.

Chronic LV dysfunction leads to **chamber dilatation**. End systolic and end diastolic dimensions (in the transgastric mid short axis view) of > 4.5 and 7 cm, respectively, suggest significant dilatation. **Spherical enlargement** of the LV is associated with longstanding aortic or mitral regurgitation or a cardiomyopathy. Ventricular wall thickness may be increased: chronic volume overload (e.g. aortic or mitral regurgitation) leads to **eccentric hypertrophy** (i.e. LV wall thickness is increased in proportion to the increase in chamber size). Chronic pressure overload (e.g. in aortic stenosis, hypertensive heart disease) leads to **concentric hypertrophy** (i.e. LV wall thickness is increased in excess of the chamber size). LV dysfunction due to myocardial infarction may be associated with asymmetrical wall thinning.

RV function is usually preserved in patients whose LV dysfunction is due to coronary artery disease or left-sided valvular heart disease – at least in the early stages of disease. In contrast, ventricular dysfunction due to a cardiomyopathy typically involves the RV as well as the LV.

Specific findings on TOE may suggest a primary diagnosis, such as valvular pathology or hypertrophic obstructive cardiomyopathy (indicated by marked septal hypertrophy in association with systolic anterior motion of the anterior mitral leaflet).

Features suggestive of coronary artery disease include the presence of an LV aneurysm or intracavity thrombus.

## Fractional area change

While ejection fraction (EF) is the most widely used measure of global systolic function, for purposes of intraoperative monitoring fractional area change (FAC) affords a reliable index of systolic performance that can be obtained more rapidly.

FAC is the proportional change in area of the LV short axis during systole and is given by the formula:

$$FAC = \frac{EDA - ESA}{EDA} \times 100 \qquad \text{(Equation 7.1)}$$

where EDA = end diastolic area and ESA = end systolic area. The normal range is 36–64%.[1]

Images are collected from the transgastric mid short axis view. Using the freeze and scroll functions the largest (EDA) and smallest (ESA) frames of a representative cardiac cycle are identified. The endocardial surfaces are then traced and the areas recorded (Figure 7.2). The papillary muscles should be excluded from the trace. The end diastolic and end systolic frames are chosen from a subjective assessment of the cavity size and not from the ECG, because the time delay between the image frames and the phase of the ECG is not always the same. The endocardial borders of the septum and the lateral walls are often poorly visualised as they lie parallel to the echo beam and therefore provide weak specular reflection. In such instances, the trace is extrapolated to form a smooth curve. In order to estimate the true location of the endocardial surface in the

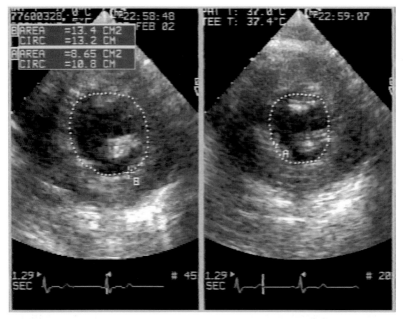

**Figure 7.2** Measurement of fractional area change (FAC): end-diastolic area (left frame) = 13.4 cm²; end systolic area (right frame) = 8.65 cm²; FAC = 35%. The papillary muscles are excluded from the trace.

region of echo dropout, it is useful to scroll rapidly back and forth between end diastolic and end systolic frames, as the endocardial border is often more obvious in systole, owing to the enhanced reflectance from a more trabeculated surface. Estimating the endocardial surface in this manner assumes normal wall motion in the region of uncertainty and will overestimate the FAC if wall motion is abnormal.

The main shortcoming of FAC measurements is that they do not take account of apical contraction. Given that the apex is commonly affected by SWMAs this is an important limitation of the method. Despite this, good agreement has been shown between FAC and EF when measured with TOE.[2]

Software that provides continuous endocardial border detection has been developed and is available with some echocardiography packages, allowing the real-time display of FAC. To detect clinically important trends, it is essential that a stable image plane is maintained and that the gain is carefully adjusted to identify the endocardium accurately.

### Ejection fraction

EF represents the proportion of diastolic volume that is ejected during ventricular contraction and is calculated as:

$$EF = \frac{EDV - ESV}{EDV} \times 100 \qquad \text{(Equation 7.2)}$$

where ESV = end systolic volume. The normal range is 55–75%.

There are numerous formulae for calculating volume from 2-D images but the two methods recommended by the American Society of Echocardiography are the **biplane method** and the **single-plane ellipsoid method**.[1]

## Biplane method

With the biplane method (also called the **modified Simpson method** or the **method of discs**) ventricular volumes are calculated using two mid-oesophageal views: the four-chamber and the two-chamber. Short loops are saved to memory and, using the scroll function, the end systolic and end diastolic frames are identified. The endocardial borders are then outlined using the trace function (Figure 7.3). In tracing the border it is important to start at one side of the mitral annulus and finish at the other; then, on pressing "return" (or "enter") on the keyboard, a horizontal line will be drawn across the mitral annulus to finish the trace. A long axis measurement will be automatically displayed, which can be adjusted if it does not intersect with the apex. In this way four areas can be estimated (the end systolic and end diastolic areas in both views). As with the FAC calculation, it is usual to extrapolate the trace in areas of echo dropout. It is important to obtain a non-foreshortened view of the LV in both planes, so that the true apex is visualised and volumes are not underestimated.

In estimating ventricular volume, the mathematical model assumes the LV cavity to be composed of a series of stacked discs of uniform thickness. The volume of each disc is calculated from its cross-sectional area and thickness; the volume of the LV cavity is then the sum of the volumes of the individual discs.

## Single-plane ellipsoid method

The single-plane ellipsoid method uses the end diastolic and end systolic frames from a single mid oesophageal four-chamber loop. The endocardial borders are traced as for the biplane method. Volume is calculated (as $8A^2/3\pi L$) assuming the shape of the LV to be ellipsoid, from the 2-D area ($A$) and length ($L$) of the cavity.

The estimation of EF may be unreliable in the presence of SWMAs and ventricular foreshortening. If the frames used for volume calculations include a SWMA, EF may be underestimated; in contrast, if a significant SWMA (e.g. an apical abnormality not visualised because of ventricular foreshortening) is not included in the volume trace, EF may be overestimated. Ventricular foreshortening due to the effects of oblique

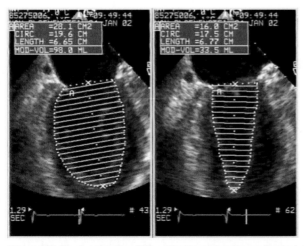

**Figure 7.3** Ejection fraction (EF) estimation using the method of discs; estimated end diastolic volume (left frame) = 98.0 ml; estimated end systolic volume (right frame) = 33.5 ml; EF = 65%. In this example EF is calculated from only a single (mid oesophageal two-chamber) view.

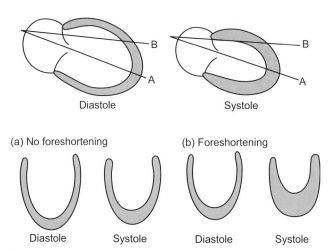

**Figure 7.4** The effect of LV foreshortening on measurements of EF and stroke volume. If the LV is fore-shortened (b) the ventricular wall may be cut obliquely, particularly at end systole. This can give the erroneous impression of increased wall thickness, reduced ventricular volume and increased EF.

imaging can also lead to overestimation of EF, even in the absence of a SWMA (Figure 7.4).

## Stroke volume and cardiac output

Stroke volume and cardiac output are important measures of the pumping function of the LV.

$$\text{Stroke volume} = \text{EDV} - \text{ESV} \qquad \text{(Equation 7.3)}$$

Thus, in the estimation of EF, stroke volume and cardiac output can also be calculated. Ventricular foreshortening will underestimate ventricular volumes, and therefore stroke volume. Furthermore, the measurements of EDV and ESV are relatively cumbersome, so stroke volume is usually derived from Doppler and 2-D data (pp.232–233).

## The effect of loading conditions

Loading conditions can affect the ejection-phase indices of systolic performance (EF, FAC and stroke volume) and must therefore be taken into account when evaluating LV function.

### Preload

The assessment of preload is discussed in Chapter 6 (pp.89–91). In the setting of normal LV contractility, EF and FAC remain relatively stable in the face of significant changes in preload.[3,4] In contrast, a reduction in stroke volume and cardiac output occurs with preload reduction.[3,4] Profound preload reduction is associated with SWMAs (p.113); in this situation, EF and FAC *are* likely to be reduced.

### Afterload

When LV contractility is normal, moderate increases in afterload have a minimal effect on ventricular performance. However, when LV contractility is depressed, even a small increase in afterload will result in a reduction in stroke volume and EF (or FAC), and an increase in EDV (or EDA). Echocardiographic measurement of afterload is possible during the perioperative period, but is complicated and rarely done.

## The relationship between stroke volume and ejection fraction

Changes in stroke volume and EF do not always occur in parallel. Thus with hypovolaemia (reduced EDV), stroke volume is decreased but EF is largely unchanged. Conversely, with chronic LV dysfunction (increased EDV), stroke volume may be normal despite a decreased EF. Acute LV dysfunction is associated with a reduction in EF (largely due to an increase in ESV) *and* stroke volume.

## Other indices of global left ventricular function

### dP/dt

The rate of rise of intraventricular pressure (d$P$/d$t$) during systole can be used as an index of systolic function, and may be less load dependent than EF or FAC.[5] This can be estimated from the CW Doppler envelope of a mitral regurgitant jet from any mid-oesophageal ventricular view (see Figure 7.5 for details). The technique has mainly been

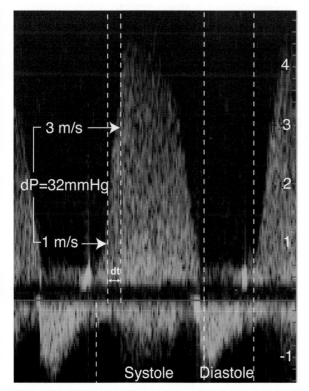

**Figure 7.5** d$P$/d$t$ of the mitral regurgitant jet velocity as a measure of systolic function. This frame shows a CW Doppler jet of mitral regurgitation taken from the mid oesophageal four-chamber view. By convention the time taken (d$t$) for the velocity to increase from 1 to 3 m/s is recorded. This corresponds to an increase in the transmitral pressure gradient (d$P$) from 4 to 36 mmHg (by the simplified Bernoulli equation). If the caliper markers are placed at the 1 and 3 m/s positions on the upstroke of the regurgitant waveform the machine software will automatically calculate the time in milliseconds. Normal systolic function is associated with a d$P$/d$t$ above 1200 mmHg/s (d$t$ < 26 ms). Severely depressed systolic function is associated with a d$P$/d$t$ less than 800 mmHg/s (d$t$ > 40 ms).[5]

used for assessment of systolic dysfunction due to mitral regurgitation and is not widely used in perioperative TOE. It cannot be used in patients with eccentric regurgitant jets, or when there is only trivial mitral regurgitation and a satisfactory Doppler profile cannot be obtained.

### Peak regurgitant jet velocity

If mitral regurgitation is present and LV function is normal, the peak velocity of the jet is typically >5 m/s, reflecting a peak transmitral pressure gradient of over 100 mmHg (pp.238–239 – the simplified Bernoulli equation). A peak velocity of ≤4.5 m/s suggests significant LV dysfunction. Note, however, that significant systolic impairment may exist despite a peak velocity within the normal range.

### Descent of mitral annulus

As the LV contracts during systole there is a reduction in the long axis dimension of the chamber, resulting in piston-like descent of the mitral annulus towards the apex. The magnitude of the annular descent can be used as an index of systolic function.

From any mid oesophageal ventricular view, the depth marker is placed through the centre of the mitral annulus and the image is frozen. The image is scrolled to an end diastolic frame (when the annulus is most basally displaced) and the position of the annular plane is noted from the depth marker. The image is then scrolled to an end systolic frame (when the annulus is most apically displaced) and the position noted. A descent of less than 0.8 cm is indicative of significant systolic dysfunction.[6]

## ASSESSMENT OF GLOBAL LV FUNCTION DURING THE PERIOPERATIVE PERIOD

While all of these methods can be used to provide information on systolic LV function, FAC is probably the most widely employed in perioperative TOE. During the prebypass period it is useful to measure FAC (or EF) formally and record it in the echo report for comparison with postbypass or later studies. However, in the busy operating room, or when the condition of the patient is unstable, most experienced echocardiographers rely on rapid subjective estimates of FAC or EF to make clinical decisions. Good correlation has been demonstrated between subjective echocardiographic assessment and radionuclide estimates of EF.[7]

## ASSESSMENT OF MYOCARDIAL ISCHAEMIA

Development of myocardial tension and fibre shortening during systole, and relaxation of tension during diastole, are energy-dependent processes requiring oxygen. Because the oxygen stores of the myocardium are low, ischaemia quickly leads to ventricular impairment; this manifests initially as diastolic dysfunction, and within a few cardiac cycles systolic dysfunction also develops (in the form of SWMAs). Ischaemia rapidly and reliably results in SWMAs. Changes in the ECG and increases in pulmonary artery wedge pressure (PAWP) occur later and may even be absent. Hence, TOE affords earlier and more reliable detection of ischaemia than the ECG or pulmonary artery catheter.[8,9]

In describing SWMAs it is important to characterise their anatomical location and severity accurately.

## Segmental analysis of the left ventricle

In order to locate the branch of the coronary artery or the bypass graft that is responsible for a wall motion abnormality it is essential to understand the blood supply to the ventricles and to have a systematic approach to the echocardiographic assessment of wall motion.

A 16-segment model is advocated in the ASE/SCA guidelines[10] (Figure 7.6). The LV is divided into three levels: **basal, mid** and **apical.** The basal and mid levels are each subdivided into six segments: **anterior, lateral, posterior, inferior, septal** and **anteroseptal.** The apex is divided into four segments: anterior, lateral, inferior and septal.

Segmental blood supply follows a predictable pattern (Figure 7.6), particularly when the dominant coronary artery is known from the angiogram. The artery that supplies the atrioventricular node, or the one that continues as the posterior descending artery (PDA), is designated the dominant artery. The PDA supplies inferior and septal walls at the basal and mid levels. In the majority (>80%) of patients the right coronary artery is dominant (i.e. the PDA is supplied by the right coronary artery); in the remaining patients the left coronary artery is dominant (i.e. the PDA is supplied by the circumflex coronary artery). In a left-dominant system, the entire LV and ventricular septum are supplied by branches of the left main coronary artery.

To visualise all 16 segments five views should be obtained: the mid oesophageal four-chamber, two-chamber and long axis views, and the transgastric basal and mid short axis views. The ASE/SCA recommendations do not include a transgastric apical short axis view but in practice this can sometimes be obtained. Thus, all segments can potentially

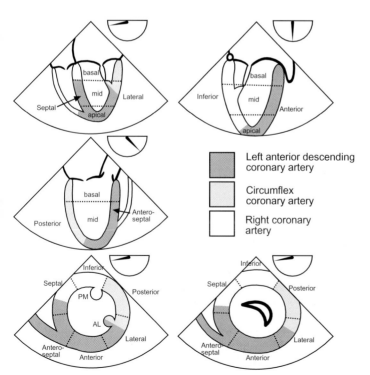

**Figure 7.6** Recommended views for assessment of segmental LV function. The 16 LV segments are shown, with their coronary blood supply (assuming right coronary dominance). Note that apical segments of the posterior and antero-septal walls are not recognised in the ASE/SCA guidelines.

be visualised in either a mid oesophageal or a transgastric window; if views in one image plane are inadequate, evaluation of any given segment should be possible in the other. In practice, the apical segments are the most difficult to visualise from both windows.

## Wall motion

Wall motion during systole consists of two components, **endocardial movement** and **wall thickening**, and may be graded as **normal, mildly hypokinetic, severely hypokinetic, akinetic** or **dyskinetic** (Table 7.1). Wall thickening is a more reliable sign than endocardial movement as an akinetic segment may appear to move because of tethering from adjacent normal myocardium. In most situations wall motion is assessed with 2-D imaging, but in the transgastric views M-mode imaging is very useful in identifying SWMAs involving the anterior and inferior walls (Figure 7.7).

## CAUSES OF SWMAs

SWMAs can result from a number of ischaemic and non-ischaemic causes (Table 7.2). An understanding of the features of the different SWMAs is important to help distinguish myocardial ischaemia from wall motion abnormalities due to other causes.

**Table 7.1** Grading of wall motion based on endocardial movement and wall thickening

| Grade | Wall motion | Endocardial movement | Endocardial thickening |
|---|---|---|---|
| 1 | Normal | Normal | >30% |
| 2 | Mild hypokinesis | Decreased | 10–30% |
| 3 | Severe hypokinesis | Slight | <10% |
| 4 | Akinesis | None | None |
| 5 | Dyskinesis | Endocardium moves outwards during systole | Endocardium thins during systole |

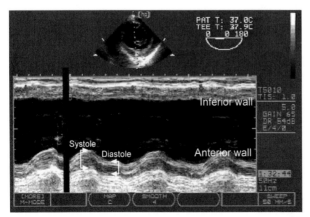

**Figure 7.7** Inferior SWMA. In this transgastric mid short axis view, an M-mode cursor has been placed across the LV. Normal thickening and movement of the anterior wall can be seen. In contrast, the inferior wall is akinetic.

| Table 7.2 Causes of segmental wall motion abnormalities |
| --- |
| Myocardial ischaemia |
| Myocardial infarction |
| Myocardial stunning |
| Intracoronary air embolus |
| Direct coronary occlusion (e.g. of coronary ostia during aortic root replacement) |
| Hypovolaemia |
| RV epicardial pacing |
| Left bundle branch block |
| Sector scan passing through membranous ventricular septum |
| Severe mitral stenosis (basal segments) |
| "Normal" postbypass finding (septal wall) |

## Myocardial ischaemia and stunning

Acute myocardial ischaemia usually results in severe hypokinesis or akinesis. Unless it occurs on a background of chronic infarction, the ventricular wall is not thinned and EDA is usually not increased.

The development of new SWMAs following bypass may represent new-onset ischaemia or **myocardial stunning**. Stunning is a condition of postischaemic ventricular dysfunction (i.e. SWMAs despite adequate blood flow) and may be related to pre-existing ischaemia, inadequate myocardial protection or both. Stunning can be difficult to distinguish from acute ischaemia. Points that can help differentiate the two conditions are:

- Ischaemia tends to produce more severe SWMAs (i.e. not mild hypokinesis).

- Stunned myocardium shows gradual improvement in function in the first minutes to hours following separation from bypass.

- Stunned myocardium may be recruited to contract with inotropic stimulation. In contrast, inotropic stimulation may have no effect, or may even worsen function, in an ischaemic segment.

## Myocardial infarction

Myocardial infarction results in akinesis or dyskinesis – in particular, no thickening occurs in a region of infarction. In the early period following infarction SWMAs can be impossible to distinguish from those due to severe ischaemia; however, with time, remodelling takes place, which results in thinning and dilatation of the ventricular wall. Occasionally, calcification may be seen within ventricular walls or papillary muscles. Marked regional deformation that is evident even in diastole is called a **true aneurysm** (Figure 7.8; p.113). Myocardial infarction, particularly involving the anterior wall, may be associated with intracavity thrombus (p.82).

## Intracoronary air

Air embolism of the coronary arteries may also cause SWMAs. This occurs most frequently with open-heart procedures (e.g. valve replacement surgery) and coronary

(a) 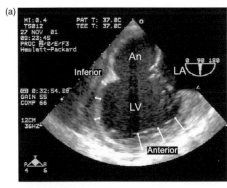 (b)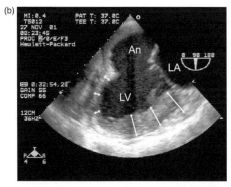

**Figure 7.8** Inferior basal LV aneurysm. (a) Transgastric two-chamber view at end diastole. The anterior and inferior walls are shown. The inferior wall is thinned at the mid and apical levels. At the basal level a large aneurysm can be seen (An); (b) The same view at end systole. Normal thickening of the anterior wall is seen, but thickening of the inferior wall is minimal. The aneurysm appears slightly larger in systole, implying dyskinesis.

revascularisation in which a LV venting device is used. The right coronary artery is more frequently affected than the left because of its anterior position. On TOE this usually manifests as acute RV distension or hypokinesis and an inferior SWMA. An air collection may also be identified within the chambers of the heart. This appears as an intense collection of echoes most commonly in the region of the pulmonary veins, LA appendage, LVOT or LV apex.

Intracoronary air produces acute myocardial ischaemia but the transient nature of the SWMAs and the benign course make the distinction from ischaemia due to coronary insufficiency important.

## Direct coronary occlusion

SWMAs due to mechanical disturbance of coronary arterial flow may be seen after specific procedures including AV replacement with occlusion of a coronary ostium, aortic root surgery with reimplantation of coronary arteries, and the Ross procedure with damage to the first septal branch of the left anterior descending coronary artery as it runs in front of the PV.

## Apparent SWMAs

These may occur for a variety of reasons. For example:

- In the transgastric basal short axis view, the sector scan may pass through the membranous ventricular septum resulting in the appearance of a wall motion abnormality in the basal septum.
- Severe mitral stenosis may result in tethering of the LV, which may impede contraction of the basal segments.
- Following cardiopulmonary bypass it is usual to see hypokinesis in the region of the septal wall; this may persist for some months following surgery. The cause is poorly understood.
- Paradoxical septal motion (in which the ventricular septum moves towards the RV in systole) may be mistaken for septal dyskinesis and occurs in the settings of RV

pressure overload, left bundle branch block and RV epicardial pacing. It can be distinguished from true dyskinesis in that systolic wall thickening occurs with paradoxical septal motion but not with a true SWMA.

- Marked hypovolaemia is associated with multiple SWMAs unrelated to myocardial ischaemia that disappear with adequate LV filling.[11] This can cause misdiagnoses during, and immediately following, separation of the patient from bypass.

# OTHER SIGNS OF MYOCARDIAL ISCHAEMIA/INFARCTION

## Mitral regurgitation

New mitral regurgitation (or worsening of existing mitral regurgitation) can occur as a direct result of acute or chronic myocardial ischaemia or infarction (p.142), particularly involving the posterior and inferior walls. (Conversely, LV dysfunction can occur as a result of severe mitral regurgitation.)

It is not possible to quantify the extent of ischaemia from the severity of mitral regurgitation, but new or worsening mitral regurgitation should raise suspicion of new ischaemia.

## Myocardial rupture

Following myocardial infarction, necrotic myocardium can become weakened or (on rare occasions) rupture. This can affect the papillary muscles, the ventricular septum or the free wall of the LV. All three conditions cause marked haemodynamic instability (Chapter 6).

- **Papillary muscle rupture** results in severe bileaflet regurgitation with flail mitral segments and haemodynamic instability. The posteromedial papillary muscle is most frequently affected (p.133). LV size is usually normal and a (usually inferior) SWMA may be identified.

- **Rupture of the ventricular septum** results in left-to-right shunting that may be seen as a turbulent jet on colour Doppler even though the actual defect in the septum may be difficult to visualise with 2-D imaging.

- **Rupture of the free wall of the LV** may result in acute pericardial tamponade (p.93). A chronic, loculated free wall rupture into the pericardial cavity is called a **false aneurysm**. Typically, a false aneurysm has a well defined neck, giving a partially "walled off" appearance. In contrast, a true aneurysm (p.111) often appears as a smooth dilatation of the LV wall in which a neck cannot be clearly identified. Sometimes this distinction is not clear.

## Diastolic dysfunction

Diastolic dysfunction frequently occurs as a consequence of LV hypertrophy, myocardial ischaemia and myocardial infarction (Chapter 8). It may coexist with systolic dysfunction or occur in the setting of normal systolic function.

# MONITORING FOR ISCHAEMIA DURING CORONARY ARTERY BYPASS GRAFT SURGERY

During the prebypass period it is important to conduct a systematic examination of all LV segments to ensure no SWMAs are missed; one or two loops should be saved for later comparison with postbypass segmental function. Wall motion in each of the LV segments visualised should be documented in the TOE report. It is also important to evaluate the presence of LV hypertrophy, mitral regurgitation and aortic atheroma, and to assess RV function.

The transgastric mid short axis view is usually used for continuous monitoring for ischaemia. In this view, segments supplied by all three coronary arteries are displayed. In addition, it is useful for the assessment of global LV function (using FAC) and volume status (using EDA). Note that only six LV segments are visualised in this image plane, and if a complete examination is not performed a significant proportion of SWMAs will be missed.[12]

Following separation of the patient from bypass, examination of the LV should be repeated to look for new SWMAs. If a new abnormality is detected it should be interpreted in the context of the following questions:

• Is the heart adequately filled?
• Is the abnormality significantly different from that in the prebypass period?
• Does the abnormality improve with time (suggesting stunning or intramyocardial air) or remain constant (suggesting ischaemia)?
• Is there evidence of trapped air within the heart?
• Does the abnormality improve (suggesting stunning) or get worse (suggesting ischaemia) with inotropic stimulation?
• Does the abnormality fit with surgical concern regarding non-revascularised myocardium or marginal graft function?
• Is the SWMA severe (severe hypokinesis or akinesis)? This is more likely to represent acute ischaemia than myocardial stunning.
• Is the patient haemodynamically unstable? This supports the diagnosis of acute ischaemia.

New SWMAs that develop at the time of chest closure suggest mechanical kinking of a graft. Early graft occlusion due to thrombus formation, particularly if temporally associated with protamine administration, should be considered if a new SWMA is noted after separation of the patient from bypass.

## CONSIDERATIONS FOR OFF-PUMP CORONARY REVASCULARISATION

In off-pump coronary artery bypass surgery the transgastric views are usually obscured when the heart is elevated to facilitate graft placement. LV function and preload must therefore be assessed in the mid oesophageal ventricular views (four-chamber, two-chamber and long axis). These views are usually well maintained, and visualisation of the LV apex may actually be improved during these manoeuvres.

During coronary occlusion (to facilitate graft placement) it is usual to see a new SWMA develop in the territory distal to the site of occlusion. However, with high-grade stenoses (>90%) this may not occur. In some situations a SWMA will occur in a site remote from the occlusion because collateral flow to the territory of a remote blocked artery is compromised. Following reperfusion, the SWMA usually disappears within 20–30 seconds.

New mitral regurgitation may occur as a consequence of myocardial ischaemia or be due to the mechanical effects of lifting the heart.

The development of *globally* reduced LV (or RV) function, ventricular dilatation, new mitral or tricuspid regurgitation and persisting SWMAs following reperfusion are all signs that should alert the anaesthetist to the potential for impending cardiovascular collapse.

# REFERENCES

1. Schiller NB, Shah PM, Crawford M, et al. Recommendations for quantitation of the left ventricle by two-dimensional echocardiography. American Society of Echocardiography Committee on Standards, Subcommittee on Quantitation of Two-Dimensional Echocardiograms. *Journal of the American Society of Echocardiography* 1989;2:358–367.

2. Ryan T, Burwash I, Lu J, et al. The agreement between ventricular volumes and ejection fraction by transesophageal echocardiography or a combined radionuclear and thermodilution technique in patients after coronary artery surgery. *Journal of Cardiothoracic and Vascular Anesthesia* 1996;10:323–328.

3. Lattik R, Couture P, Denault AY, et al. Mitral Doppler indices are superior to two-dimensional echocardiographic and hemodynamic variables in predicting responsiveness of cardiac output to a rapid intravenous infusion of colloid. *Anesthesia and Analgesia* 2002;94:1092–1099.

4. Preisman S, DiSegni E, Vered Z, et al. Left ventricular preload and function during graded haemorrhage and retranfusion in pigs: analysis of arterial pressure waveform and correlation with echocardiography. *British Journal of Anaesthesia* 2002;88:716–718.

5. Loutfi H, Nishimura RA. Quantitative evaluation of left ventricular systolic function by Doppler echocardiographic techniques. *Echocardiography* 1994;11:305–314.

6. Simonson JS, Schiller NB. Descent of the base of the left ventricle: an echocardiographic index of left ventricular function. *Journal of the American Society of Echocardiography* 1989;2:25–35.

7. Amico AF, Lichtenberg GS, Reisner SA, et al. Superiority of visual versus computerized echocardiographic estimation of radionuclide left ventricular ejection fraction. *American Heart Journal* 1989;118:1259–1265.

8. Wohlgelernter D, Cleman M, Highman HA, et al. Regional myocardial dysfunction during coronary angioplasty: evaluation by two-dimensional echocardiography and 12 lead electrocardiography. *Journal of the American College of Cardiology* 1986;7:1245–1254.

9. van Daele ME, Sutherland GR, Mitchell MM, et al. Do changes in pulmonary capillary wedge pressure adequately reflect myocardial ischemia during anesthesia? A correlative preoperative hemodynamic, electrocardiographic, and transesophageal echocardiographic study. *Circulation* 1990;81:865–871.

10. Shanewise JS, Cheung AT, Aronson S, et al. ASE/SCA guidelines for performing a comprehensive intraoperative multiplane transesophageal echocardiography examination: recommendations of the American Society of Echocardiography Council for Intraoperative Echocardiography and the Society of Cardiovascular Anesthesiologists Task Force for Certification in Perioperative Transesophageal Echocardiography. *Anesthesia and Analgesia* 1999;89:870–884.

11. Seeberger MD, Cahalan MK, Rouine-Rapp K, et al. Acute hypovolemia may cause segmental wall motion abnormalities in the absence of myocardial ischemia. *Anesthesia and Analgesia* 1997;85:1252–1257.

12. Rouine-Rapp K, Ionescu P, Balea M, et al. Detection of intraoperative segmental wall-motion abnormalities by transesophageal echocardiography: the incremental value of additional cross sections in the transverse and longitudinal planes. *Anesthesia and Analgesia* 1996;83:1141–1148.

# 8

# Left Ventricular Diastolic Dysfunction

*David Sidebotham*
*Marian Hussey*

Patients presenting for cardiac surgery are at risk of diastolic dysfunction or frank diastolic heart failure and this may be responsible for, or contribute to, perioperative haemodynamic instability. Until recently, the echocardiographic assessment of diastolic function has primarily involved the interpretation of transmitral and pulmonary venous Doppler waveforms. Newer Doppler techniques are now changing our approach to the evaluation of diastole.

In this chapter the application of these techniques to the practice of perioperative TOE is outlined.

## THE PHYSIOLOGY OF DIASTOLE[1,2]

### The phases of diastole

The pressure changes in the LA and the LV and the volume change in the LV throughout the cardiac cycle are shown in Figure 8.1. Diastole extends from closure of the AV to closure of the MV and is composed of four phases:

1. isovolumetric relaxation;
2. early filling;
3. diastasis;
4. atrial systole.

Many factors influence ventricular filling during these phases, but in the end the LA to LV pressure gradient is the driving force for ventricular filling.

### Isovolumetric relaxation

This commences with closure of the AV and extends to opening of the MV. Ventricular volume remains unchanged and there is a rapid fall in intracavity pressure due to active relaxation. The isovolumetric relaxation time (IVRT) is prolonged in any condition that impairs active relaxation (e.g. myocardial ischaemia); it is shortened by a raised LA pressure, because this causes earlier opening of the MV.

### Early diastolic filling

Early diastolic filling begins with opening of the MV. Ventricular pressure continues to decline despite ventricular filling because of ongoing active relaxation. The pressure gradient from the LA to the LV is greatest during this phase, resulting in as much as 80% of ventricular filling. The main determinants of diastolic filling at this time are the rate of active relaxation, the recoil of the elastic myocardial elements and the LA pressure. Early diastolic filling can be characterised (invasively) by the rate of volume change of the LV (dV/dt).

### Diastasis

Ventricular filling slows in mid diastole as the transmitral pressure gradient declines. This phase is known as **diastasis** and is perhaps the most complicated phase of diastole. The

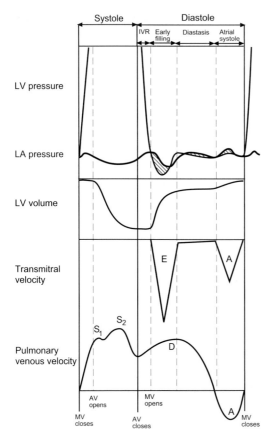

**Figure 8.1** Changes in pressure, volume and flow throughout the cardiac cycle. The four phases of diastole are shown: isovolumetric relaxation (IVR), early filling, diastasis and atrial systole. The shaded area shows the periods of diastole in which LA pressure exceeds LV pressure, and represents the transmitral "filling pressure". Filling pressure is maximal during early filling (leading to the E wave), with a second smaller peak in late diastole due to atrial systole (leading to the A wave). The periods of maximal filling pressure correspond to the two peaks seen on the transmitral PW Doppler velocity waveform. On the pulmonary venous PW Doppler velocity waveform two systolic peaks ($S_1$ and $S_2$), a diastolic peak (D) and a reversed A wave (A) are shown. See text for explanations of the Doppler waveforms.

main determinant of ventricular filling at this time is LV chamber compliance (dV/dP) or its inverse, chamber stiffness (see Figure 6.1).

Chamber compliance is determined by a number of factors including intrinsic myocardial stiffness, ventricular mass, pericardial restraint, RV volume and loading conditions. Chamber compliance is also a function of ventricular volume; a distended chamber will have a lower compliance than an empty one. Loading conditions and ventricular mass may affect chamber compliance without altering myocardial stiffness.

### Atrial systole
Atrial systole increases the transmitral pressure gradient, and under normal circumstances accounts for 15–20% of ventricular filling. In conditions that impair active myocardial relaxation, such as aortic stenosis, the contribution of atrial systole to ventricular filling may increase substantially.

## Active versus passive diastolic dysfunction
Abnormalities of diastole can be divided into those affecting the early, active, part of relaxation and those affecting the later passive filling phases.

Active diastolic dysfunction is due to delayed re-uptake of calcium ions into the sarcoplasmic reticulum and causes **prolongation of relaxation**, which affects isovolumetric relaxation and the first part of early filling. Passive diastolic dysfunction is due to **reduced chamber compliance** (or increased chamber stiffness) and affects the later part of early filling, diastasis and atrial systole.

Most forms of diastolic dysfunction in their early clinical course are of the abnormal relaxation type (e.g. in myocardial ischaemia, hypertension, aortic stenosis and hypertrophic cardiomyopathy). Reduced chamber compliance is the predominant finding in infiltrative processes (e.g. amyloidosis) and myocardial fibrosis (e.g. widespread myocardial infarction). The natural history of diastolic dysfunction is that, with time as the disease advances, abnormal relaxation progresses to reduced chamber compliance.

# ECHOCARDIOGRAPHIC ASSESSMENT OF DIASTOLIC DYSFUNCTION

The echocardiographic assessment of diastolic function is largely based on the careful assessment of the transmitral and pulmonary venous **PW Doppler waveforms**. **Colour M-mode** and **tissue Doppler imaging** are becoming the methods of choice for assessing diastolic function. Important information on ventricular function and volume status can also be obtained from 2-D imaging.

## 2-D imaging

**LV hypertrophy** is a frequent finding in patients with diastolic dysfunction. Ventricular hypertrophy can be either **concentric** (wall thickness increased out of proportion to chamber size) or **eccentric** (wall thickness increased in proportion to the increase in chamber size). Pressure overload (from aortic stenosis or hypertension) produces concentric hypertrophy and is associated with impaired relaxation and, eventually, reduced chamber compliance. Reduced LV compliance associated with LV hypertrophy may contribute to haemodynamic instability during the perioperative period (p.90). Volume overload (from mitral and aortic regurgitation) produces eccentric hypertrophy. Concentric hypertrophy may be asymmetrical, frequently involving the anterior septum in preference to other segments (the anteroseptal "knuckle" seen in elderly hypertensive patients).

Ventricular wall thickness should be assessed at end diastole in the transgastric mid short axis view using either 2-D or M-mode imaging. Hypertrophy of the anterior septum is best appreciated in the mid oesophageal long axis view. With TOE, it is difficult to avoid obliquely imaging this region using M-mode, therefore 2-D measurements should be used. Normal values are provided in Appendix 2.

In patients with severe diastolic dysfunction or mitral stenosis, prolonged diastolic filling can be appreciated on 2-D imaging. A presystolic "kick" may be observed due to atrial systole.

Occasionally specific causes of diastolic dysfunction may be identified on 2-D imaging, such as aortic stenosis or hypertrophic cardiomyopathy.

## PW Doppler imaging

Ventricular filling depends on the LA to LV pressure gradient, which also determines the transmitral diastolic velocity profile. For this reason the transmitral PW Doppler waveform has become an important tool in the assessment of diastolic function. As the transmitral pressure gradient is also influenced by *atrial* filling, additional information is gained by evaluation of the pulmonary venous PW Doppler waveform. A number of comprehensive reviews deal with the PW Doppler evaluation of diastolic function.[3-5]

## Transmitral PW Doppler waveforms

Normal and pathological transmitral PW Doppler waveforms are shown in Figures 8.1 and 8.2; reference values are provided in Table 8.1.

### Normal waveforms

Following isovolumetric relaxation and opening of the MV, diastolic filling commences. The normal transmitral velocity waveform consists of two peaks; a larger E wave due to early diastolic filling and a smaller A wave due to atrial systole. A number of variables can be measured from the Doppler signal including the IVRT, maximum E wave velocity ($E_{max}$), E wave velocity–time-integral (area under the velocity–time curve: $E_{VTI}$), E wave deceleration time ($E_{dec}$), maximum A wave velocity ($A_{max}$), A wave velocity–time integral ($A_{VTI}$) and the ratio of $E_{max}$ to $A_{max}$ (E/A ratio).

Three patterns of abnormal transmitral flow are recognised: **impaired relaxation, pseudonormalisation** and **restrictive filling**.

### Impaired relaxation

With impaired ventricular relaxation IVRT is prolonged and MV opening is slightly delayed. LV pressure is maintained longer than normal in diastole, which diminishes the transmitral pressure gradient and reduces early diastolic flow resulting in a prolonged, low-velocity E wave ($\downarrow E_{max}$, $\downarrow E_{VTI}$, $\uparrow E_{dec}$). Active relaxation is complete by late diastole and therefore a greater proportion of filling occurs with atrial systole ($\uparrow A_{max}$, $\uparrow A_{VTI}$). The E/A ratio is typically reduced to <1.

The extent to which impaired relaxation produces this transmitral Doppler waveform depends on the LA pressure. A low LA pressure will exaggerate the pattern of abnormal relaxation and an elevated LA pressure will tend to minimise it, producing a more normal-looking waveform (pseudonormalisation – see below).

### Measurement of IVRT

The IVRT is the time between the closing click of the AV and opening click of the MV. It can theoretically be estimated by positioning a CW Doppler signal so that aortic systolic and mitral diastolic waveforms are visualised simultaneously. This can sometimes be achieved in the deep transgastric long axis view, but in practice it is frequently difficult to obtain a clear signal of both flow patterns at once.

### Pseudonormal filling

Most disease processes that are associated with diastolic dysfunction initially produce a pattern of impaired relaxation with a normal LA pressure. However, as the disease progresses LA pressure tends to rise. As atrial pressure rises, the MV opens earlier, shortening the IVRT. The gradient for early filling is greater, which will tend to increase $E_{max}$ and $E_{VTI}$. This in turn leads to a large rise in mid diastolic ventricular pressure, which shortens $E_{dec}$ and reduces $A_{max}$. These changes tend to minimise the effects of impaired relaxation on the transmitral Doppler waveform, producing a normal-looking pattern. Further disease progression is associated with a reduction in chamber compliance and a true restrictive filling pattern (see below). The transition phase between abnormal relaxation and restrictive filling is known as **pseudonormalisation** and represents intermediate disease severity.

### Restrictive filling

This transmitral Doppler pattern is seen in patients with reduced chamber compliance in association with an elevated LA pressure.

During early filling elevated LA pressure results in an increased transmitral pressure gradient and therefore a rapid rise in E wave velocity, producing an increased $E_{max}$ and $E_{VTI}$. Later in diastole the reduced compliance results in a rapid increase in ventricular pressure as the ventricle fills. This acts to shorten $E_{dec}$ and decrease the magnitude of the A wave ($\downarrow A_{max}$, $\downarrow A_{VTI}$). The E/A ratio is typically >2.

## Pulmonary venous Doppler waveforms

Interrogation of the pulmonary venous Doppler waveform provides additional information and may help clarify the pattern of diastolic dysfunction (Figures 8.1 and 8.2, and Table 8.1).

### Normal waveforms

Forward flow occurs throughout most of the cardiac cycle and forms distinct peaks in systole (S wave) and diastole (D wave). There is a brief reversal of flow in late diastole associated with atrial systole (A wave). The S wave represents flow into the LA during ventricular systole and is due to atrial relaxation and the suction effect of the base to apex movement of the heart as it contracts and twists. Typically it has two components, $S_1$ and $S_2$, but for the purposes of evaluating diastolic dysfunction the systolic wave is treated as a single component. The D wave is related to a fall in atrial pressure secondary to ventricular filling, which promotes forward flow in the pulmonary veins. Parameters of clinical interest include the maximum height of the S, D and A waves and the S/D ratio. The normal S/D ratio is approximately 1.

### Abnormal waveforms

Abnormal relaxation causes a reduction in size of the D wave. This is because diastolic pulmonary venous flow mirrors early diastolic transmitral flow. Thus a decrease in transmitral $E_{max}$ is associated with a decrease in the pulmonary venous D wave. The S/D ratio is increased to >1.

Pseudonormalisation and restrictive filling produce a progressive increase in the D wave in parallel with the increase in LA pressure and increase in transmitral $E_{max}$. The S/D ratio is decreased with <1. In addition, the increase in LA pressure seen with pseudonormalisation and restrictive filling increases the reverse flow into the pulmonary veins during atrial systole, producing an increase in the reversed A wave. A pulmonary venous A wave >0.35 m/s, in the presence of a normal transmitral waveform, is a marker of pseudonormalisation.

## Factors that influence the Doppler waveforms

Transmitral and pulmonary venous flow patterns are dependent not only on diastolic function but on many physiological, pathological and technical factors, and more than one may contribute to the pattern seen at any one time.

### Position of the sample volume

The position of the sample volume is important. The appropriate position for the assessment of diastolic function is at the level of the open leaflet tips in diastole, in contrast to the measurement of stroke volume in which the sample volume should be placed at the level of the annulus. This distinction is important; if the sample volume is placed at the level of the mitral annulus, or withdrawn into the LA, the peak velocities will be lower and the E/A ratio may change.

**Table 8.1** Normal and abnormal values for transmitral and pulmonary venous indices of diastolic function. Data from European Study Group report on diagnosing diastolic heart failure,[3] Benjamin et al,[6] Garcia et al[7] and de Marchi et al.[8]

| | Normal values | Abnormal relaxation | Pseudonormal filling | Restrictive filling |
|---|---|---|---|---|
| IVRT | <100 ms | Increased >100 | Decreased 60–100 | Decreased <60 |
| Transmitral $E_{max}$ | 0.71 ± 0.14 m/s$_{(<30\ years)}$<br>0.63 ± 0.10 m/s$_{(40-49\ years)}$<br>0.55 ± 0.11 m/s$_{(60-69\ years)}$ | Decreased | Normal | Increased |
| Transmitral $A_{max}$ | 0.35 ± 0.06 m/s$_{(20-29\ years)}$<br>0.45 ± 0.08 m/s$_{(40-49\ years)}$<br>0.55 ± 0.10 m/s$_{(60-69\ years)}$ | Increased | Normal | Decreased |
| E/A ratio | 2.08 ± 0.55$_{(20-29\ years)}$<br>1.44 ± 0.26$_{(40-49\ years)}$<br>1.03 ± 0.26$_{(60-69\ years)}$ | Decreased <1 | Normal 1–2 | Increased >2 |
| $E_{dec}$ | 179 ± 20 ms$_{(<50\ years)}$<br>210 ± 36 ms$_{(>50\ years)}$ | Increased >220 ms | Normal 150–200 ms | Decreased <150 ms |
| Pulmonary venous S wave | 0.49 ± 13 m/s$_{(20-29\ years)}$<br>0.58 ± 15 m/s$_{(40-49\ years)}$<br>0.64 ± 19 m/s$_{(>60\ years)}$ | Increased | Decreased | Decreased |
| Pulmonary venous D wave | 0.61 ± 10 m/s$_{(20-29\ years)}$<br>0.53 ± 10 m/s$_{(40-49\ years)}$<br>0.44 ± 13 m/s$_{(>60\ years)}$ | Decreased | Increased | Increased |
| S/D ratio | 0.81 ± 0.19$_{(20-29\ years)}$<br>1.13 ± 0.4$_{(40-49\ years)}$<br>1.57 ± 0.57$_{(>60\ years)}$ | Increased >1 | Decreased <1 | Decreased <1 |
| Peak Pulmonary Venous A wave reversal | 0.23 ± 0.08 m/s$_{(20-29\ years)}$<br>0.24 ± 0.09 m/s$_{(40-49\ years)}$<br>0.25 ± 0.06 m/s$_{(>60\ years)}$ | Normal <0.35 m/s | Increased >0.35 m/s | May be decreased |

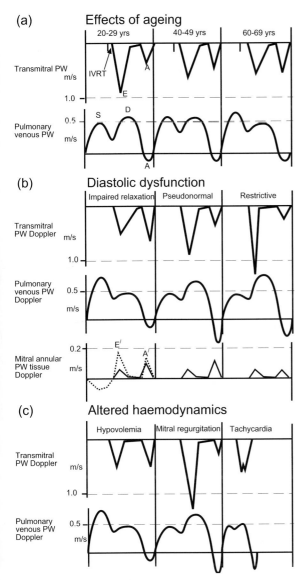

**Figure 8.2** Transmitral and pulmonary venous waveforms seen with increasing age (a), diastolic dysfunction (b), and hypovolaemia, mitral regurgitation and tachycardia (c). Normal (dotted line) and abnormal mitral annular PW tissue Doppler waveforms are also shown (see p.125). Data from Appleton et al[4] and Oh et al[5].

## Increasing age[9]

In children and young adults relaxation is rapid and largely complete by the first part of early filling. The predominant effect of increasing age is a decreased rate of myocardial relaxation, which produces a pattern of decreased $E_{max}$, increased $A_{max}$, decreased E/A ratio and prolonged $E_{dec}$. The E and A velocities equalise at around 60 years of age. There is a progressive decrease in the pulmonary venous D wave with increasing age.

## Loading conditions[10–12]

An increase in preload increases the transmitral pressure gradient because of an increase in LA pressure. The working position of the LV on the diastolic pressure–volume curve is shifted to the right, to the steeper, less compliant part of the curve (see Figure 6.1). This will produce a pattern of transmitral filling similar to that seen with restrictive diastolic dysfunction ($\uparrow E_{max}$, $\downarrow A_{max}$, $\downarrow E_{dec}$, $\uparrow$E/A ratio >2). The pulmonary venous waveform shows an increase in both the S and D waves and an increase in the reverse A wave.

Preload reduction (due to hypovolaemia or venodilatation) decreases the transmitral gradient and therefore reduces $E_{max}$ and $E_{dec}$. The effect on the A wave is variable (increased, decreased or no effect). The E/A ratio is generally reduced but not reversed. The pulmonary venous D wave and reverse A waves are reduced.

Increased afterload is associated with reduced active ventricular relaxation, which acts to decrease $E_{max}$, prolong the $E_{dec}$ time and increase $A_{max}$.

## Heart rate and rhythm

With tachycardia the transmitral E wave decreases relative to the A wave, resulting in a reduced E/A ratio. There is less delay between the E and A waves, and at heart rates above 100 beats per minute fusion of the E and A waves occurs. On the pulmonary venous Doppler trace, tachycardia causes an increase in the S wave and a decrease in the D wave. Bradycardia increases the transmitral E/A ratio.

With atrial fibrillation, transmitral and pulmonary venous A waves are absent. The pulmonary venous S wave will be decreased as it is partly dependent on atrial relaxation (as well as mitral annular descent). $E_{max}$ and $E_{dec}$ will depend on the cardiac cycle length.

Atrioventricular dissociation, complete heart block or VVI pacing will produce dissociated transmitral E and A waves, depending on the underlying rhythm.

RV epicardial pacing causes asynchronous and prolonged LV myocardial relaxation which results in a reduced $E_{max}$.

## Aortic and mitral valve disease

Mitral regurgitation and stenosis both produce important effects on the transmitral and pulmonary venous waveforms and are discussed in Chapter 9 (pp.146 and 152).

Aortic regurgitation results in an elevated LA pressure and a rapid early diastolic rise in ventricular pressure, due to regurgitation of blood into the LV. On the transmitral waveform this produces a pattern similar to that of restrictive diastolic dysfunction ($\uparrow E_{max}$, $\downarrow E_{dec}$, $\downarrow A_{max}$).

## The effects of spontaneous and mechanical ventilation

During spontaneous breathing inspiration is associated with a fall in intrathoracic pressure, which augments systemic venous return and causes an increase in *tricuspid* E and A wave velocities (<20%). There is a small (<5%) inspiratory reduction in transmitral E and A wave velocities, probably due to pooling of blood in the pulmonary circulation. These changes are reversed during expiration. The E/A ratios are largely unchanged. Certain conditions are associated with an exaggeration of these normal respiratory variations, including constrictive pericarditis, pericardial tamponade, acute asthma and pneumothorax.

The pattern seen with positive pressure ventilation is incompletely understood. There is some evidence, at least in neonates, that the normal pattern of respiratory variation is reversed.[13] The effects of positive end expiratory pressure (PEEP) are complex. A progressive increase in PEEP is associated with a decrease in tricuspid and mitral E wave velocities during both inspiration and expiration. The A wave velocity remains unchanged or reduces slightly. The E/A ratio is typically decreased.[14-16]

### Rules of thumb for interpretation of transmitral and pulmonary venous waveforms

In cardiac surgical patients who are mechanically ventilated, undergo large fluid shifts, are paced, and may have associated cardiovascular disease, the interpretation of transmitral and pulmonary venous waveforms is complicated. The following rules of thumb may be useful:

- The "normal" pattern in patients over 60 years of age is one of impaired relaxation (E/A ratio <1). However, an E/A ratio <0.6 is never normal, and suggests significantly impaired relaxation in any age group.
- Pseudonormalisation should be suspected when a normal transmitral waveform is seen in association with the following:
  - Age >60 years.
  - An elevated pulmonary artery wedge pressure (PAWP).
  - Echocardiographic evidence of LV hypertrophy.
- A transmitral E/A ratio >1.8 (particularly in an older patient) suggests:
  - Restrictive or pseudonormal diastolic dysfunction.
  - Volume overload.
  - Mitral or aortic regurgitation.
- If the transmitral E/A ratio is greater than 1.8 and $E_{dec}$ is below 180 ms, suspect pseudonormalisation. Seek confirmation from the pulmonary venous waveform (an S/D ratio < 1 and a reversed A wave > 0.35 m/s).

## NEWER DOPPLER TECHNIQUES[17]

Over the last few years there has been increasing interest in the techniques of colour M-mode flow propagation velocity and tissue Doppler imaging in the assessment of diastolic function. The main advantages of these techniques over conventional PW Doppler is that they appear to be less load dependent, and do not display a biphasic response to increasing disease severity. Colour M-mode flow propagation velocity is relatively easy to measure, and colour M-mode is available on most TOE systems. Not all echocardiography systems are currently equipped for tissue Doppler imaging. Both of the techniques are useful when used in combination with conventional PW Doppler to differentiate normal from pseudonormal filling.

### Colour M-mode flow propagation velocity[17]

M-mode imaging displays the position of structures along a vertical scan line over time (see Figure 2.9). Colour M-mode superimposes colour-encoded blood velocity data onto the same scan line. The information displayed on a colour M-mode recording of LV inflow can be used to assess diastolic function. The **propagation velocity** (Vp) of blood within the LV is the slope of any isovelocity line connecting the mitral leaflets to some point within the ventricle (Figure 8.3) and is normally >55 cm/s (M-mode displays distance (metres) versus time (seconds) and therefore the slope of a line is in units of velocity). Diastolic dysfunction (impaired relaxation, pseudonormalisation, and restrictive filling) is associated with a low Vp (<55 cm/s).

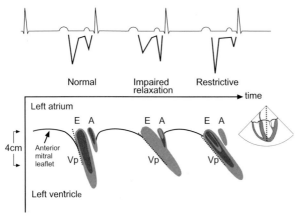

**Figure 8.3** Schematic of the LV inflow colour M-mode filling patterns seen with normal diastolic function, impaired relaxation and restrictive filling. The ECG and corresponding transmitral PW Doppler profiles are also shown. From any mid oesophageal ventricular view an M-mode cursor is placed through the MV and directed towards the LV apex. Using colour M-mode, two-colour waveforms can usually be identified corresponding to the PW Doppler E and A waves. The velocity at which blood flow propagates within the LV (the propagation velocity – Vp) is given by the slope of any isovelocity line on the "colour E wave". An isovelocity line occurs at the colour/no colour transition, or along *any* zone of colour aliasing, and can be measured using the caliper function. The colour scale can therefore be altered to produce aliasing as desired without changing Vp. The slope should be measured from the mitral annulus to a point 4 cm into the LV. Vp is reduced with diastolic dysfunction. The degree of aliasing of the colour E wave is reduced with impaired relaxation and increased with restrictive filling (compare the maximum E wave velocities on the respective PW Doppler signals).

## Tissue Doppler imaging[4,18]

Tissue Doppler imaging is a recently developed ultrasound modality based on the same principles as standard PW Doppler imaging. In contrast to conventional Doppler imaging, which measures the velocity of blood, tissue Doppler measures the velocity of the *myocardium* which is then displayed as a spectral PW signal or as a colour map.

Diastolic filling can be assessed using tissue Doppler interrogation of mitral annular motion, displayed as a conventional PW Doppler map. Mitral annular motion is of lower velocity but higher amplitude than blood flow, therefore the Doppler gain setting must be reduced (often to 0%) and the scale set to detect velocities <20 cm/s. A PW sample volume is placed within the mitral annulus in a mid oesophageal ventricular view, ensuring that longitudinal mitral motion is parallel with the Doppler signal. Motion is in the opposite direction to transmitral blood flow (the annulus moves towards the probe during diastole due to longitudinal expansion of the LV). This produces an early diastolic E wave ($E_m$) and a late diastolic A wave ($A_m$). The $E_m/A_m$ ratio is similar to the standard PW Doppler E/A ratio. Normal diastolic function is associated with an $E_m$ >8 cm/s, abnormal diastolic function (impaired relaxation, pseudonormalisation, and restrictive filling) with an $E_m$ < 8 cm/s. Abnormal $E_m$ and $A_m$ patterns are shown in Figure 8.2.

## THE ESTIMATION OF LEFT ATRIAL PRESSURE

Central to the diagnosis of severe diastolic dysfunction is the finding of an elevated LA pressure. In theory it is possible to estimate LA pressure quantitatively from the velocity of a jet of aortic regurgitation and the diastolic arterial pressure (p.241), but in practice this is technically difficult with TOE.

A number of semiquantitative parameters have been investigated in an attempt to estimate LA pressure using echocardiography. However, all are subject to confounding influences such as the effect of loading conditions, atrial and ventricular compliance, systolic function, and chronicity of the elevated LA pressure. It follows that the signs of elevated LA pressure derived from TOE must be interpreted in the context of other clinical information. Nevertheless the following may be helpful.

### Abnormal motion of the interatrial septum

Normally the interatrial septum bows predominantly from left to right, reflecting the pressure difference between the right and left atria. In ventilated patients with normal atrial pressures, mid systolic reversal (i.e. bowing from right to left) occurs during both inspiration and expiration. This reversal is lost with elevation of LA pressure. If the LA pressure lies between 10 and 15 mmHg, the reversal occurs only at end expiration. Above 15 mmHg no reversal is seen. False positives occur in the presence of severe tricuspid regurgitation, and false negatives with low ventilatory pressures and severe mitral regurgitation.[19]

### Transmitral and pulmonary venous Doppler waveforms

The relationship between LA pressure and various parameters derived from the transmitral and pulmonary venous PW Doppler waveforms has been investigated.[20,21] For practical purposes, three useful signs suggestive of an increased LA pressure are:

- Increased pulmonary venous A wave (i.e. reversal velocity >0.35 m/s);
- Pulmonary venous A wave duration > transmitral A wave duration (i.e. opposite to normal);
- S wave velocity < D wave velocity in the pulmonary venous wave form (again, opposite to normal in most age groups, but see Table 8.1).

### Tissue Doppler imaging

The ratio of the transmitral E wave to the mitral annular $E_m$ wave ($E/E_m$) is related to mean LV diastolic pressure (a surrogate for mean LA pressure); an $E/E_m < 8$ suggests that LA pressure is normal, and an $E/E_m > 15$ suggests elevated LA pressure.[22]

## DIASTOLIC DYSFUNCTION DURING THE PERIOPERATIVE PERIOD

Diastolic dysfunction is a common problem, particularly in patients undergoing cardiac surgery; the main risk factors and clinical features are outlined in Table 8.2. It may occur in conjunction with systolic dysfunction or as an isolated phenomenon. In one study approximately 50% of patients presenting with acute pulmonary oedema had normal systolic function on 2-D echocardiography; in most of these cases the underlying cause was thought to be diastolic dysfunction.[23]

For a number of conditions, notably hypertension (particularly if associated with LV hypertrophy), myocardial ischaemia or infarction and aortic stenosis, prolonged relaxation is an early finding. In each case, as the disease progresses a pseudonormal or restrictive filling pattern may develop.

Congestive cardiac failure due to systolic dysfunction results in a restrictive filling pattern. Following acute myocardial infarction, the early development of a restrictive filling

**Table 8.2** Diastolic heart failure: risk factors and clinical features

| Risk factors |
| --- |
| Advancing age (>65 years) |
| Female gender |
| Renal failure |
| Diabetes |
| Hypertension |
| Aortic stenosis |
| LV hypertrophy |
| Coronary artery disease |
| **Clinical features** |
| History of acute pulmonary oedema |
| $S_4$ gallop |
| Radiographic evidence of pulmonary congestion and normal heart size |
| ECG evidence of LV hypertrophy |
| Normal or increased ejection fraction |
| Increased end diastolic pressure on preoperative angiogram |

pattern ($E_{dec}$ < 140 ms) is strongly predictive of the development of congestive cardiac failure and sudden death.[24]

In addition to coexisting pathology, cardiopulmonary bypass itself is responsible for an acute prolongation of ventricular relaxation during the early postoperative period,[25] an abnormality that has largely resolved by 24 hours.[26]

As outlined in Chapter 6 (p.90), reduced LV compliance can complicate the echocardiographic diagnosis of hypovolaemia and contribute to perioperative haemodynamic instability.

## REFERENCES

1. Pagel PS, Grossman W, Haering JM, et al. Left ventricular diastolic function in the normal and diseased heart: perspectives for the anesthesiologist (first of two parts). *Anesthesiology* 1993;79:836–854.
2. Schmidt MA, Starling MR. Physiologic assessment of left ventricular systolic and diastolic performance. *Current Problems in Cardiology* 2000;25:827–910.
3. European Study Group on Diastolic Heart Failure. How to diagnose diastolic heart failure. *European Heart Journal* 1998;19:990–1003.
4. Appleton CP, Firstenberg MS, Garcia MJ, et al. The echo-Doppler evaluation of left ventricular diastolic function. A current perspective. *Cardiology Clinics* 2000;18:513–546.
5. Oh JK, Appleton CP, Hatle LK, et al. The noninvasive assessment of left ventricular diastolic function with two-dimensional and Doppler echocardiography. *Journal of the American Society of Echocardiography* 1997;10:246–270.
6. Benjamin E, Levy D, Anderson KM, et al. Determinants of Doppler indexes of left ventricular diastolic function in normal subjects (the Framingham Heart Study). *American Journal of Cardiology* 1992; 70:508–515.
7. Garcia MJ. Diastolic dysfunction and heart failure: causes and treatment options. *Cleveland Clinic Journal of Medicine* 2000;67:727–738.
8. de Marchi SF, Bodenmüller M, Lai DL, et al. Pulmonary venous flow velocity patterns in 404 individuals without cardiovascular disease. *Heart* 2001;85:23–29.
9. Klein AL, Burstow DJ, Tajik AJ, et al. Effects of age on left ventricular dimensions and filling dynamics in 117 normal persons. *Mayo Clinic Proceedings* 1994;69: 212–224.

10. Nishimura RA, Abel MD, Hatle LK, et al. Relation of pulmonary vein to mitral flow velocities by transesophageal Doppler echocardiography: effect of different loading conditions. *Circulation* 1990;81:1488–1497.

11. Berk MR, Xie G, Kwan OL, et al. Reduction of left ventricular preload by lower body negative pressure alters Doppler transmitral filling patterns. *Journal of the American College of Cardiology* 1990;16:1387–1392.

12. Stoddard MF, Pearson AC, Kern MJ, et al. Influence of alteration in preload on the pattern of left ventricular diastolic filling as assessed by Doppler echocardiography in humans. *Circulation* 1989;79:1226–1236.

13. Maroto E, Fouron J-C, Teyssier G, et al. Effect of intermittent positive pressure ventilation on diastolic ventricular filling patterns in premature infants. *Journal of the American College of Cardiology* 1990;16:171–174.

14. Hoffmann R, Lambertz H, Jütten H, et al. Mitral and pulmonary venous flow under influence of positive end-expiratory pressure ventilation analyzed by transesophageal pulsed Doppler echocardiography. *American Journal of Cardiology* 1991;68:697–701.

15. Yamada T, Takeda J, Satoh M, et al. Effect of positive end-expiratory pressure on left and right ventricular diastolic filling assessed by transoesophageal Doppler echocardiography. *Anaesthesia and Intensive Care* 1999;27:341–345.

16. Poelaert JIT, Reichert CLA, Koolen JJ, et al. Transesophageal echo-Doppler evaluation of the hemodynamic effects of positive-pressure ventilation after coronary artery surgery. *Journal of Cardiothoracic and Vascular Anesthesia* 1992;6:438–443.

17. Garcia MJ, Thomas JD, Klein AL. New Doppler echocardiographic applications for the study of diastolic function. *Journal of the American College of Cardiology* 1998;32:865–875.

18. Gorcsan J 3rd. Tissue Doppler echocardiography. *Current Opinion in Cardiology* 2000;15:323–329.

19. Kusumoto FM, Muhiudeen IA, Kuecherer HF, et al. Response of the interatrial septum to transatrial pressure gradients and its potential for predicting pulmonary capillary wedge pressure: an intraoperative study using transesophageal echocardiography in patients during mechanical ventilation. *Journal of the American College of Cardiology* 1993;21:721–728.

20. Vanoverschelde J-LJ, Robert AR, Gerbaux A, et al. Noninvasive estimation of pulmonary arterial wedge pressure with Doppler transmitral flow velocity pattern in patients with known heart disease. *American Journal of Cardiology* 1995;75:383–389.

21. Giannuzzi P, Imparato A, Temporelli PL, et al. Doppler-derived mitral deceleration time of early filling as a strong predictor of pulmonary capillary wedge pressure in postinfarction patients with left ventricular systolic dysfunction. *Journal of the American College of Cardiology* 1994;23:1630–1637.

22. Ommen SR, Nishimura RA, Appleton CP, et al. Clinical utility of Doppler echocardiography and tissue Doppler imaging in the estimation of left ventricular filling pressures: a comparative simultaneous Doppler-catheterization study. *Circulation* 2000;102:1788–1794.

23. Gandhi SK, Powers JC, Nomeir A-M, et al. The pathogenesis of acute pulmonary edema associated with hypertension. *New England Journal of Medicine* 2001;344:17–22.

24. Poulsen SH, Jensen SE, Egstrup K. Longitudinal changes and prognostic implications of left ventricular diastolic function in first acute myocardial infarction. *American Heart Journal* 1999;137:910–918.

25. Öwall A, Anderson R, Brodin LÅ, et al. Left ventricular filling as assessed by pulsed Doppler echocardiography after coronary artery bypass grafting. *Journal of Cardiothoracic and Vascular Anesthesia* 1992;6:573–577.

26. Gorcsan J 3rd, Diana P, Lee J, et al. Reversible diastolic dysfunction after successful coronary artery bypass surgery: assessment by transesophageal Doppler echocardiography. *Chest* 1994;106:1364–1369.

# 9

# The Mitral Valve

*David Sidebotham*
*Malcolm Legget*

The MV is ideally suited to examination with TOE as it lies in close proximity to the oesophagus and is separated from the probe by the blood-filled LA, which acts as a superb acoustic window. The valvular structures can be positioned easily in the centre of the sector scan, permitting the plane of the scan to be rotated 180° through the mid-point of the valve and allowing full visualisation of the leaflets. In systole, the leaflets lie perpendicular to the ultrasound beam, enhancing the quality of the 2-D image. Flow through the valve is nearly parallel to the ultrasound beam, creating excellent conditions for Doppler analysis. These factors, combined with the importance of mitral pathology in the cardiac surgical patient, have contributed substantially to the greatly increased use of perioperative TOE over the last decade.

## MITRAL ANATOMY[1-3]

The **MV apparatus** is a term used to describe the structures associated with valve function and includes the fibrous skeleton of the heart, annulus, leaflets, chordae tendinae, papillary muscles and the adjacent myocardium.

### Fibrous skeleton, annulus and leaflets

The fibrous skeleton of the heart provides the structural framework for the four heart valves and is based on the three U-shaped **cords** that form the aortic annulus (Figure 9.1). Extensions of these cords form the left and right **trigones**, which together form the **mitral annulus**. The mitral annulus is weakest posteriorly where the extensions of the two trigones join.

The mitral annulus is a three-dimensional, saddle-shaped, ellipsoid structure which alters shape and decreases in area as it descends during systole (Figure 9.2). The "low" (more apical) axis is along the intercommissural line (seen in the mid oesophageal commissural view); this is also the "longer" axis. The "high" (more basal) axis is along the anterior–posterior line (seen in the mid oesophageal long axis view); this is also the "shorter" axis. Note that the "shorter axis" of the mitral annulus is imaged in the mid oesophageal "long axis" view.

Annular dimensions should be assessed at end systole in both the mid-oesophageal commissural and long axis views.[4] In the long axis view, an end systolic annular dimension of >3.6 cm indicates dilatation (Appendix 2).

The diagnosis of MV prolapse should be made only with reference to the "high" axis (mid oesophageal long axis view) as the presence of leaflet prolapse will be overdiagnosed if the "low" axis is used.

The MV is bileaflet, consisting of an anterior and a posterior cusp (Figure 9.3). Each leaflet inserts at its base into the mitral annulus. The leaflets do not lie in a strictly anterior–posterior orientation; the anterior mitral leaflet lies somewhat medial and the posterior mitral leaflet somewhat lateral. The posterior leaflet has twice the annular

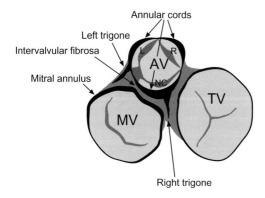

**Figure 9.1** The fibrous skeleton of the heart consists of three annular cords, which form the aortic annulus, and two fibrous trigones, which form the mitral annulus. The left trigone extends from the left annular cord (L) and the right trigone from the non-coronary annular cord (NC). The intertrigonal space is known as the aortic curtain or intervalvular fibrosa, and merges with the anterior mitral leaflet. The mitral annulus is weakest posteriorly where the trigones join.

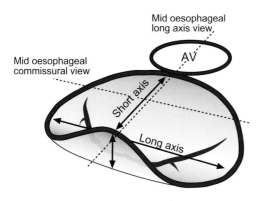

**Figure 9.2** The mitral annulus is an ellipsoid, saddle-shaped structure. The "high", "short" axis is imaged in the mid oesophageal long axis view (130°) and the "low", "long" axis in the mid oesophageal commissural view (60°).

attachment but only half the base-to-tip length of the anterior leaflet (i.e. the posterior leaflet is longer and thinner) but each leaflet has approximately the same surface area.

The valve leaflets join at two **commissures**: the anterolateral and posteromedial. During systole, when the leaflet tips are opposed, a curved **coaptation line** forms between the two commissures. There is normally 3–5 mm of leaflet overlap along the coaptation line during systole. The anterior leaflet is in fibrous continuity with the non-coronary leaflet and, to a lesser extent, the left cusp of the AV.

The posterior leaflet is divided into three distinct anatomical **scallops** or **segments**: the anterolateral, middle and posteromedial. Small scallops may be identified in the region of the commissures. Carpentier and Duran have each developed systems of classification of the mitral leaflets (Figure 9.4). The ASE/SCA guidelines use the Carpentier nomenclature and their approach has been adopted throughout this chapter.

## Papillary muscles and chordae tendinae
The MV is supported by two **papillary muscles**: the anterolateral and posteromedial. Their orientation is similar to that of the commissures of the same names (Figure 9.3). The larger, anterolateral papillary muscle usually consists of a single trunk, whereas the smaller posteromedial papillary muscle often consists of two or three distinct pillars.

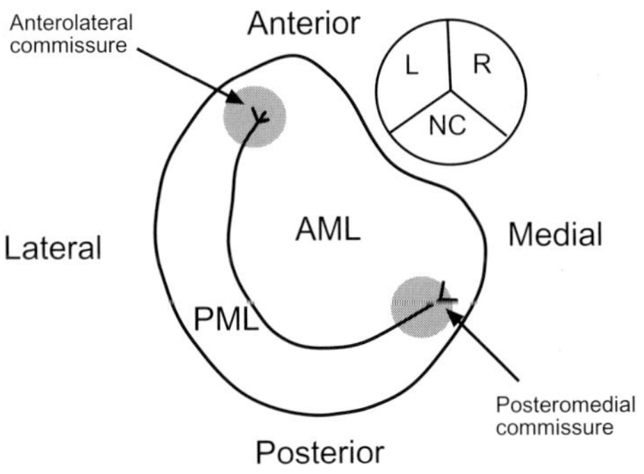

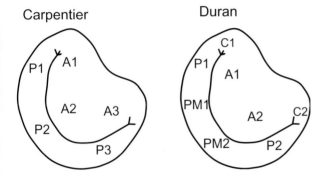

**Figure 9.3** Anatomical view of the MV showing the leaflets, commissures and orientation of the papillary muscles. The MV is viewed from the base of the heart looking towards the LV apex (p.134). AML = anterior mitral leaflet, PML = posterior mitral leaflet. The position of the left (L), right (R) and non-coronary (NC) AV leaflets relative to the MV is also shown.

**Figure 9.4** The Carpentier and Duran naming systems for the mitral segments. Carpentier divides the posterior leaflet into P1, P2 and P3, corresponding to the anterolateral, middle and posteromedial scallops respectively. Duran subclassifies the middle scallop into lateral (PM1) and medial (PM2) components. The anterior leaflet is divided into three (Carpentier) or two (Duran) segments. Duran classifies the commissural scallops into C1 (anterolateral) and C2 (posteromedial).

The papillary muscles attach to the valve leaflets via thin fibrous structures, the **chordae tendinae**. First-order chordae attach to the leaflet tip, second-order to the undersurface of the leaflet and third-order to the base of the leaflet as it inserts into the mitral annulus. Third-order chordae are unusual in that they arise not from the papillary muscles but from the ventricular wall and are present only on the posterior leaflet (see Figure 9.13). A substantial amount of blood normally passes through the interchordal space during diastole, therefore chordal fusion may contribute to mitral stenosis by causing subvalvular obstruction.[1]

The anterolateral papillary muscle supports the anterolateral segments of each leaflet (A1/P1 and part of A2/P2) and the posteromedial papillary muscle supports the posteromedial segments of each leaflet (A3/P3 and part of A2/P2). The anterolateral papillary muscle has a dual blood supply, from branches of the left anterior descending and circumflex arteries, whereas the posteromedial papillary muscle is usually supplied entirely by the right coronary artery. For this reason the posteromedial muscle is more prone to infarction and subsequent rupture.

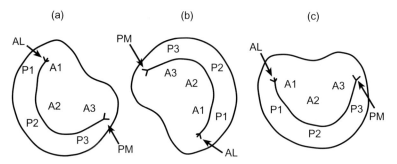

**Figure 9.5** Orientation of the MV: (a) anatomical view; (b) TOE view; (c) surgeon's view. AL = anterolateral commissure, PM = posteromedial commissure.

## ORIENTATION OF THE MITRAL VALVE

Orientation of the MV can be confusing. Three views may be used (Figure 9.5).

### Anatomical view

The valve is viewed from the base of the heart (behind the valve) with the atria cut away. This is the most intuitive of the views as the patient's left and right correspond to the observer's left and right, and the anterior and posterior leaflets appear in their appropriate positions. The lateral aspect of the valve is on the left and the medial (or septal) aspect on the right.

The anatomical orientation is used in line drawings throughout this chapter.

### TOE view

Rotation of the anatomical view through 180° produces the TOE view, in which the observer's left and right are reversed relative to the patient. This corresponds to the orientation of the MV as it appears in the transgastric basal short axis view.

### Surgeon's view

This is the view the surgeon has, standing on the patient's right, examining the valve through the opened LA.

## SYSTEMATIC EXAMINATION OF THE MITRAL VALVE

The ability to relate TOE images of the MV to specific anatomical regions is crucial for accurate diagnosis of valvular pathology. In this section a sequence of examination is described based on the ASE/SCA guidelines[5] and two other reports.[2,6]

The examination consists of four standard mid oesophageal views (four-chamber, commissural, two-chamber and long axis) and two transgastric views (basal short axis, two-chamber). Details on how to obtain these images are outlined in Chapter 4. In each view the valve should be examined with 2-D imaging; colour flow Doppler should also be used in at least the mid oesophageal long axis view, but more extensive colour flow imaging will be needed if significant mitral pathology is detected. From a practical point of view it is preferable to use both modalities in the mid oesophageal views before moving on to the transgastric views. Complete examination of the MV also involves evaluation of the transmitral and pulmonary venous Doppler waveforms.

The key echocardiographic–segmental relationships are summarised in Table 9.1.

**Table 9.1** Mitral segments seen in the mid oesophageal views

| TOE view | Mitral segment visualised (left to right across the screen) |
| --- | --- |
| Four-chamber | A2, A1/P1 |
| Commissural | P3/A3, A2, A1/P1 |
| Commissural and left turn of probe | P3, P2, P1 |
| Commissural and right turn of probe | A3, A2, A1 |
| Two-chamber | P3/A3, A2, A1 |
| Long axis | P2/A2 |
| Long axis with left turn of probe | P1/A1 |
| Long axis with right turn of probe | P3/A3 |

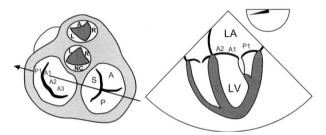

**Figure 9.6** Mid oesophageal four-chamber view. The image on the left is for orientation purposes and shows the four valves from the base of the heart with the atria cut away. In the mid oesophageal views the TOE probe sits behind the heart with the same "view" as the reader. The arrow indicates the left to right orientation of the leaflets as they appear on the TOE image.

## Mid-oesophageal four-chamber view (0–20°; Figure 9.6)

### Echocardiographic anatomy
The anterior leaflet is displayed on the left and the posterior leaflet on the right. With the transducer rotated to 15–20° the scan plane typically cuts the coaptation line obliquely, passing through A2, A1/P1. With the transducer at 0° the scan plane may cut the coaptation line more perpendicularly, passing through A2/P2.

### Additional views
Slight withdrawal (or anteflexion) of the probe moves the sector scan further towards the anterolateral commissure and cuts through the LVOT (mid-oesophageal five-chamber view). Slight advancement (or retroflexion) of the probe moves the sector scan towards the posteromedial commissure.

### Main utility
The mid oesophageal four-chamber view is a convenient starting place for examination of the MV and gives a general idea of leaflet pathology. With the transducer at 0°, the probe

may be advanced and withdrawn to scan along the coaptation line. However, even with the transducer at 0° it can be difficult to be sure that the coaptation line is cut perpendicularly. It is therefore preferable to use the mid oesophageal long axis view for this purpose (pp.137–138). If the coaptation line *is* cut obliquely the assessment of leaflet length and vena contracta may be unreliable. Also, it is less easy to be sure which leaflet segment is visualised as the probe is advanced and withdrawn.

## Mid-oesophageal commissural view (60°; Figure 9.7)
### Echocardiographic anatomy
This view is transitional between views in which the anterior leaflet appears on the left (<60°) and those in which it appears on the right (>60°). The scan passes through the intercommissural line and therefore cuts the (curved) coaptation line twice: P3/A3 on the left and A1/P1 on the right. The body of A2 appears to flick in and out of the centre of the annulus as the MV opens and closes. The LA appendage is not usually seen but both papillary muscles are usually visible. This is also known as the "seagull view".

### Additional views
Turning the probe to the left (anticlockwise) sweeps the sector scan through the body of the posterior leaflet (P3, P2, P1). Turning to the right (clockwise) sweeps the sector scan through the body of the anterior leaflet (A3, A2, A1).

### Main utility
The commissural view is very useful for assessment of which *segments* are regurgitant. On colour flow Doppler, regurgitation arising from the left coaptation point indicates involvement of the posteromedial segments (P3/A3); regurgitation arising from the right coaptation point implies involvement of the anterolateral segments (A1/P1). Regurgitation appearing from both coaptation points suggests that it is occurring along a substantial length of the coaptation line.

This view is not useful for assessing which *leaflet* is involved, or for the evaluation of the vena contracta, which may be significantly overestimated (see below). Care is needed when assessing regurgitation in this view as two distinct jets, one from each coaptation point, may appear as a single jet, leading to an overestimation of severity. Two distinct jets may, alternatively, give the erroneous impression of a mitral cleft or perforation.

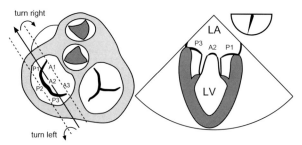

**Figure 9.7** Mid oesophageal commissural view.

## Mid oesophageal two-chamber view (90°; Figure 9.8)
Echocardiographic anatomy
The sector scan cuts through P3 on the left and all three segments of the anterior leaflet on the right (A3, A2, A1). The coaptation line is cut at P3/A3. The coronary sinus is seen on the left and the LA appendage on the right. The posteromedial papillary muscle is usually visible on the left. The segmental anatomy is similar to that seen when the probe is turned to the right from the commissural view.

Main utility
This view is useful for assessing the coaptation line at the level of the posteromedial segments (P3/A3) and gives a good view of the entire anterior leaflet. This is usually the best view in which to see the LA appendage.

## Mid oesophageal long axis view (120–150°; Figure 9.9)
Echocardiographic anatomy
The mid-oesophageal long-axis view can be identified by the echocardiographer's ability to visualise both the mitral and aortic valves but neither papillary muscle. In most patients this occurs with the sector scan between 120° and 150°. This view cuts the coaptation line perpendicularly through P2/A2.

Additional views
Turning the probe sweeps the sector scan perpendicularly along the coaptation line. Turning to the right (clockwise) sweeps the image plane towards the posteromedial commissure (P3/A3); turning to the left (anticlockwise) sweeps the image plane towards the anterolateral commissure (P1/A1). The anterolateral commissure may be identified by being able to visualise the LA appendage; the posteromedial commissure may be

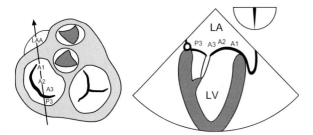

**Figure 9.8** Mid oesophageal two-chamber view.

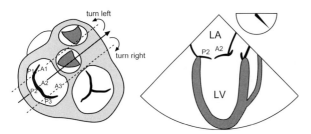

**Figure 9.9** Mid oesophageal long axis view.

identified by visualising the coronary sinus or the RA. During this manoeuvre, to maintain a true long axis orientation it may also be necessary to advance the probe when turning to the right and to withdraw it when turning to the left.

## Main utility
The mid oesophageal long axis view is very useful for assessment of mitral pathology for the following reasons:

- Since the image plane cuts the coaptation line perpendicularly, the observed base-to-tip leaflet length accurately reflects the true leaflet length. For the same reason it is the appropriate view for the assessment of the width of the vena contracta (see below).
- This image plane passes through the "high" (more basal) axis of the mitral annulus and is therefore the appropriate view in which to assess leaflet prolapse.
- The scan cuts the posterior leaflet through the P2 scallop, which is the mitral segment most likely to be affected in myxomatous degeneration, annular dilatation and regurgitation.
- The image plane can be swept along the coaptation line by turning the shaft of the probe, allowing a detailed assessment of all segments of each leaflet.

## Transgastric basal short axis view (0°; Figure 9.10)
### Echocardiographic anatomy
This view shows the MV *en face* and allows visualisation of all six mitral segments. P3 is closest to the apex of the sector scan, the posteromedial commissure is in the upper left and the anterolateral commissure in the lower right of the image. It is also called the "fishmouth" view.

### Additional views
The transgastric mid short axis view should also be obtained to assess the papillary muscles and adjacent myocardium.

### Main utility
Using colour flow Doppler this view is, in theory, useful for assessing where along the coaptation line regurgitation is occurring. A loop can be saved in memory and slowly scrolled through to assess where the systolic colour disturbance is taking place. However, in practice it is frequently difficult to localise the origin of the jet. This is partly due to the fact that the image plane is perpendicular to the direction of regurgitation, making colour flow Doppler difficult to interpret.

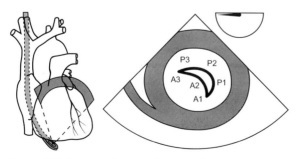

**Figure 9.10** Transgastric basal short axis view.

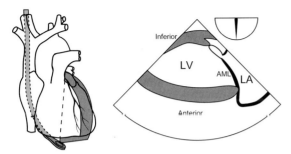

**Figure 9.11** Transgastric two-chamber view.

In the mid short axis view it is important to look for segmental wall motion abnormalities and ventricular dilatation, which may contribute to MV dysfunction.

### Transgastric two-chamber view (90°; Figure 9.11)
Echocardiographic anatomy and main utility
The posterior mitral leaflet appears in the near field and the anterior mitral leaflet in the far field. It can be difficult to be sure of segmental leaflet anatomy in this view, but a clear view of the papillary muscles and chordae is usually obtained.

## MITRAL VALVE PATHOLOGY

Until recently the most common lesion affecting the native MV was **rheumatic heart disease** and in many developing countries this is still the case. Rheumatic heart disease is primarily a disease of the MV, and may or may not involve other valves. The predominant lesion is usually mitral stenosis; mitral regurgitation frequently coexists but is not usually the haemodynamically significant lesion.

The most frequent cause of native mitral regurgitation in most industrialised nations is **myxomatous degeneration**. Rarely, myxomatous degeneration is associated with systemic diseases such as Marfan and Ehlers–Danlos syndromes. Mitral regurgitation also develops as a consequence of **LV dysfunction, endocarditis** and rarely as a complication of **acute myocardial infarction** with **papillary muscle rupture**.

**Mitral annular calcification** is a relatively common degenerative process involving the annulus and rarely causes significant valve dysfunction. The major implication of this condition is that it can create difficulties for the surgeon during valve removal and suturing in of a mitral prosthesis or annuloplasty ring. Additionally, on TOE the calcification may cause shadowing and echo dropout, which obscures the far field. Table 9.2 summarises the common causes and mechanisms of native MV dysfunction.

## MITRAL REGURGITATION

The following points need to be addressed during echocardiographic assessment of mitral regurgitation:

- The *pathological process* underlying the regurgitation (myxomatous degeneration, ventricular dysfunction, endocarditis, rheumatic disease).
- The *mechanism* of regurgitation (prolapse, flail, restriction, perforation or cleft of a leaflet).

| Table 9.2 The causes and mechanisms of native MV dysfunction | | | |
|---|---|---|---|
| Pathology | Lesion | Mechanism of valve dysfunction | Direction of regurgitant jet |
| Rheumatic disease | Stenosis ± regurgitation | Leaflet restriction; chordal shortening | Eccentric: towards side of lesion; may be central if both leaflets equally affected |
| Myxomatous degeneration | Regurgitation | Prolapse; flail; chordal stretch or rupture; annular dilatation | Eccentric: away from side of lesion |
| Ventricular dysfunction | Regurgitation | Altered papillary/leaflet orientation; increased ventricular sphericity; papillary dysfunction or rupture; tethering and leaflet restriction; annular dilatation; systolic anterior motion (hypertrophic obstructive cardiomyopathy) | Cardiomyopathy: central; ischaemic: typically eccentric towards side of lesion if main effect is leaflet restriction; hypertrophic obstructive cardiomyopathy: eccentric posteriorly directed |
| Endocarditis | Regurgitation | Leaflet destruction; perforation | Often multiple jets, variable direction |

- The *location and extent* of the lesion (which segments are involved and whether the lesion involves the commissures).
- Associated abnormalities.

Despite the important role of colour flow Doppler in the assessment of mitral regurgitation, most of this information is gained from careful 2-D imaging.

# ECHOCARDIOGRAPHIC FEATURES OF MITRAL REGURGITATION

## Myxomatous degeneration
This is a degenerative process in which the valve leaflets become thickened and elongated. There is redundant leaflet tissue and stretching of the chordae leading to excessive leaflet motion, which creates a characteristic appearance on 2-D imaging (Figure 9.12). Regurgitation develops from either leaflet prolapse or flail. The annulus is usually significantly dilated.

### Leaflet prolapse
Prolapse is said to occur when the body of the leaflet domes above the level of the mitral annulus in systole (by more than 2 mm, using transthoracic echocardiographic criteria[7]). This should be assessed in the mid oesophageal long axis view at end systole. The leaflet tip is directed towards the LV and a coaptation defect may be visible (Figure 9.13). Prolapse occurs as a consequence of leaflet redundancy and chordal stretch; significant myxomatous change is usually evident. Regurgitation usually develops slowly and ranges in severity from trivial to severe.

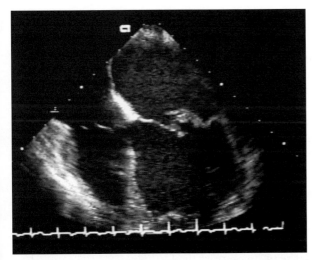

**Figure 9.12** Myxomatous degeneration of the MV. In this systolic frame taken from the mid oesophageal four-chamber view, the posterior mitral leaflet shows the typical features of myxomatous degeneration: increased leaflet thickness and length, a visible coaptation defect and evidence of a flail segment. Note the dilated LA and LV.

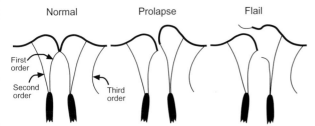

**Figure 9.13** Mitral leaflets: normal, prolapse and flail. The classification of chordae tendinae is also shown (see p.133).

Mild prolapse in the presence of normal leaflet morphology can be considered a variation of normal and is usually associated with trivial regurgitation.[8]

### Flail leaflet
A flail leaflet results in a visible coaptation defect with the leaflet tip directed towards the LA throughout systole (Figure 9.13). The cause is usually torn chordae in association with marked myxomatous change but can also be papillary muscle rupture. The freeze and scroll modes, can be very helpful in visualising the ruptured chordae flicking into the LA during systole. In general, regurgitation due to a flail leaflet is more severe and develops more rapidly than that associated with leaflet prolapse.

### Location and direction of the regurgitant jet
Leaflet prolapse and flail most commonly develop in the posterior leaflet, particularly the P2 segment.[9]

With either prolapse or flail the direction of the regurgitant jet is *away* from the side of the lesion and, since it is rare for both leaflets to be affected equally, these jets are usually eccentric and appear to hug the wall of the LA.

## Ventricular dysfunction

The mechanisms underlying mitral regurgitation due to global LV dysfunction are incompletely understood but are thought to be primarily related to an altered geometric relationship between the papillary muscles and the mitral leaflets. The severity of mitral regurgitation is more dependent on the degree of LV sphericity (with loss of the normal ellipsoid shape) than the magnitude of the reduction in ejection fraction.[10] Increased LV sphericity results in widening of the interpapillary angle and tethering or restriction of leaflet motion, leading to regurgitation.[11]

On 2-D imaging the valve may appear morphologically normal but with loss of the usual systolic leaflet overlap or with a visible coaptation defect. With dilated cardiomyopathy the regurgitant jet is usually central. For ischaemic mitral regurgitation there may be dilatation of specific areas of myocardium leading to asymmetrical leaflet tethering and an eccentric regurgitant jet. In this situation the regurgitant jet is directed *towards* the side of the lesion.

Dilatation of the annulus may also contribute to regurgitation, particularly in the region of the P2 segment, but in most cases this is not the major mechanism of regurgitation.

In hypertrophic obstructive cardiomyopathy the regurgitant jet is usually directed posteriorly and the anterior leaflet tends to obstruct the LVOT.

## Papillary muscle rupture

Occasionally, as a complication of myocardial infarction, papillary muscle rupture occurs. This most frequently affects the posteromedial muscle (see above) and results in torrential bileaflet regurgitation involving A3/P3 and A2/P2. The papillary muscle and chordae can usually be seen flicking in and out of the LA.

## Native valve endocarditis

Endocarditis results in mitral regurgitation due to destruction, perforation and deformity of the valve leaflets. Typically vegetations develop on the upstream, or low-pressure, side of a valve. Thus in mitral endocarditis lesions are most commonly seen on the LA surface of the valve. Mitral stenosis is rare.

If mitral endocarditis is suspected a careful search for vegetations on the other heart valves must be undertaken.

Leaflet perforation is characterised by the presence of one or more regurgitant jets that do not appear to arise from the coaptation line. The presence of two separate proximal convergence zones should alert the operator to the possibility of perforation.

## Rheumatic heart disease

The mechanism of regurgitation in rheumatic mitral disease involves leaflet restriction, chordal shortening and tethering which result in a failure of leaflet coaptation. The regurgitant jet is directed *towards* the side of the lesion.

## **Features associated with mitral regurgitation**

In addition to abnormalities of the valve itself, other echocardiographic findings are usually seen in patients with significant (at least moderate) mitral regurgitation:[12]

- LA dilatation. This is common with chronic severe regurgitation but is not a feature of acute regurgitation.
- Pronounced left-to-right bowing of the interatrial septum due to elevated LA pressure. This is best seen in the mid oesophageal four-chamber or bicaval views.
- Spherical enlargement of the LV with eccentric hypertrophy (i.e. wall thickness is increased in proportion to the increase in LV size; p.119). End diastolic volume increases before end systolic volume.

- Hypercontractile LV. This is a normal finding in severe mitral regurgitation. Normal or mildly reduced LV systolic function (ejection fraction < 55% and an end systolic short axis diameter > 4–4.5 cm) suggests significant LV impairment.
- Signs of pulmonary hypertension, consistent with LV decompensation. These include a tricuspid regurgitation jet velocity >3 m/s and enlargement of the RV and the RA.

## Grading mitral regurgitation[12,13]

There are a number of ways of assessing the severity of mitral regurgitation. These need to be considered collectively and in context as they may provide conflicting data (Table 9.3).

| Table 9.3 The 2-D, colour flow and spectral Doppler signs of severe mitral regurgitation | |
|---|---|
| **TOE sign** | **Value** |
| **Colour flow Doppler** | |
| Diameter of vena contracta > 6 mm (mid oesophageal long axis view) | +++ |
| LV PISA radius > 1 cm (alias velocity at 40 cm/s) | +++ |
| Wall-hugging jet that encircles the LA | +++ |
| Jet enters a pulmonary vein | ++ |
| Jet enters LA appendage | ++ |
| **Spectral Doppler** | |
| Systolic flow reversal in contralateral pulmonary vein | ++++ |
| E wave height exceeds 1.4 m/s on transmitral Doppler (do not use after MV repair) | +++ |
| Intensity of regurgitant jet is similar to diastolic jet on transmitral Doppler | ++ |
| V wave cut-off sign | ++ |
| **2-D imaging** | |
| Flail leaflet | +++ |
| End systolic LV dimension > 4.5 cm or ejection fraction < 55% | ++ |
| Spherical dilatation of the LV | ++ |
| Enlarged LA | + |
| Hypercontractile LV | + |
| Rightward bulging of interatrial septum | + |
| RV and RA dilatation | + |
| Pulmonary hypertension | + |
| **Signs suggesting severe regurgitation is unlikely** | |
| A wave dominance on transmitral Doppler profile | ++ |
| Spontaneous echo contrast in the LA | ++ |
| The utility of each sign is rated from one (+) to four (++++) Modified from Schiller et al[12] and Patel et al[13] | |

## Semiquantitative versus quantitative Doppler

Quantitative Doppler can provide an objective assessment of the severity of regurgitation (pp.233–237), but in the intraoperative setting the necessary measurements are relatively time consuming to make, and there is considerable potential for inaccuracy. However, a number of semiquantitative techniques have been well validated and are applicable to TOE. These are discussed below.

## Colour flow Doppler

A number of grading systems based on different aspects of the colour flow map have been described, including:

• Jet length.
• Jet area (including mosaic jet area).
• Jet area as a percentage of LA area.
• Width of the vena contracta.

Jet area as a percentage of atrial area is widely used and has been reasonably well validated with angiography[14] (Table 9.4) but tends to underdiagnose the severity of eccentric jets. This is because a jet that impinges on the atrial wall entrains less blood than a central jet (see the Coanda effect – p.230) and therefore generates a reduced flow disturbance and a smaller colour map.

The most useful colour flow Doppler grading system is based on the width of the vena contracta.[15,16] The vena contracta is the narrowest point of the jet as it passes through the valve and is in effect the diameter of the effective regurgitant orifice (ERO; see Figure 16.1). It should be estimated in the mid oesophageal long axis view to avoid cutting the coaptation line obliquely and potentially overestimating the diameter of the jet.[15] In this view the probe should be turned to the left and to the right to identify the point along the coaptation line where the diameter of the vena contracta is at its maximum. A diameter of 6 mm or more identifies angiographically severe mitral regurgitation with a sensitivity of 95% and specificity of 98% (Table 9.4).[15]

Unfortunately, all methods based on colour flow Doppler are susceptible to misinterpretation due to changes in machine settings and loading conditions (Table 9.5). These problems are most marked with grading systems based on jet length or absolute jet area and are least troublesome with the vena contracta method.

### Proximal flow acceleration

In the presence of mitral regurgitation a proximal isovelocity surface area (PISA) may be seen on the LV side of the valve in systole, and may be used in the quantitative

**Table 9.4** Grading mitral regurgitation using colour flow Doppler, on the basis of width of the vena contracta and maximal jet area as a percentage of LA area[14–16]

| Severity | Width of vena contracta (mm) | Maximal jet area as a percentage of LA area |
|---|---|---|
| Mild | 2–4 | <20 |
| Moderate | 4–6 | 20–40 |
| Usually severe | ≥5.5–6 | >40 |
| Always severe | ≥10 | |

assessment of the ERO (pp.236–237). As a rule of thumb, when the alias velocity is set to 40 cm/s a PISA radius greater than 1 cm suggests severe regurgitation (p.237).[17]

## Other signs on colour flow Doppler

In addition to the criteria listed above two other features on colour flow Doppler suggest severe regurgitation:

- Wall-hugging jets.
- Jets that enter the LA appendage or pulmonary veins. These provide visual evidence of pulmonary venous flow reversal (see below).

## Spectral Doppler

Both transmitral CW Doppler and pulmonary venous PW Doppler provide important information on the severity of mitral regurgitation and should form part of the routine assessment of the MV. Normal waveforms are described on pp.120–121.

### Intensity and shape of the regurgitant jet

The intensity or brightness of the transmitral regurgitant jet on CW Doppler is determined by both the regurgitant blood flow and the Doppler gain setting. By comparing the intensity of the map in systole with that in diastole a qualitative assessment of the severity of mitral regurgitation can be made that is independent of the gain setting (Figure 9.14):

- A systolic signal that is complete, and of equal intensity to the diastolic signal, suggests severe regurgitation.
- A systolic signal that is complete but less intense than the diastolic signal suggests moderate regurgitation.
- An incomplete systolic signal suggests mild regurgitation.

An additional clue to the presence of severe mitral regurgitation is given by the shape of the regurgitant Doppler waveform. Regurgitation of a large volume of blood into the LA causes a late systolic reduction in the transmitral gradient due to a sharp rise in the LA pressure (seen as a V wave on the LA pressure trace). This causes a late systolic reduction in regurgitant jet velocity, which gives the Doppler map an asymmetrical shape and is known as the **V wave cut-off sign**[12] (Figure 9.14). This sign is most obvious with acute regurgitation into a non-dilated LA and may not be seen with chronic regurgitation where the LA is more compliant.

| **Table 9.5** Factors that lead to a reduction in the dimensions of the regurgitant colour flow map |
| --- |
| Reduction in colour gain setting (reduces the size of the colour map) |
| Increase in colour scale setting (reduces aliasing within the colour map) |
| Eccentric or wall-hugging jet (minimal effect on the vena contracta) |
| Reduction in preload* |
| Reduction in afterload* |
| *Associated with a reduction in the severity of the mitral regurgitation |

## Regurgitant jet velocity

The regurgitant jet velocity is determined by the LV to LA systolic pressure gradient and not directly by the severity of the regurgitation. It is normally >5 m/s, reflecting a pressure gradient higher than 100 mmHg (by the simplified Bernoulli equation; p.238). Assuming a velocity of 5 m/s, normal AV function and a systolic arterial pressure of 110 mmHg, LA pressure will be 10 mmHg. A peak velocity of 4 m/s equates to a pressure gradient of 64 mmHg. Assuming a systolic arterial pressure of 90 mmHg and normal AV function, the LA pressure will be 26 mmHg. Thus a lower regurgitant velocity may be associated with more advanced disease.

## Transmitral E wave velocity

Mitral regurgitation creates a volume load on the LA, which increases the peak early diastolic filling velocity ($E_{max}$; Figure 9.14). An $E_{max} > 1.2$ m/s is indicative of severe mitral regurgitation with a sensitivity of 86% and specificity of 86%.[18] To reduce the likelihood of a false-positive result, a value above 1.4 m/s can be used as a marker of severe regurgitation. Note that this sign is unreliable in the presence of a hyperdynamic circulation or even minor degrees of mitral stenosis (e.g. following MV repair).

A wave dominance ($A_{max} > E_{max}$) virtually rules out severe mitral regurgitation.

## Pulmonary venous Doppler profile

Alterations in the systolic (S wave) and diastolic (D wave) patterns on the pulmonary venous PW Doppler waveforms are extremely useful in quantifying the severity of mitral regurgitation. Trivial or mild regurgitation is generally associated with a normal flow pattern (S wave > D wave). Moderate regurgitation is associated with systolic blunting (S wave < D wave) and severe regurgitation with systolic flow reversal[19] (Figure 9.14). Note the following caveats:

- Elevated LA pressure can cause systolic blunting in the absence of mitral regurgitation.
- Systolic blunting or reversal may not affect all pulmonary veins equally. This is intuitive for eccentric jets but may also occur with central jets.[20] Therefore at least one

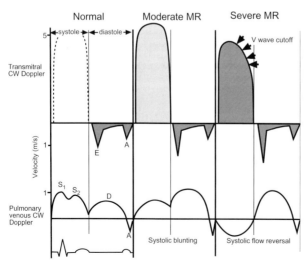

**Figure 9.14** The changes seen in the transmitral CW and pulmonary venous PW Doppler waveforms with moderate or severe mitral regurgitation (MR). See text for details of waveforms.

pulmonary vein from each side should be interrogated. For eccentric jets, the contra-lateral pulmonary vein (i.e. on the opposite side from the direction of the jet) should be used to grade the severity of the regurgitation.

# VALVE REPAIR FOR MITRAL REGURGITATION

Prebypass identification of the location, mechanism and extent of the regurgitant defect can guide surgical decision making. After bypass the quality of the repair and the development of any complications can be immediately assessed. TOE has been shown to improve surgical outcome in this setting, and mitral valve repair has been classified as a category I indication for perioperative TOE (see Table 1.1).

## Indications for valve repair

The most common indication for mitral repair is myxomatous degeneration; this has the highest chance of success. An isolated flail segment involving P2 is the most favourable lesion[9]; the rate of successful repair is lower for lesions involving the anterior leaflet (either isolated anterior leaflet or bileaflet lesions).

Mitral repair is also used for regurgitation secondary to ventricular dysfunction, rheumatic heart disease and endocarditis.

## The prebypass examination

In most cases the severity of the mitral regurgitation will have been carefully assessed with preoperative transthoracic echocardiography, and perhaps with TOE as well. Furthermore, the effects of general anaesthesia (afterload and preload reduction) tend to minimise the severity of mitral regurgitation, complicating the intraoperative assessment. For these reasons, grading the **severity** is not usually the main priority of the prebypass examination. Rather, it is important to assess the **location** and **mechanism** of the jet as these two factors will have a direct bearing on the surgical repair and may not have been fully elucidated preoperatively. All mitral segments should be systematically examined, following the sequence outlined above. The TV and both ventricles should also be carefully examined for evidence of ventricular decompensation.

## Surgical techniques

A number of techniques are used depending on the underlying pathology. Only a brief description of each is given here.

### Quadrangular resection

Used for isolated lesions, typically of the P2 segment, with or without chordal rupture. A segment of leaflet is resected and the defect directly sutured.

### Sliding valvuloplasty

Used for extensive myxomatous lesions of the posterior leaflet with significant prolapse or flail. As for quadrangular resection, but in addition a strip of leaflet along the posterior mitral annulus is resected to reduce the base-to-tip length of the posterior leaflet and minimise the risk of systolic anterior motion (see below).

### Commissural plication

Used to control excessive leaflet tissue in the region of the commissures.

## Chordal shortening
May be used in combination with one of the above procedures when excessive leaflet tissue or chordal stretching occurs.

## Chordal transfer
Used for myxomatous degeneration of the anterior leaflet where a direct quadrangular resection with subsequent loss of chordal tissue may lead to insufficient leaflet support. A combined procedure involving quadrangular resection of the posterior and anterior leaflets is performed. The resected segment of the posterior leaflet and its associated chordae are transferred to the anterior leaflet.

## Annuloplasty ring
An annuloplasty ring is widely used in mitral repair procedures to provide support to the repair and reduce annular size. The ring is usually incomplete as no support is required to the thickened intervalvular fibrosa. Annuloplasty rings are strongly echogenic.

## The postbypass examination
Before the success of the repair is assessed the patient should have fully separated from bypass with any venting devices that pass through the MV removed. Immediately after separating from bypass it is normal for patients to be relatively vasodilated, and at times hypovolaemic, and it is usually necessary to administer fluids and vasoconstricting agents to match the awake haemodynamic state. During the immediate postbypass period the hyperdynamic, underfilled heart can make colour Doppler very difficult to interpret. In this situation the colour sample volume and gain should be reduced, the colour scale increased, the ventricle filled and the situation reviewed a few minutes later. An additional problem, which may complicate echocardiographic interpretation in the immediate postbypass period, involves the presence of significant regurgitation caused by ventricular dysfunction (usually due to stunning). It is important to allow the LV time to recover from the effects of cardiopulmonary bypass and institute appropriate inotropic therapy before a definitive assessment of mitral regurgitation is made.

An annuloplasty ring is easily visible on 2-D examination. If the patient has undergone a quadrangular resection, the posterior leaflet may appear shorter and less mobile than it did preoperatively – indeed the valve will appear to have only a single leaflet (Figure 9.15).

The postbypass assessment must determine the extent and location of any **residual regurgitation, systolic anterior motion** (SAM) and valvular **stenosis**.

### Residual regurgitation
Residual regurgitation requiring a second bypass run occurs in approximately 5% of all mitral repairs and is due to either an incomplete repair or suture dehiscence.[21] Suture dehiscence may appear as a leaflet perforation with the origin of the regurgitant jet displaced from the coaptation line.

In most cases the regurgitation is either trivial or (rarely) severe and the management decision is clear. In contrast, the distinction between mild and moderate regurgitation can be difficult. It is important to examine the valve in multiple planes and to use a range of criteria to grade the severity (see Table 9.3). The two most useful criteria are the width of the vena contracta and flow in the contralateral pulmonary veins. Careful examination of the valve in the mid oesophageal long axis view is particularly useful as it allows the

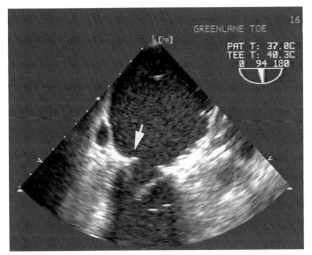

**Figure 9.15** MV following valve repair. In this diastolic frame taken from the mid oesophageal two-chamber view the posterior mitral leaflet is barely visible (arrow). This is a normal finding following a quadrangular resection of the posterior leaflet. Note the coronary sinus to the left of the arrow.

entire coaptation line to be scanned and is the appropriate view for assessing both the width of the vena contracta and the presence of leaflet prolapse.

It is not unusual to see a maximum E wave velocity of more than 1.2 m/s due to mild mitral stenosis and a hyperdynamic circulation. This criterion is therefore unreliable following MV repair.

Accurately categorising the severity of any residual regurgitation does not, however, answer the question as to what should be done for patients with mild-to-moderate regurgitation after mitral repair. The decision to reoperate must take into account the likelihood of improvement with a further attempt at repair, the patient's ability to tolerate a second (or even third) bypass run, and the desirability of repair versus replacement in a particular individual.

## Systolic anterior motion

SAM involves prolapse of the anterior mitral leaflet into the LVOT during systole, causing outflow tract obstruction and mitral regurgitation. Risk factors for the development of SAM following mitral repair include:

- A small non-dilated LV.
- Use of a small annuloplasty ring.
- Excessive posterior mitral leaflet tissue causing anterior displacement of the coaptation line.

The sliding valvuloplasty repair technique is designed to reduce the risk of SAM by decreasing the base-to-tip length of the posterior leaflet and therefore displacing the coaptation line posteriorly.

SAM is best appreciated in the mid oesophageal five-chamber and long axis views, and has a distinctive appearance on TOE (Figure 9.16); during systole the distal anterior mitral leaflet can be seen bending into the LVOT and is usually kinked at the mid portion. There is loss of leaflet coaptation and (usually) a posteriorly directed jet of regurgitation, which is typically moderate to severe. A greatly increased velocity across

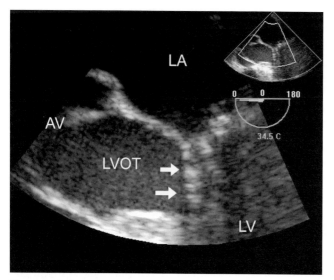

**Figure 9.16** Systolic anterior motion (SAM) following MV repair. The image shows a close-up view of the LVOT from the mid oesophageal five-chamber view, in mid systole. The AV is seen in an open position on the left of the image. The distal portion of the anterior mitral leaflet can be seen obstructing the LVOT (arrows). In this particular patient, no coaptation defect is seen between the two mitral leaflets, although this often occurs.

the LVOT is apparent on CW Doppler (3–5 m/s), best seen in the transgastric long-axis or deep transgastric views. This appears as intense aliasing on colour flow Doppler.

In its most severe form SAM prevents separation from bypass and requires immediate surgical revision. However, in most cases, particularly those in which SAM involves only the distal anterior leaflet and chordae, it gradually resolves with appropriate medical therapy (volume loading, vasoconstrictors, β-blockers, stopping inotropic and vasodilating drugs).

The surgical approaches to persistent or severe SAM involve removal of the annuloplasty ring, revision of the sliding valvuloplasty or valve replacement. Recently it has been suggested that reduction in the base-to-tip length of the *anterior* leaflet may be beneficial.[22]

### Valvular stenosis

This is very rare following repair. The extent of diastolic leaflet excursion on 2-D imaging will usually give a qualitative guide to the extent of any mitral stenosis. It is usual in most institutions to measure the pressure gradient and calculate the pressure half-time to rule out significant stenosis (see below), but these measurements have not been validated in this setting. A peak E wave velocity above 2 m/s, or a shallow deceleration slope, should alert the examiner to the possibility of mitral stenosis and corroborative evidence should be sought.

## MITRAL STENOSIS

The vast majority of haemodynamically significant native MV stenoses are due to **rheumatic heart disease**. In most cases these can be successfully managed with percutaneous mitral balloon valvuloplasty. Therefore, patients presenting for surgical correction are those who have valvular features unsuitable for this technique, including extensive leaflet and subvalvular calcification, mitral or tricuspid regurgitation and LA thrombus.

Surgery involves either valve repair (open commissurotomy) or valve replacement. The intraoperative echocardiographic examination should not focus on the severity of the stenosis as, in most cases, this will have been carefully assessed preoperatively. It is more important to evaluate the following:

- The presence of LA thrombus, particularly within the LA appendage.
- The presence and severity of tricuspid regurgitation.
- LV and RV function.
- The degree of residual stenosis or regurgitation following valve repair.
- Prosthesis function following valve replacement.

## Echocardiographic features of rheumatic mitral stenosis

The hallmarks of rheumatic mitral stenosis include:

- Leaflet thickening, particularly of the commissures and leaflet edges.
- Loss of leaflet mobility. This occurs as a consequence of commissural fusion, and chordal shortening and tethering, and creates the appearance of **diastolic doming** of the body of the anterior mitral leaflet (the "hockey stick sign; Figure 9.17).
- Leaflet calcification.
- Subvalvular involvement. The chordae appear shortened, tethered and, on occasion, calcified.

Leaflet morphology and diastolic doming are best appreciated in the mid oesophageal five-chamber and long axis views. The subvalvular involvement is usually best visualised from the transgastric two-chamber view. In the transgastric basal short axis view there is loss of the open "fishmouth" appearance and calcification may be seen in the region of the commissures.

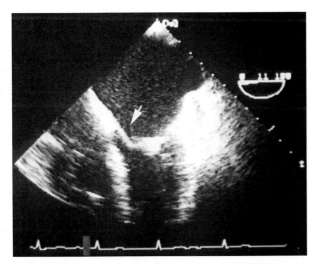

**Figure 9.17** Diastolic doming of the anterior mitral leaflet (arrow) in a patient with severe rheumatic mitral stenosis. Note the marked thickening and echogenicity of the tip of the anterior and posterior leaflets, typical of rheumatic MV disease.

On colour flow Doppler some degree of mitral regurgitation may be seen. This may be eccentric or (if both leaflets are equally affected) central. Eccentric jets are directed *towards* the side of the predominant lesion. Marked colour aliasing and PISA formation can usually be seen on the LA side of the valve during diastole.

## Associated features of mitral stenosis
A number of non-valvular features of mitral stenosis may be seen, including:

- Atrial dilatation. There is usually pronounced left-to-right bowing of the interatrial septum.
- Spontaneous echo contrast in the LA. This sign is strongly suggestive of significant mitral stenosis.
- LA thrombus. This is a frequent finding, particularly in the LA appendage. Within the atrial appendage thrombus must be differentiated from pectinate muscle (see Figures 5.4 and 5.16). If thrombus is detected it may be removed by the surgeon while on bypass.
- RV dysfunction. Severe mitral stenosis is associated with the signs of RV failure: tricuspid regurgitation, RA enlargement and pulmonary hypertension.
- LV dysfunction. Despite being protected from pressure and volume overload the LV is frequently abnormal. It may appear small and underfilled. A rigid mitral annulus may impede systolic contraction. Diastolic filling may appear to be prolonged (the 2-D equivalent of prolonged E wave deceleration).

## Grading mitral stenosis
The severity of mitral stenosis may be assessed by a number of methods. The grading of severity, on the basis of valve area and pressure gradient, is summarised in Table 9.6.

### Transmitral pressure gradient
Pressure gradients across the MV are easily estimated from the transmitral CW Doppler waveform. Once a representative Doppler envelope has been saved, peak and mean transmitral pressure gradients can be estimated using the caliper and trace functions respectively. Note that the transmitral pressure gradient will be increased with elevated cardiac output (p.238), mitral regurgitation (p.146) and restrictive diastolic filling (p.120).

### Pressure half time
Calculation of the pressure half time $(Pt_{1/2})$ is the most useful technique for the rapid estimation of valve area in patients with mitral stenosis. The $Pt_{1/2}$, in milliseconds, refers to the rate of diastolic pressure decline across the MV (pp.241–243). On transmitral CW

| Table 9.6 Grading of mitral stenosis on the basis of mean transvalvular pressure gradient and valve area | | |
|---|---|---|
| | Mean transvalvular pressure gradient (mmHg) | Mitral valve area (cm²) |
| Normal | | 4–6 |
| Mild | <6 | >1.5 |
| Moderate | 6–12 | 1.0–1.5 |
| Severe | >12 | <1.0 |

Doppler, the E wave normally undergoes rapid deceleration due to the abrupt fall in transmitral pressure gradient as the LV fills during early diastole. In mitral stenosis the pressure gradient is maintained much later in diastole, resulting in a greatly prolonged E wave deceleration and $Pt_{1/2}$ (see Figure 16.4). Experimentally, a mitral valve area of 1 cm$^2$ has been shown to equate to a $Pt_{1/2}$ of 220 ms (see Equation 16.24).

In practice this is a very simple and rapid method of estimating MV area. Once a representative Doppler profile has been saved, the E wave descent is evaluated at two points and the $Pt_{1/2}$ and valve area calculated using the automated machine software. The technical considerations, caveats and factors that influence $Pt_{1/2}$ are outlined on p.243.

## Mitral planimetry

Planimetry is a well described technique for the evaluation of MV area by transthoracic echocardiography but is not recommended with TOE. Although it is usually possible to obtain a satisfactory *en face* view of the valve from the transgastric basal short-axis view, it is difficult to be sure that the scan cuts the valve at right angles to the valve leaflets. An oblique cut will tend to overestimate valve area. Similarly, the scan must pass through the tip rather than the body of the leaflets to avoid overestimating valve area.

## Proximal flow convergence (PISA method)

Haemodynamically significant mitral stenosis is associated with colour aliasing and PISA formation on the LA side of the valve during diastole. The MV area may be calculated on the basis of PISA radius and velocity and the transmitral $E_{max}$ (p.236).

## Continuity equation

The estimation of valve area in mitral stenosis by means of the continuity equation is outlined on p.234.

## **Valve repair for mitral stenosis**

Patients with rheumatic mitral stenosis who are unsuitable for balloon valvotomy and who do not have significant mitral regurgitation may be considered for open commissurotomy. This procedure is performed on cardiopulmonary bypass and involves commissurotomy, chordal splitting, decalcification, removal of LA thrombus (if present) and excision of the LA appendage. Before bypass the echocardiographer should primarily examine the LA and appendage for thrombus and assess the severity of any regurgitation. After bypass the most common problem is significant mitral regurgitation, which usually necessitates valve replacement.

## **REFERENCES**

1. Roberts WC. Morphologic features of the normal and abnormal mitral valve. *American Journal of Cardiology* 1983;51:1005–1028.
2. Bollen BA, Luo HH, Oury JH, et al. Case 4 – 2000: a systematic approach to intraoperative transesophageal echocardiographic evaluation of the mitral valve apparatus with anatomic correlation. *Journal of Cardiothoracic and Vascular Anesthesia* 2000;14:330–338.
3. Fenster MS, Feldman MD. Mitral regurgitation: an overview. *Current Problems in Cardiology* 1995;20: 193–280.
4. Fyrenius A, Engvall J, Janerot-Sjöberg B. Major and minor axes of the normal mitral annulus. *Journal of Heart Valve Disease* 2001;10:146–152.
5. Shanewise JS, Cheung AT, Aronson S, et al. ASE/SCA guidelines for performing a comprehensive intraoperative multiplane transesophageal echocardiography examination: recommendations of the American Society of Echocardiography Council for Intraoperative Echocardiography and the Society of Cardiovascular Anesthesiologists Task Force for Certification in Perioperative Transesophageal Echocardiography. *Anesthesia and Analgesia* 1999;89:870–884.
6. Shah PM, Raney AA, Duran CMG, et al. Multiplane transesophageal echocardiography: a roadmap for mitral valve repair. *Journal of Heart Valve Disease* 1999;8:625–629.
7. Freed LA, Levy D, Levine RA, et al. Prevalence and clinical outcome of mitral-valve prolapse. *New England Journal of Medicine* 1999;341:1–7.

8. Nishimura RA, McGoon MD. Perspectives on mitral-valve prolapse. *New England Journal of Medicine* 1999;341:48–50.

9. Muratori M, Berti M, Doria E, et al. Transesophageal echocardiography as predictor of mitral valve repair. *Journal of Heart Valve Disease* 2001;10:65–71.

10. Nass O, Rosman H, Al-Khaled N, et al. Relation of left ventricular chamber shape in patients with low (< or = 40%) ejection fraction to severity of functional mitral regurgitation. *American Journal of Cardiology* 1995;76:402–404.

11. Otsuji Y, Handschumacher MD, Schwammenthal E, et al. Insights from three-dimensional echocardiography into the mechanism of functional mitral regurgitation: direct in vivo demonstration of altered leaflet tethering geometry. *Circulation* 1997;96:1999–2008.

12. Schiller NB, Foster E, Redberg RF. Transesophageal echocardiography in the evaluation of mitral regurgitation: the twenty-four signs of severe mitral regurgitation. *Cardiology Clinics* 1993;11:399–408.

13. Patel AR, Mochizuki Y, Yao J, et al. Mitral regurgitation: comprehensive assessment by echocardiography. *Echocardiography* 2000;17:275–283.

14. Helmcke F, Nanda NC, Hsiung MC, et al. Color Doppler assessment of mitral regurgitation with orthogonal planes. *Circulation* 1987;75:175–183.

15. Grayburn PA, Fehske W, Omran H, et al. Multiplane transesophageal echocardiographic assessment of mitral regurgitation by Doppler color flow mapping of the vena contracta. *American Journal of Cardiology* 1994;74:912–917.

16. Tribouilloy C, Shen WF, Quéré J-P, et al. Assessment of severity of mitral regurgitation by measuring regurgitant jet width at its origin with transesophageal Doppler color flow imaging. *Circulation* 1992;85:1248–1253.

17. Pu M, Prior DL, Fan X, et al. Calculation of mitral regurgitant orifice area with use of a simplified proximal convergence method: initial clinical application. *Journal of the American Society of Echocardiography* 2001;14:180–185.

18. Thomas L, Foster E, Schiller NB. Peak mitral inflow velocity predicts mitral regurgitation severity. *Journal of the American College of Cardiology* 1998;31:174–179.

19. Enriquez-Sarano M, Dujardin KS, Tribouilloy CM, et al. Determinants of pulmonary venous flow reversal in mitral regurgitation and its usefulness in determining the severity of regurgitation. *American Journal of Cardiology* 1999;83:535–541.

20. Mark JB, Ahmed SU, Kluger R, et al. Influence of jet direction on pulmonary vein flow patterns of severe mitral regurgitation. *Anesthesia and Analgesia* 1995;80:486–491.

21. Marwick TH, Stewart WJ, Currie PJ, et al. Mechanisms of failure of mitral valve repair: an echocardiographic study. *American Heart Journal* 1991;122:149–156.

22. Raney AA, Shah PM, Joyo CI. The 'Pomeroy procedure': a new method to correct post-mitral valve repair systolic anterior motion. *Journal of Heart Valve Disease* 2001;10:307–311.

# 10

# The Aortic Valve and Left Ventricular Outflow Tract

*Malcolm Legget*
*David Sidebotham*

The AV, LVOT and aortic root are positioned in the centre of the heart in close proximity to the mid oesophagus and are separated from it by the LA, which acts as an excellent acoustic window. Thus, 2-D and colour flow Doppler imaging of this region is usually of a high quality, and the information provided by TOE can have a significant impact on the management of a number of important disease states.

Conditions affecting the LVOT and AV are addressed in this chapter; conditions that specifically involve the aortic root (e.g. sinus of Valsalva aneurysm) are discussed in Chapter 11. Prosthetic valves in the aortic position are discussed in Chapter 12.

## ANATOMY

The entire LVOT comprises:

1. the subvalvular LVOT, which is the funnel-shaped portion of the LV extending from the free edges of the mitral leaflets to the aortic annulus (commonly referred to as the "LVOT");
2. the AV;
3. the aortic root and the proximal ascending aorta. The **aortic root** is the part of the aorta between the AV annulus and the **sinotubular junction**.

The aortic annulus is formed by three cords, which together form the basis of the fibrous skeleton of the heart (see Figure 9.1). The AV is composed of three similarly sized, crescent-shaped leaflets, which are each attached to the aortic wall along a U-shaped line with its upper attachments along the sinotubular junction.

Behind each leaflet is the respective **sinus of Valsalva**, a dilatation of the aortic root that functions as a reservoir for coronary blood flow in diastole, and ensures separation of the leaflet from the ostium of the coronary artery in systole. Each sinus and leaflet is named according to the adjacent coronary artery (left, right or non-). The right leaflet is situated anteriorly and rightward, the left leaflet posteriorly and leftward, and the non-coronary leaflet posteriorly and rightward. Each leaflet is separated by a commissure and coapts with its adjacent leaflet along a closure (or coaptation) line. Usually the leaflet tips overlap by 2–3 mm in systole, but in disease states that cause the aortic sinuses to dilate the degree of coaptation is reduced allowing regurgitation to occur. The apex or central portion of the free edge of each leaflet has a localised thickening called the **nodule of Arantius** (Figure 10.1).

The walls of the LVOT comprise the **anterior mitral leaflet**, the **membranous inter-ventricular septum** and the **anterior LV wall** (Figure 10.1). The left and non-coronary leaflets are in continuity with the base of the anterior leaflet of the MV and the **inter-valvular fibrosa** (see Figure 9.1).

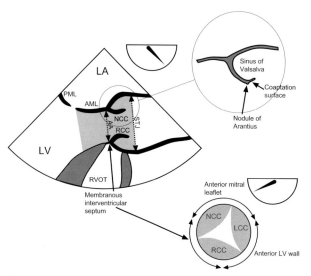

**Figure 10.1** Anatomy of LV outflow region as seen in the mid oesophageal AV long axis view. The appropriate positions in which to measure the diameters of the aortic annulus (AA) and sinotubular junction (STJ) are shown. The magnified schematic of the non-coronary cusp (NCC) (right) shows the sinus of Valsalva and nodule of Arantius. The lower inset shows the orientation of the AV leaflets to the walls of the LVOT, as they appear in the mid oesophageal AV short axis view. RCC = right coronary cusp, LCC = left coronary cusp, AML = anterior mitral leaflet, PML = posterior mitral leaflet.

# ECHOCARDIOGRAPHIC EXAMINATION

Four standard views are needed for a systematic examination of the AV, root and LVOT:

1. mid oesophageal AV short axis view;
2. mid oesophageal AV long axis view;
3. deep transgastric long-axis view;
4. transgastric long axis view.

Details of how to obtain the views and the important echocardiographic anatomy are provided in Chapter 4. Summarised below are details specific to the assessment of the AV and LVOT.

## Mid oesophageal AV short axis view (40°; Figure 4.4)

This view usually provides excellent images of all three AV leaflets and is consequently the ideal view in which to assess leaflet morphology. To improve visualisation of the leaflets it may be necessary to rotate the transducer backwards or forwards so that the sinuses appear to be of equal size, and to advance or withdraw the probe so that the image plane passes through the leaflet tips. Off-axis imaging may cause one leaflet to appear larger and falsely thickened, or give the erroneous impression of a diastolic coaptation defect.

From the standard position the probe may be advanced to examine the LVOT or withdrawn to visualise the origin of the coronary arteries (Figure 10.2), sinuses and sinotubular junction.

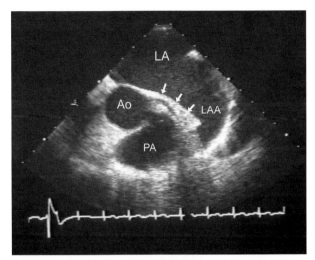

**Figure 10.2** Left main coronary artery. The probe has been withdrawn slightly from the mid oesophageal AV short axis view so that the scan plane passes just above the AV. The left main and proximal left anterior descending coronary arteries (arrows) can be seen exiting the aorta (Ao) and passing between the left atrial appendage (LAA) and pulmonary artery (PA).

With 2-D imaging the presence of specific leaflet pathology, such as bicuspid valve or calcific degeneration, may be identified. The view is useful for identification of the presence of a diastolic coaptation defect and, with colour flow Doppler, the location of and severity of any aortic regurgitation.

## Mid oesophageal AV long-axis view (130°; Figures 4.5 and 10.1)

This is the appropriate view for assessing the dimensions of the AV annulus, sinuses and sinotubular junction. The dimensions of the annulus and sinotubular junction are of particular interest as they are indicative of the size of prosthetic AV required. The AV annulus should be measured at the points where the leaflets insert into the aorta.

To measure these diameters accurately it is essential that the image plane passes through the centre of the aorta (see Figure 16.6); this may require turning the shaft of the probe to the left or right to ensure the maximum aortic diameter is visualised. A clue that the image is off-axis is a thickened appearance to one of the AV cusps or one of the aortic walls. All measurements should be at the same phase of the cardiac cycle. The inner edge to inner edge technique is usual (p.244).

From the standard position, withdrawing the probe and turning it to the right can aid in visualisation of more of the ascending aorta; advancing the probe may improve visualisation of the LVOT.

This view is also useful for assessment of the presence of diastolic leaflet prolapse (suggesting regurgitation) or impaired systolic opening (suggesting stenosis). The LVOT may be examined for evidence of fixed or dynamic obstruction. Colour flow Doppler can be used to look for turbulent flow (suggesting obstruction or stenosis) in the LVOT or proximal ascending aorta, and to assess aortic regurgitation.

## The transgastric views

Both the deep transgastric long axis and transgastric long axis views (see Figures 4.21 and 4.22) provide windows with which to image the LVOT and AV from the ventricular aspect. In patients with prosthetic aortic or mitral valves, imaging the LVOT from the mid oesophageal windows may be impossible owing to echo dropout and far field shadowing. In such a situation the transgastric views may provide some details of this region.

The main utility of these views is the Doppler interrogation of the LVOT and AV, as they provide the only images of the AV in which reasonable alignment with a spectral Doppler signal may be obtained using TOE.

Unfortunately, both views are difficult to obtain in some patients, and even if a view can be obtained adequate alignment with the Doppler signal is not always possible. Furthermore, the depth of the LVOT may be beyond the maximum depth that can be unambiguously resolved with PW Doppler, particularly if the LVOT velocity is increased (p.38).

# AORTIC STENOSIS

Aortic stenosis may occur as a consequence of calcific degeneration of a normal trileaflet valve, rheumatic aortic disease or a congenital valve abnormality, particularly a bicuspid AV.

## Calcific aortic stenosis

This is the most common form of aortic stenosis and tends to occur in patients over the age of 70 years. It is characterised by fibrocalcific changes in the body and along the free edges of the leaflets, resulting in a marked increase in echogenicity and restriction of leaflet motion (Figure 10.3). The leaflets may be affected asymmetrically

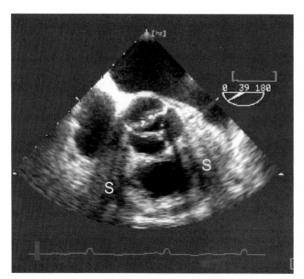

**Figure 10.3** Calcific aortic stenosis of a trileaflet AV. The valve is shown in the mid oesophageal AV short axis view in mid-systole. Heavy calcification can be seen along the free edges of the leaflets causing far field shadowing (S). Some commissural fusion is present. Systolic opening is reduced, suggesting significant stenosis.

and there may be fusion of one or more of the commissures. Calcification may extend down into the LVOT (**teardrop calcification**) and onto the base of the anterior mitral leaflet.

## Bicuspid aortic valve

This is the most common congenital cardiac malformation. It occurs in approximately 2% of the normal population and may be familial.[1] Secondary calcification occurs in a significant number of cases, and usually leads to the onset of symptoms in the fourth to sixth decades of life. The characteristic echocardiographic sign is that of two leaflets opening in systole, resulting in an elliptical rather than a star-shaped orifice. A **raphe** or fibrous ridge is usually present on one of the leaflets, perpendicular to the orifice, and is typically more sclerotic than the leaflets themselves. A calcified raphe may have the appearance of a commissure (or closure line) in diastole, so the diagnosis of a bicuspid AV can reliably be made only in systole (Figure 10.4).

The most common form of congenitally bicuspid AV is that of a larger anterior cusp and a smaller posterior cusp. A raphe is usually seen on the anterior cusp and may give the appearance of fused left and right cusps. The two coronary arteries arise from the sinus of Valsalva adjacent to the anterior cusp. Less commonly, there is a large rightward leaflet and a smaller leftward leaflet. A raphe may be seen on the rightward leaflet, giving the appearance of fused right and non-coronary cusps. A severely calcified bicuspid valve may be indistinguishable from a trileaflet valve.

When examining an AV that appears to be bicuspid the following points should be considered:

- Off-axis imaging in the AV short axis view can be misleading and give the appearance of a trileaflet valve.
- A doming appearance to the valve leaflets in diastole in the AV long axis view may be due to eccentric closure of the leaflets, and is not necessarily due to prolapse.
- If a bicuspid AV is detected it is important to rule out other associated abnormalities, including coarctation of the aorta, subaortic obstruction and dilatation of the aortic root.

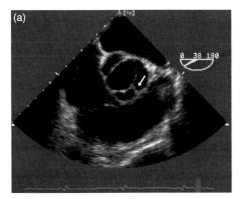 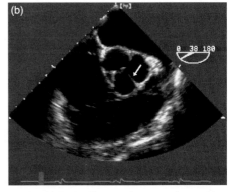

**Figure 10.4** Bicuspid AV. (a) The open valve in systole. An elliptical orifice can be seen along with a calcified raphe (arrow). (b) The same valve in diastole. The raphe (arrow) now gives the appearances of a closed trileaflet valve. This type of bicuspid valve, with a large anterior cusp and a small posterior cusp, is the most common.

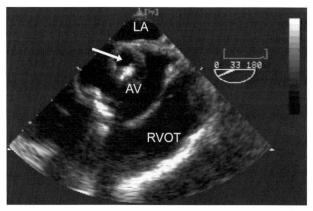

**Figure 10.5** Unicuspid AV. In this mid oesophageal AV short axis view, a unicuspid AV is shown in systole. The valve is heavily calcified and the valve orifice (arrow) extremely narrowed, suggesting significant stenosis.

Very occasionally an AV may be congenitally **unicuspid** (Figure 10.5) or **quadracuspid**. Unicuspid valves virtually always become stenotic in childhood or early adulthood.

### Rheumatic aortic stenosis
Rheumatic valvulitis tends to produce thickening of the free edges of the AV leaflets and fusion of the commissures, causing a circular rather than a star-shaped orifice, which may be eccentric. It is usually associated with a degree of aortic regurgitation due to retraction of the aortic leaflets, and is almost always associated with significant rheumatic changes of the mitral leaflets and chordae tendinae.

## ECHOCARDIOGRAPHIC ASSESSMENT OF AORTIC STENOSIS

The severity of aortic stenosis may be graded on the basis of calculated valve area, transvalvular velocities and transvalvular pressure gradients (Table 10.1).

The two main methods for evaluating AV area are **direct planimetry** and use of the **continuity equation**.

### 2-D imaging
A detailed 2-D examination of the valve is an important first step. If the valve leaflets are thin and mobile then significant valvular stenosis can be excluded. The *absence* of valvular calcification makes significant stenosis unlikely, but the *presence* of calcification does not necessarily imply severe stenosis. An increased velocity across the valve detected with CW Doppler, in the absence of significant AV pathology on 2-D imaging, should alert the echocardiographer to the possibility of LVOT obstruction (p.169).

With transthoracic echocardiography in the parasternal long axis view, a maximal cusp separation <8 mm on 2-D imaging is strongly suggestive of severe stenosis, and a maximal cusp separation >12 mm indicates that stenosis is no more than mild.[2] With TOE, a similar view of the AV can be obtained from the mid oesophageal long axis view.

An additional feature which may be present is post-stenotic dilatation of the aortic root and proximal ascending aorta.

**Table 10.1** Grading aortic stenosis

|  | $V_{max}$ (m/s) | $P_{max}$ (mmHg) | $P_{mean}$ (mmHg) | Valve area (cm$^2$) |
|---|---|---|---|---|
| Normal | <1.5 |  |  | >2.5 |
| Mild | 2.5–3.5 | 25–50 | 12–25 | 1.2–1.8 |
| Moderate | 3.5–4.5 | 50–80 | 25–40 | 0.8–1.2 |
| Severe | >4.5 | >80 | 40–50 | 0.6–0.8 |
| Critical | >5.5 | >100 | >50 | <0.6 |

$V_{max}$ = peak velocity across AV, $P_{max}$ = maximum gradient across AV, $P_{mean}$ = mean pressure gradient across AV

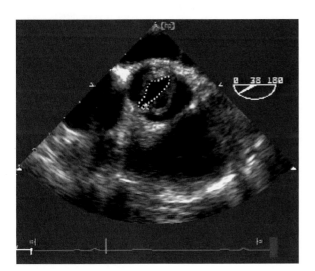

**Figure 10.6** AV planimetry.

## Planimetry of the aortic valve

Direct planimetry of the AV orifice can be used to determine severity of stenosis with TOE[3,4] (Figure 10.6), but a detailed knowledge of the method and possible pitfalls of this technique are essential. Key points are outlined below:

**Step 1.** Obtain the optimal short axis of the AV so that the free edges of the leaflets can be visualised in systole.

**Step 2.** Carefully advance and withdraw the probe while anteflexing or retroflexing, to obtain a view of the restricted valve orifice parallel to the image plane.

**Step 3.** Reduce the 2-D gain to a minimum to facilitate visualisation of the leaflet edges and to reduce reverberation.

**Step 4.** Use the zoom mode to magnify the image, and then use the freeze and scroll functions to obtain the maximum orifice in systole at the leaflet tips.

**Step 5.** Trace the area of the restricted valve orifice along the inner edge but not inside the leaflets. Smooth over irregularities in the leaflet edges due to areas of significant leaflet thickening.

**Step 6.** Repeat the measurement three times and take an average of the result.

Direct planimetry may be difficult in the following circumstances:

- When there is severe thickening or calcification of the aortic leaflets or root, particularly posteriorly, causing shadowing of the valve orifice.[5,6]
- When a true short axis view of the AV is difficult to obtain, because of distortion or marked dilatation of the aortic root.
- When there is markedly accentuated cardiac motion (e.g. in high cardiac output states) causing the valve to move in and out of the image plane.

The validity of AV planimetry with TOE has been extensively studied and compared with valve area obtained by invasive catheter-based measurements and by the use of the continuity equation. None of these methods is a "gold standard". The limits of agreement in published studies vary widely (from 0.5 to 1.2 cm²).[7]

Planimetry by TOE cannot be used to differentiate moderate from severe aortic stenosis and the information obtained is therefore adjunctive to other data.

## Colour flow Doppler imaging

While colour flow Doppler cannot be used to quantify the severity of aortic stenosis directly, the presence of intense aliasing in the proximal aorta implies turbulent, high-velocity flow in this region, consistent with a poststenotic flow pattern.

## Spectral Doppler imaging and the continuity equation

Doppler echocardiography has been well validated as a means of assessing AV area by transthoracic echocardiography using the continuity equation.[8,9] The technique is outlined in Chapter 16; in particular see Equations 16.6 and 16.7 and Examples 16.2 and 16.3.

With TOE it is necessary to acquire the following:

1. the AV velocity–time integral ($VTI_{AV}$) – this can be obtained by tracing the outline of a CW Doppler envelope directed through the AV from a transgastric view;
2. the area of the LVOT – this can be obtained from the diameter of the AV annulus in the AV long axis view;
3. the VTI at the level of the LVOT ($VTI_{LVOT}$). To measure the $VTI_{LVOT}$ place a PW sample volume at the level of the AV then withdraw it into the LVOT until a smooth Doppler envelope is obtained with minimal spectral broadening. Colour Doppler can be used to direct the spectral signal to the region of maximal flow.

For the assessment of AV area by the continuity equation, maximum velocity has been shown to be a valid substitute for VTI. This has been further simplified to the ratio of the peak velocities across the AV and LVOT (termed the **Doppler velocity index** – p.233) and has been used to follow the progression of prosthetic AV stenosis (p.197).

An alternative method, which avoids the requirement to measure VTI at the AV and LVOT separately and has been validated for TOE, is the **double-envelope technique**. The velocity profiles of the LVOT and AV are measured simultaneously from a single CW Doppler envelope. In many patients the outline of the $VTI_{LVOT}$ can be identified as a brighter, lower velocity region of the envelope (Figure 10.7). This technique has the advantages of simplicity and of minimising error due to beat-to-beat variability in blood flow. Using TOE, the double-envelope technique provides better agreement than planimetry with transthoracic and invasive estimates of AV area.[10]

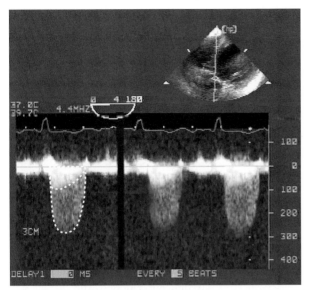

**Figure 10.7** Double envelope technique. A spectral Doppler envelope through the LV outflow has been taken from the deep transgastric long-axis view. There is an increased gradient (36 mmHg, calculated by the modified Bernoulli equation from the velocity, which is approximately 3 m/s) consistent with mild aortic stenosis. The brighter, low-velocity (approximately 1 m/s) region represents flow through the LVOT. Simultaneous evaluation of the VTIs across the AV and LVOT allows the AV area to be estimated. The rounded shape of the outer waveform suggests that the velocities may have been underestimated. See text for details.

## Considerations and caveats

The major limitation of continuity equation methods with TOE relates to the difficulties associated with the deep transgastric and transgastric long axis views (pp.157–158). Note that it is impossible to *overestimate* the true velocity using spectral Doppler (p.35); therefore a number of waveforms should be obtained and the highest velocity used (not the average). A clue to the fact that the true velocity has been underestimated is a rounded shape to the Doppler waveform, as shown in Figure 10.7; the AV Doppler profile ought to have a sharply peaked appearance, particularly in the presence of aortic stenosis.

If the LVOT diameter is inaccurate a large measurement error will occur as the value is squared to estimate this area.

The $VTI_{LVOT}$ is normally in the range of 15–25 cm. A high value may indicate increased transvalvular flow such as occurs with high cardiac output or aortic regurgitation; alternatively it may indicate the presence of subvalvular obstruction (p.169) or that the sample volume has been placed too close to the AV and in a region of flow acceleration. A low value suggests low cardiac output or that the alignment between the Doppler beam and LVOT is poor.

## Transvalvular velocity and pressure gradients

Transvalvular velocities and pressure gradients can be estimated from a CW Doppler envelope directed through the AV, and provide a rapid estimate of the severity of aortic stenosis. However, it is important to recognise the limitations of this approach:

Firstly, there is no universally accepted numerical grading system, and the values given in Table 10.1 are somewhat arbitrary. Secondly, the relationship between valve area and velocity (and pressure gradient) is predicated on flow. A high transvalvular flow (such as occurs with elevated cardiac output or aortic regurgitation) will increase the transvalvular velocity for a given valve area. Conversely, a low cardiac output will reduce the transvalvular velocity. Thirdly, the simplified Bernoulli equation assumes a low velocity (<1 m/s) proximal to the orifice (in this case the LVOT); this may not always be the case (p.238). Finally, as outlined above, accurate measurement of aortic transvalvular velocity is difficult with TOE.

### Assessment of aortic stenosis during the perioperative period

In most situations the diagnosis of aortic stenosis will have been made preoperatively. In addition, given the caveats outlined above, the intraoperative period is not the ideal time to assess the severity of aortic stenosis.

On occasion, a degree of aortic stenosis may be discovered as an unexpected finding and may influence perioperative decision making (e.g. the discovery of mild-to-moderate aortic stenosis may lead the surgeon to reconsider performing coronary revascularisation off-pump).

During planned AV replacement for aortic stenosis the echocardiographer should focus on associated conditions such as the presence of aortic regurgitation (which has implications for the conduct of bypass; p.167), LV and RV function, the presence of aortic atheroma, coexisting valvular disease and (after bypass) prosthesis function.

# AORTIC REGURGITATION

Aortic regurgitation may result from abnormalities of the AV and the aortic root, and may be acute or chronic. Acute aortic regurgitation most commonly results from aortic dissection (p.178) or endocarditis. Endocarditis causes regurgitation by leaflet distortion or perforation, or by the development of an aortic root abscess which may distort the sinotubular junction.

The valvular abnormalities described above (bicuspid AV, rheumatic disease or calcific degeneration) can all cause chronic regurgitation to a variable extent. Leaflet prolapse can occur in myxomatous AV disease (which usually affects the MV as well) and in the presence of a conal ventricular septal defect (p.225).

Dilatation of the aorta resulting in loss of the sinotubular angle may cause aortic regurgitation by reducing the overlap between the cusps in diastole. Causes include annuloaortic ectasia (idiopathic destruction of the elastic fibres and smooth muscle of the media), hypertensive heart disease, connective tissue disease (e.g. Marfan syndrome, Ehlers–Danlos syndrome) and sinus of Valsalva aneurysm.

# ECHOCARDIOGRAPHIC ASSESSMENT OF AORTIC REGURGITATION

Quantitative Doppler can provide an objective assessment of the severity of aortic regurgitation, in particular estimation of the **regurgitant fraction** (p.235). However, because these calculations are relatively time consuming and have considerable potential for error, they are not well suited to perioperative use. In contrast, a number of semiquantitative methods based on colour flow and spectral Doppler imaging have been described, which are applicable to intraoperative use with TOE.

| Table 10.2 The 2-D, colour flow and spectral Doppler signs suggestive of severe aortic regurgitation |
| --- |
| **Colour Doppler imaging** |
| Jet area >60% of LVOT area (MO AV short axis view) |
| Jet width >40% of LVOT width (MO AV long axis view) |
| Vena contracta >6 mm (MO AV long axis view) |
| Jet extension beyond insertion of papillary muscles (MO AV long axis view) |
| PISA radius >0.7 cm (on aortic side of valve in diastole, with aliasing velocity of 33 cm/s, MO AV long axis view) |
| Presystolic closure of the MV and diastolic mitral regurgitation |
| **Spectral Doppler imaging (deep TG long axis and TG long axis views)** |
| Intensity of regurgitant jet = intensity of systolic ejection |
| Peak velocity of systolic ejection >2 m/s |
| Holodiastolic flow reversal in descending thoracic aorta |
| **2-D imaging** |
| Diastolic coaptation defect (MO AV short axis view) |
| Diastolic leaflet prolapse (MO AV long axis view) |
| LV dilatation: LV end systolic dimension >4.5 cm (TG mid short axis view) |
| MO = mid oesophageal, TG = transgastric. |

The signs suggestive of severe regurgitation are summarised in Table 10.2.

## 2-D imaging
The AV should be examined for specific pathology such as congenital abnormalities (e.g. bicuspid AV) and acquired defects (e.g. vegetations, abscess formation or myxomatous change). The leaflets should be inspected for thickening, asymmetry or distortion of the cusps, and abnormalities in coaptation. If a regurgitant jet is identified with colour flow Doppler imaging in the AV short axis view, toggling the colour map on and off will usually reveal a coaptation defect on 2-D imaging. However, if the scan plane passes through the body rather than the tips of the leaflets, the appearance may resemble a defect even with a normal valve.

In the AV long axis view, the leaflets should be inspected for evidence of prolapse and the sinotubular junction examined for evidence of dilatation. Significant regurgitation is unlikely in the absence of identifiable pathology on 2-D imaging.

LV volume overload is a consistent finding in chronic severe aortic regurgitation.

## Colour flow Doppler
Mid oesophageal AV short axis view
In this view, colour flow Doppler is useful for determination of the origin of the jet. A small central jet is consistent with mild regurgitation and one that extends down between the free edges of the leaflets is usually indicative of more severe disease. The **area of the regurgitant jet** can be estimated from this view and compared with the area of the LVOT by tracing the two areas on the same frame in mid diastole. On

transthoracic echocardiography a ratio of jet area to LVOT area of <25% is consistent with mild regurgitation, while an area >60% is consistent with severe regurgitation.[11] If the plane of the scan passes below the level of the coaptation point the severity of the regurgitation will be overestimated, as the jet typically "sprays out" and widens in the LVOT.

## Mid oesophageal AV long axis view

This view can be used for the determination of the **width of the regurgitant jet**, which correlates reasonably well with the severity of regurgitation. A **ratio of jet width to outflow tract diameter** >40% indicates severe aortic regurgitation.[12] This ratio is best measured using colour M-mode. An extension of the jet width and jet area concept involves measurement of the **vena contracta width**, which is the narrowest portion of the jet located just distal to the regurgitant orifice. The cross-sectional area of the vena contracta is proportional to the effective regurgitant orifice area. A vena contracta wider than 6 mm on TOE is associated with a regurgitant fraction of >50% (i.e. severe regurgitation).[13]

**Jet length** can also be used to assess the severity of aortic regurgitation, although this method is less reliable than other Doppler methods. In general, a jet that extends past the level of the papillary muscles is likely to be severe, and one that extends less than 2 cm beyond the level of the AV is likely to be mild.

Quantification of the size of the PISA (p.236) on the aortic side of the valve in diastole is a useful method for assessment of the severity of aortic regurgitation, particularly when the jet is eccentric. If a large proximal convergence zone is noted, severe regurgitation is usually present; for example, in one study a PISA radius > 0.7 cm, at an aliasing velocity of approximately 33 cm/s, was always associated with severe regurgitation.[14]

An additional sign suggestive of severe aortic regurgitation is the presence of **presystolic closure of the MV**. Severe aortic regurgitation leads to a rapid diastolic rise in LV pressure, which can cause closure of the MV before the onset of systole. This can be detected by capturing short colour flow loops from the AV long axis view, and then (using the scroll function) seeking evidence of MV closure (in late diastole) before the aortic regurgitant jet disappears. Occasionally, **diastolic mitral regurgitation** may also be identified with colour flow Doppler.

## Spectral Doppler

Spectral Doppler sampling of the regurgitant jet can be achieved from the transgastric views. Flow is towards the transducer (and therefore displayed above the baseline) and has an early peak velocity of 3–5 m/s, due to the high pressure gradient between the aorta and LV. The **intensity of the regurgitant jet** is proportional to the blood flow across the AV in diastole and can be used for grading severity. It is helpful to compare the regurgitant jet with the antegrade flow signal to eliminate the confounding effect of differences in the Doppler gain setting (Figure 9.14 shows the same principle for mitral regurgitation).

**The slope of the regurgitant Doppler envelope** is indicative of the rate of pressure equalisation between the aorta and LV, and is dependent on the severity of the regurgitation. In acute or severe regurgitation the slope may be steeper. In practice, this index of severity (the **pressure half time**) is not well suited to use with TOE in the perioperative setting (pp.243–244).

The **peak velocity across the AV in systole** is another sign of the severity of aortic regurgitation. A velocity of >2 m/s indicates that regurgitation is likely to be at least moderate (assuming normal cardiac output and the absence of aortic stenosis).

## Flow reversal in the thoracic aorta

Early diastolic flow reversal within the descending thoracic aorta is a normal finding, and can be readily evaluated from the descending aortic long axis view. Increasing severity of aortic regurgitation is associated with more prolonged reversal of diastolic flow. In the proximal abdominal aorta, holodiastolic flow reversal has a sensitivity of 100% and specificity of 97% for severe regurgitation.[15] With TOE it is not always possible to visualise the abdominal aorta; holodiastolic flow reversal in the descending thoracic aorta usually indicates severe regurgitation, but may occur in the presence of moderate regurgitation.

## Assessment of aortic regurgitation during the perioperative period

As with aortic stenosis, the diagnosis of significant aortic regurgitation will usually have been made preoperatively. However, TOE has an important role as the primary assessment tool in specific situations, notably in the critical-care setting when transthoracic windows may be suboptimal (e.g. in the assessment of AV endocarditis), in the assessment of aortic dissection, and in the evaluation of AV repair or prosthesis function following replacement. Furthermore, aortic regurgitation may be discovered as an incidental finding in the operating room. Even the presence of mild aortic regurgitation is important as it can complicate the administration of antegrade cardioplegia and may necessitate the placement of a LV venting device before arresting the heart. This is particularly important when the heart is not visible (e.g. during repair of a descending thoracic aneurysm through a left thoracotomy).

# OTHER AORTIC VALVE PATHOLOGY

## Masses

Masses attached to the AV leaflets are reasonably common and may first be noted during a perioperative TOE examination (Table 10.3).

The mid oesophageal AV long axis view is usually best for identifying the presence of a mass, but the short axis view is then usually better for identifying its exact location and point(s) of attachment. It is important to remember that with ageing the closure lines and bodies of the leaflets tend to thicken and the **nodules of Arantius** become more prominent. **Valvular strands** (see Figure 5.11), **Lambl's excrescences** and **papillary fibroelastomas** may be identified from time to time on the AV (Chapter 5).

## Endocarditis of the aortic valve

TOE is more sensitive and specific for the detection of AV vegetations and associated complications than transthoracic echocardiography,[16] and consequently is the investigation of choice for the evaluation of suspected AV endocarditis.

AV vegetations typically appear as echogenic masses with soft tissue reflectance (p.82) attached to the ventricular side of the leaflet. They typically prolapse into the LVOT during diastole. Their motion typically has a fluttering quality. There is often a pre-existing abnormality of the AV, and vegetations may be more difficult to detect with a significantly calcified or disorganised valve.

## Complications of endocarditis

Complications related to the AV itself include **leaflet perforation, rupture** and **aneurysm formation**. Cusp perforation is seen as an interruption in the continuity of leaflet tissue

**Table 10.3** Classification of AV masses that may be identified with TOE

| Nodular thickening of leaflets |
| --- |
| Calcific degeneration |
| Rheumatic thickening and nodules |
| Nodules of Arantius |
| Lambl's excrescences |
| Papillary fibroelastomas |
| Vegetations |
| Thrombi |
| Rheumatoid nodules |
| **Linear masses** |
| Lambl's excrescences |
| Thrombi |
| Vegetations |
| **Papillary or pedunculated masses** |
| Vegetations |
| Papillary fibroelastomas |
| Thrombi |

at a site remote from the commissures, but within the aortic annulus. The presence of an eccentrically positioned proximal flow convergence zone on the aortic side of the valve strongly suggests the presence of a leaflet perforation. Aneurysm of a cusp appears as a thinning or bulging of a portion of the leaflet. Both of these complications may lead to leaflet rupture, where a flail portion of the valve prolapses into the LVOT in diastole. This is almost always associated with torrential aortic regurgitation.

Complications remote from the valve include the development of **metastatic vegetations**, and the formation of **abscesses** or **fistulae**[7] (Figure 10.8). Metastatic vegetations may occur within the LVOT – the site will depend on the direction of the regurgitant jet. Abscesses appear as echolucent or echo-free spaces surrounding the aortic annulus, and may extend into the proximal aorta, the interventricular septum or the intervalvular fibrosa. Abscesses may rupture, creating fistulae between adjacent chambers. Off-axis imaging with colour flow Doppler is often required to track the path of the communication.

## LEFT VENTRICULAR OUTFLOW TRACT

The optimal image plane for the assessment of the LVOT is the mid oesophageal AV long axis view. In addition, a short axis view of the LVOT can be obtained by advancing the probe slightly from the mid oesophageal AV short axis view.

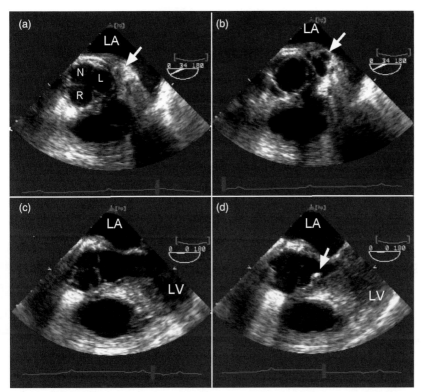

**Figure 10.8** Complications of AV endocarditis. The top two frames show an aortic root abscess from the mid oesophageal AV short axis view. In diastole (a) the aortic root appears thickened (arrow), particularly in the region of the left coronary cusp. In systole (b) a series of loculated fluid-filled spaces can be seen. The two lower frames are taken from the same patient and show a close-up of the LVOT from the mid oesophageal five-chamber view. In diastole (c) the LVOT appears normal, but in late systole (d) a metastatic vegetation can be seen in the region of the interventricular septum (arrow).

## Left ventricular outflow tract obstruction

LVOT obstruction may be **fixed** or **dynamic**. Fixed obstruction is usually secondary to a subaortic narrowing, which may be due to a thin, discrete fibrous membrane or a thick fibrous ring associated with marked septal hypertrophy. Fixed obstruction should be suspected when there is an increased velocity within the LVOT (>1.5 m/s), peaking in early to mid systole, with apparently unrestricted AV motion. On colour flow Doppler there will be colour aliasing proximal to the AV, with coarse fluttering and early closure of the aortic leaflets in systole. Aortic regurgitation may coexist due to the jet from the subaortic stenosis impinging on the AV from below. Other outflow tract abnormalities such as **bicuspid AV** and **aortic coarctation** may be present. The gradient across the subaortic obstruction may be obtained using PW Doppler from a transgastric window. Intraoperative TOE can guide the surgeon to the site of the stenosis, the degree of resection required and the adequacy of repair. Following resection it is important to rule out any residual obstruction, ventricular septal defect or valvular regurgitation.

Dynamic LVOT obstruction is due to a reduction in the distance between the anterior leaflet of the MV and the interventricular septum in systole. This may occur when there is severe **septal hypertrophy** (e.g. in hypertrophic cardiomyopathy or severe hypertensive heart disease) or following **MV repair**. When surgical myectomy is undertaken, TOE can identify the region of maximal obstruction and the presence of complications such as a ventricular septal defect or worsened mitral regurgitation.[17] Myectomy is now routinely performed percutaneously using alcohol injection into the basal interventricular septum.

Dynamic LVOT obstruction is also discussed in Chapters 6 and 9.

# REFERENCES

1. Roberts WC. The congenitally bicuspid aortic valve. A study of 85 autopsy cases. *American Journal of Cardiology* 1970;26:72–83.
2. Godley RW, Green D, Dillon JC, et al. Reliability of two-dimensional echocardiography in assessing the severity of valvular aortic stenosis. *Chest* 1981;79:657–662.
3. Stoddard MF, Arce J, Liddell NE, et al. Two-dimensional transesophageal echocardiographic determination of aortic valve area in adults with aortic stenosis. *American Heart Journal* 1991;122:1415–1422.
4. Kim CJ, Berglund H, Nishioka T, et al. Correspondence of aortic valve area determination from transesophageal echocardiography, transthoracic echocardiography, and cardiac catheterization. *American Heart Journal* 1996;132:1163–1172.
5. Cormier B, Iung B, Porte JM, et al. Value of multiplane transesophageal echocardiography in determining aortic valve area in aortic stenosis. *American Journal of Cardiology* 1996;77:882–885.
6. Bernard Y, Meneveau N, Vuillemenot A, et al. Planimetry of aortic valve area using multiplane transoesophageal echocardiography is not a reliable method for assessing severity of aortic stenosis. *Heart* 1997;78:68–73.
7. Shively BK. Transesophageal echocardiographic (TEE) evaluation of the aortic valve, left ventricular outflow tract, and pulmonic valve. *Cardiology Clinics* 2000;18:711–729.
8. Skjaerpe T, Hegrenaes L, Hatle L. Noninvasive estimation of valve area in patients with aortic stenosis by Doppler ultrasound and two-dimensional echocardiography. *Circulation* 1985;72:810–818.
9. Otto CM, Pearlman AS, Comess KA, et al. Determination of the stenotic aortic valve area in adults using Doppler echocardiography. *Journal of the American College of Cardiology* 1986;7:509–517.
10. Maslow AD, Mashikian J, Haering JM, et al. Transesophageal echocardiographic evaluation of native aortic valve area: utility of the double-envelope technique. *Journal of Cardiothoracic and Vascular Anesthesia* 2001;15:293–299.
11. Perry GJ, Helmcke F, Nanda NC, et al. Evaluation of aortic insufficiency by Doppler color flow mapping. *Journal of the American College of Cardiology* 1987;9:952–959.
12. Zarauza J, Ares M, Vilchez FG, et al. An integrated approach to the quantification of aortic regurgitation by Doppler echocardiography. *American Heart Journal* 1998;136:1030–1041.
13. Willett DL, Hall SA, Jessen ME, et al. Assessment of aortic regurgitation by transesophageal color Doppler imaging of the vena contracta: validation against an intraoperative aortic flow probe. *Journal of the American College of Cardiology* 2001;37:1450–1455.
14. Sato Y, Kawazoe K, Nasu M, et al. Clinical usefulness of the proximal isovelocity surface area method using echocardiography in patients with eccentric aortic regurgitation. *Journal of Heart Valve Disease* 1999;8:104–111.
15. Takenaka K, Dabestani A, Gardin JM, et al. A simple Doppler echocardiographic method for estimating severity of aortic regurgitation. *American Journal of Cardiology* 1986;57:1340–1343.
16. Shapiro SM, Young E, De Guzman S, et al. Transesophageal echocardiography in diagnosis of infective endocarditis. *Chest* 1994;105:337–382.
17. Grigg LE, Wigle ED, Williams WG, et al. Transesophageal Doppler echocardiography in obstructive hypertrophic cardiomyopathy: clarification of pathophysiology and importance in intraoperative decision making. *Journal of the American College of Cardiology* 1992;20:42–52.

# 11.

# The Thoracic Aorta

*Colin Royse*

The examination of the thoracic aorta is an essential component of a routine perioperative examination with TOE, and when combined with epiaortic scanning provides detailed information on a range of surgical pathologies. In particular, dislodgement of aortic atheroma is the most common cause of stroke and neurocognitive dysfunction following cardiac surgery. Since the development of aortic atheroma is closely associated with advanced age, and given the increasing age of patients presenting for cardiac surgery, accurate assessment of this problem is essential.

## ANATOMY

The thoracic aorta is divided into the **ascending aorta**, **arch** and **proximal descending aorta**.

The ascending aorta arises from the aortic annulus and extends towards the right, around the main pulmonary artery, crossing the right pulmonary artery anteriorly. It is 4–5 cm in length and ends at the pericardial reflection.

The aortic arch starts at the pericardial reflection and the origin of the right brachio-cephalic artery, and extends to the origin of the left subclavian artery. It lies anterior to the trachea, superior to the pulmonary artery and posterior to the innominate vein; it is 4–5 cm in length.

The proximal descending aorta arises at the origin of the left subclavian artery and extends to the level of the diaphragm. It starts to the left of the vertebral column and moves to the right as it descends.

The normal dimensions of the ascending and descending aorta are provided in Appendix 2.

## ECHOCARDIOGRAPHIC CLASSIFICATION

The thoracic aorta can be divided into six zones, which correspond to regions of potential manipulation during cardiac surgery. The ascending aorta is divided into zones 1–3 (the proximal, mid and distal ascending aorta), the arch into zones 4 and 5 (proximal and distal halves), and the entire proximal descending aorta forms zone 6.[1] Zone 1 is the site of aortotomy for valve replacement; zone 2 is the site of the proximal anastomoses of coronary grafts; zone 3 is the site of aortic cross-clamping and antegrade cardioplegia cannulation; zone 4 is the site of aortic cannulation; zone 5 is not manipulated directly but can be affected by the jet stream of cardiopulmonary bypass flow; zone 6 is the site for a correctly positioned intra-aortic balloon pump. Only zone 1, part of zone 2, and zones 5 and 6 can be reliably imaged with TOE.

# ECHOCARDIOGRAPHIC EXAMINATION

It is important to use a systematic approach to the examination of the thoracic aorta; the image sequence should follow the outline given in Chapter 4. When imaging the arch and descending aorta, it is helpful to reduce the sector depth to 6 cm and reduce the gain setting. This provides a more detailed image of the aorta and helps differentiate the intima (grey) from the media (white).

## Ascending aortic views

A useful starting point is the **mid oesophageal AV short axis view** (see Figure 4.4). Pathology involving the ascending aorta is frequently associated with abnormalities of the AV and aortic root. In particular, note the presence of a bicuspid AV (which is associated with ascending aortic dilatation) and the presence of aortic regurgitation. In the **mid oesophageal AV long axis view** (see Figure 4.5) the dimensions of the aortic annulus and sinotubular junction can be measured (see Figure 10.1). This view is also useful for assessment of aortic regurgitation and identification of aortic root pathology such as sinus of Valsalva aneurysm and aortic dissection.

The **mid oesophageal ascending aortic short axis and long axis views** (see Figures 4.6 and 4.7) are useful for the identification of aortic atheroma and dissection, and for the measurement of the diameter of the proximal ascending aorta. As a rough guide, the aorta should be about the same diameter as the pulmonary artery.

## Descending aortic and aortic arch views (see Figure 4.23)

The **upper oesophageal aortic arch long axis and short axis views** allow visualisation of the distal aortic arch. In the short axis view (90°), the origin of the left subclavian artery can usually be identified. This is an important landmark that has implications in a number of clinical situations. The tip of an intra-aortic balloon pump catheter should be distal to the left subclavian artery. The origin of a patent ductus arteriosus lies opposite the origin of the subclavian artery, and this is the most common site for aortic coarctation and aortic rupture. Finally, whether the origin of a descending thoracic aneurysm occurs above or below the left subclavian artery will determine the appropriate cardiopulmonary bypass technique to facilitate surgical repair (see below).

The descending thoracic aorta is usually well seen in the **descending aortic short and long axis views**. In short axis it is frequently necessary to turn the shaft of the probe to the left or right to keep the aorta centred on the screen. The image is usually lost or becomes poor as the stomach is entered. These views are useful for the identification of aortic atheroma, aortic dissection and left pleural effusion.

## Limitations of TOE in the assessment of the aorta

Imaging of the distal ascending aorta (zone 3) and proximal arch (zone 4) is limited by interposition of the trachea and left main bronchus between the oesophagus and the aorta. Consequently these regions cannot be visualised with TOE in most patients. Imaging of the proximal ascending aorta (zone 2) also suffers because it is an anterior structure and lies in the far lateral position (on the right) of the sector scan. In addition, posterior aortic calcification will lead to ultrasound dropout, further degrading the quality of the anterior wall image. For these reasons, **epiaortic imaging** is required for accurate assessment of the distal ascending aorta and proximal aortic arch.

TOE examination of the thoracic aorta is affected by **reverberation artifacts** which can occur from calcification in the aortic wall or from vascular catheters. A curved

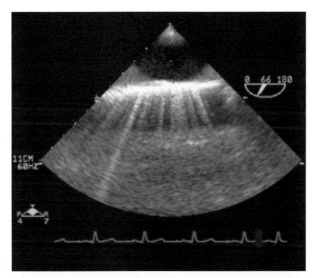

**Figure 11.1** Reverberation artifact in the descending thoracic aorta.

artifact in the ascending aorta is often seen from a pulmonary artery catheter; this can be misdiagnosed as a dissection. In the descending aorta a reverberation artifact of the whole aorta is often seen (Figure 11.1) and may resemble an aneurysm or dissection. What is particularly disconcerting is that colour Doppler is often seen in the reverberation artifact, although with less intensity than in the true image. Reverberation artifacts should be twice or half the distance from the probe to the true image (p.28). Occasionally **side-lobe artifacts** (p.21) can also give the appearances of a dissection flap within the aorta.

Inaccuracy in the measurement of aortic dimensions can arise owing to the effects of oblique or off-axis imaging (see Figure 16.6). In short axis (e.g. the ascending aortic short axis view) the aorta may appear oval due to the effects of oblique imaging, leading to *overestimation* of the aortic diameter. In long axis imaging (e.g. the descending aortic long axis view) the diameter may be *underestimated* by off-axis imaging, which fails to cut through the centre of the aorta. An oblique cut through the aortic wall can make it appear falsely thickened. This effect is most apparent in the aortic arch long axis view. The curved shape of this structure can give the erroneous impression of atheromatous thickening in the lateral parts of the sector scan. These problems are all less likely with epiaortic scanning.

The aorta expands slightly in systole causing a small increase in diameter. To eliminate this effect all measurements should be made at the same time during the cardiac cycle (the aortic dimensions provided in Appendix 2 are from end diastole) from inner edge to inner edge (p.244).

## AORTIC ATHEROMA

Dislodgement of aortic atheroma has been identified as the leading cause of stroke following cardiac surgery and is increasingly recognised as an important cause of stroke in the non-surgical population.[2] Severe adverse neurological outcome occurs in 1–6% of patients following cardiac surgery,[3] but this represents only the tip of the iceberg of neurological injury. More subtle cognitive damage may be caused by multiple small emboli to the brain, leading to personality changes, memory difficulty, affective disorder or intellectual deterioration. This occurs in 30–70% of patients undergoing conventional aortocoronary graft surgery using cardiopulmonary bypass.[4]

Severe ascending aortic atheroma is an unlikely finding in patients less than 50 years of age but it increases proportionally with age – occurring in one-third of patients over 80.[5] The proportion of moderate or severe atheroma is greater in the arch and descending aorta than in the ascending aorta.[1,3] There are two key steps to reducing neurological morbidity from aortic atheroma: firstly, detecting the atheroma accurately, and secondly, avoiding dislodging it from the aortic wall during surgical manipulations.

## Classification of atheroma

Atheroma is identified by thickening of the intima – normal intima is smooth and less than 2 mm thick. Initially atheroma appears as smooth intimal thickening but as it progresses it becomes more extensive, complex in shape (hills and valleys) and rough in appearance (Figure 11.2). In its most severe form, atheroma is mobile and frond-like, extending well into the aortic lumen (Figure 11.3). Two widely used grading systems for atheroma are shown in Table 11.1.

## The role of TOE

Despite the limitations of TOE in visualising atheroma in the distal ascending aorta and proximal arch, there is evidence that mobile atheroma detected in the *descending thoracic aorta* is predictive of postoperative stroke.[7] Furthermore, in one study, the absence of moderate-to-severe atheroma in the parts of the aorta that were visible with TOE was associated with a very low risk of stroke.[8]

However, moderate-to-severe atheroma is far more common in the descending thoracic aorta than in the ascending aorta or aortic arch. Therefore atheroma in the descending aorta is a poor predictor of atheroma in the ascending aorta or arch.[9]

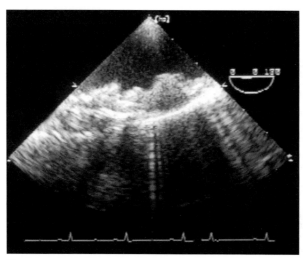

**Figure 11.2** Extensive aortic atheroma seen in the aortic arch long-axis view. The atheroma is nearly 1 cm thick.

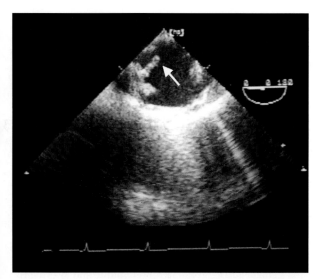

**Figure 11.3** Mobile atheroma (arrow) seen in the descending aortic short axis view.

| Table 11.1 Classification of aortic atheroma | |
|---|---|
| **Royse et al[1]** | |
| Normal | Smooth intima, <2 mm thick |
| Mild | Smooth intima, 2–4 mm thick |
| Moderate | Smooth intima, >4 mm thick |
| Severe | Complex shape or mobile, >4 mm thick |
| **Katz et al[6]** | |
| Grade 1 | Normal or mild intimal thickening |
| Grade 2 | Severe intimal thickening, no protruding atheroma |
| Grade 3 | Atheroma protruding <5 mm into lumen |
| Grade 4 | Atheroma protruding >5 mm into lumen |
| Grade 5 | Atheroma of any size with a mobile component |

## Epiaortic scanning

Epiaortic scanning involves the direct application of a high-frequency probe to the aortic wall. The surgeon can manipulate the probe while the anaesthetist adjusts the settings on the machine. Probes with a frequency in the 5–7.5 MHz range have the problem of near-field crowding, and it is necessary to use a spacer (e.g. a sterile bag containing saline as a coupling medium) to offset the probe from the aorta. Alternatively, purpose-designed high-frequency probes are now commercially available (e.g. the Phillips Medical System 15 MHz intraoperative probe). Zones 1–4 can be completely visualised, including the origins of the brachiocephalic and left common carotid arteries. With practice the entire epiaortic scan can be completed in a matter of minutes.

TOE is able to identify fewer than 30% of patients shown with epiaortic scanning to have moderate or severe atheroma in the ascending aorta or arch.[9] Therefore epiaortic scanning is the method of choice for the reliable determination of atheroma burden in this region and should be used routinely on high-risk patients (e.g. patients over 70 years of age), or if significant atheroma is detected with TOE.

### Therapeutic options

Screening for atheroma is of little value unless coupled with proactive interventions to avoid displacement of atheroma during surgical manipulations. The simplest technique is to select sites for aortic manipulation that are distant from the sites of atheroma. However, it may not be technically possible to do this. In conventional aortocoronary bypass graft surgery the proximal anastomoses are placed on the mid ascending aorta (zone 2). They cannot be moved more proximally because the risk of kinking the graft increases. One option that provides "more room to move" is the use of an exclusive pedicle arterial technique such as a Y graft, in which a proximal radial artery graft is attached to the left internal mammary artery. In one study this technique was associated with a lower incidence of neurocognitive dysfunction than conventional aortocoronary grafting.[10] Other strategies include using a single aortic cross-clamp technique and altering the position of the aortic cannulation site.

Off-pump coronary artery bypass (OPCAB) surgery eliminates the need for aortic cannulation and reduces the need for aortic cross-clamping. When combined with an exclusive pedicle Y graft technique, OPCAB surgery eliminates the need for *any* aortic manipulation.

## AORTIC ANEURYSM

An aneurysm is a dilatation of the aorta to 50% or more above normal size (Figure 11.4). Aetiology includes atheroma, hypertension, cystic medial necrosis, connective tissue disorders (e.g. Marfan syndrome, Ehlers–Danlos syndrome), trauma, infection and

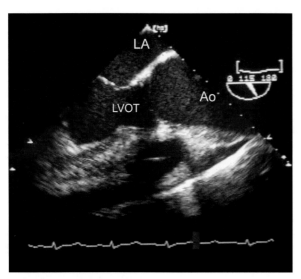

**Figure 11.4** Aortic aneurysm involving the ascending aorta (Ao): mid oesophageal AV long axis view. There is loss of the sinotubular junction, which increases the likelihood of aortic regurgitation. Centimetre markers are shown on the right of the sector display.

annuloaortic ectasia (idiopathic destruction of the elastic fibres of the media affecting the aortic annulus and proximal ascending aorta).

Dissection may occur within aneurysms and aneurysmal dilatation may be associated with dissections or ruptures.

The main indications for surgery are increasing size and progressive aortic regurgitation. The decision to operate will vary amongst surgeons and institutions but as a rough guide a fusiform aneurysm >5 cm, a marfanoid aneurysm >4.5 cm, or a saccular aneurysm >3–5 cm may warrant surgery.

Caution should be used when diagnosing an aneurysm with TOE if the image is poor, or if the dimensions are at the upper limits of normal. If there is any doubt, or in the case of an unexpected finding in the operating room, epiaortic imaging should be used.

Aortic aneurysms can be divided into those involving the ascending aorta and those involving the descending aorta.

## Ascending aortic aneurysms

These often occur in combination with AV pathology. Dilatation of the aortic root may be seen distal to a stenotic AV (particularly a bicuspid valve). Conversely, aortic dilatation that involves the sinotubular junction is a common cause of AV regurgitation (p.164). In this situation it is important to differentiate between normal and abnormal aortic leaflet morphology, as the former may be suitable for an AV sparing procedure.[11]

For operations involving reimplantation of coronary arteries it is useful to identify flow in the coronary ostia with either TOE or epiaortic imaging. Abnormal flow (such as occurs with a kinked artery) will be of high velocity and associated with a mosaic pattern on colour flow Doppler. This is best appreciated by withdrawing the probe slightly from the mid oesophageal AV short axis view until the origin of the left and (sometimes) the right coronary systems is seen. Following repair it is important to rule out new segmental wall motion abnormalities, which are suggestive of coronary insufficiency.

## Descending aortic aneurysms

Aneurysms of the descending aorta have been classified by Crawford according to site of origin and degree of distal involvement. Types I and II extend from the proximal descending thoracic aorta to above or below the renal arteries respectively; type III begin more distally, but above the diaphragm, and extend into the abdomen; type IV are confined to the aorta below the diaphragm.

A key surgical issue is whether the aneurysm arises above or below the origin of the left subclavian artery. If the neck of the aneurysm is proximal to the left subclavian (i.e. within the arch), then deep hypothermic circulatory arrest will be required for repair. In contrast, if the origin is distal to the left subclavian artery (i.e. within the descending aorta), it may be possible to clamp the aorta distal to the left common carotid artery and perform the operation with left-heart bypass. The upper oesophageal aortic arch views are helpful in defining the origin of the aneurysm.

In patients undergoing repair of a descending thoracic aneurysm via a left thoracotomy, the heart cannot be directly inspected during cardiopulmonary bypass, and TOE may be invaluable in detecting unexpected ventricular dilatation secondary to aortic regurgitation.

## Sinus of Valsalva aneurysm

The right coronary sinus is most commonly affected by a saccular dilatation projecting into the RA, and may assume a billowing "windsock" appearance (Figure 11.5). This is best appreciated in the mid oesophageal AV short axis view. The aetiology is usually

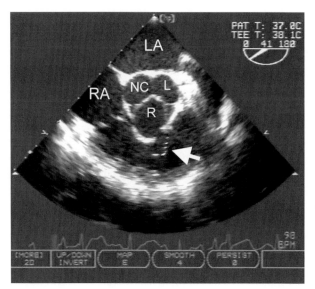

**Figure 11.5** Ruptured aneurysm of the sinus of Valsalva: mid oesophageal AV short axis view. A thin flap of tissue can be seen extending from the right sinus of Valsalva (R). These appearances are very similar to a perimembranous or conal ventricular septal defect (see Figure 15.1(d)).

congenital, but can occur with cystic medial degeneration, Marfan syndrome, endocarditis or penetrating injury. Presentation may be dramatic if there is rupture into an adjacent structure, with chest pain and cardiac failure. Associated findings with TOE include aortic regurgitation, ventricular septal defects, valvular or subvalvular pulmonary stenosis, compression of the RVOT and conduction abnormalities.[12] If rupture occurs it is most commonly into the RA producing a left-to-right shunt.

## AORTIC DISSECTION

In many centres TOE is the tool of choice for the diagnosis of aortic dissection and the evaluation of its complications. The sensitivity and specificity of TOE is similar to that of magnetic resonance imaging, computed tomography or aortography.[13] It has the advantage of being accessible in the emergency department, and offers superior evaluation of cardiac function and detection of pericardial effusions.

Dissection is said to occur when the media of the aorta has been split and contains extraluminal blood within a "false" lumen. This occurs with medial degenerative disease and/or hypertension. Connective tissue diseases are frequently associated with dissections, notably Marfan syndrome.

### Classification and management of dissections

The Stanford and DeBakey systems are commonly used to classify dissections of the thoracic aorta.

- Stanford Type A dissections involve the ascending aorta regardless of the site of origin.
- Stanford Type B includes all dissections not involving the ascending aorta.
- DeBakey Type I dissections involve the ascending aorta and extend at least to the arch.
- DeBakey Type II dissections are confined to the ascending aorta.

- DeBakey Type III dissections originate in the descending aorta, can involve the arch, but do not extend into the ascending aorta.

The objectives of surgery for dissection include prevention of rupture, obliteration of the false lumen, and reperfusion of key organs. In general, Stanford Type A dissections are operated on urgently, whereas Type B dissections are usually managed conservatively, unless associated with a complicating factor such as aneurysm formation.

## Echocardiographic findings

Dissection is identified by the presence of an intimal flap. The TOE appearances are usually dramatic: the intimal flap can be seen moving freely within the proximal ascending aorta and not infrequently may prolapse through the AV into the LVOT (Figure 11.6). This is best seen in the mid oesophageal AV long axis view. The diagnosis is less clear if the false lumen contains haematoma; in this situation thickening of the aortic wall may be the only clue to dissection.

Entry and exit points may be identified by colour flow Doppler. Type A dissections usually have entry points in the ascending aorta (zones 1–3), typically just above the sino-tubular junction. They are best seen in the mid oesophageal AV long axis view (zone 1) or with epiaortic scanning (zones 2 and 3). In most patients with Type A dissections the intimal flap can be seen to extend into the aortic arch and descending thoracic aorta.

It can sometimes be difficult to differentiate the true and false lumens but the following clues may help:

- The true lumen is often round when viewed in short axis.
- The true lumen typically expands during systole.
- The true lumen often has normal flow patterns on colour Doppler.
- The false lumen is often crescent-shaped when viewed in short axis.
- The false lumen is commonly larger than the true lumen.
- The false lumen may show spontaneous echo contrast, suggestive of sluggish flow.
- Differentiation of the true and false lumen in the distal ascending aorta may be helped by epiaortic scanning, which should be performed if aortic cannulation is planned in this region.

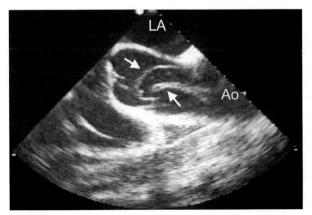

**Figure 11.6** Aortic dissection. An intimal flap (arrows) can be seen in the ascending aorta (Ao) in this mid oesophageal AV long axis view.

Besides identification of the site and extent of the dissection itself, the following must also be considered:

- The presence and severity of aortic regurgitation (see below).
- The presence of a pericardial effusion and tamponade.
- Involvement of the coronary ostia.
- Left and right global and segmental ventricular function.
- The presence of a left pleural effusion.
- True lumen flow during commencement of cardiopulmonary bypass to detect "malperfusion" syndrome.
- The identification of dissection within major aortic branches, with TOE or epiaortic imaging.

Various imaging artifacts can resemble aortic dissection. In addition to the artifacts described on pp.172–173, the presence of the innominate vein in the upper oesophageal aortic arch view can give the erroneous impression of a dissection flap (see Figure 5.15).

Aortic regurgitation is common in patients with a Type A dissection. The usual mechanism is separation of the leaflet commissures from the aortic wall into the lumen of the aorta, resulting in leaflet prolapse and regurgitation. The non-coronary and right cusps are most frequently affected. In this situation the presence of even severe regurgitation is not a contraindication to valve preservation as reapposition of the commissures to the aortic wall usually corrects the regurgitation. In contrast, regurgitation in association with annular dilatation, Marfan syndrome or a bicuspid valve typically necessitates valve replacement.

Following repair, TOE is useful for assessing residual aortic incompetence, checking flow in the coronary ostia, and identifying new segmental wall motion abnormalities.

## AORTIC RUPTURE

Aortic rupture is associated with deceleration injury, and is a frequent cause of death in motor vehicle accidents. The site of the rupture is most commonly the isthmus just distal to the left subclavian artery, where the aorta is tethered by the ligamentum arteriosum. The heart and the diaphragm also fix the aorta and these sites are also associated with rupture, although less commonly.

On TOE an intimal flap may be seen which characteristically has a free edge (unlike a dissection flap, it does not typically extend across the aortic wall). The aorta is usually surrounded with haematoma, and a false aneurysm may be seen (Figure 11.7). The presence of haematoma can degrade the image quality, making conclusive diagnosis very difficult. There are several tips to aid in diagnosing this condition:

- Image quality of the distal arch should be very good; poor image quality suggests surrounding haematoma.
- The size of the aorta should decrease from the arch to the proximal descending aorta. Even a small increase in diameter points to a rupture.
- Intimal disruption can resemble severe atheroma, but atheroma is very rare in a young person. "Severe atheroma" in a person under 50 years of age is suggestive of rupture.
- The site of rupture can vary according to the nature of trauma. The whole length of the aorta should be examined from the arch to the diaphragm.

Because of these difficulties, in most centres, when aortic rupture is suspected aortography is used.

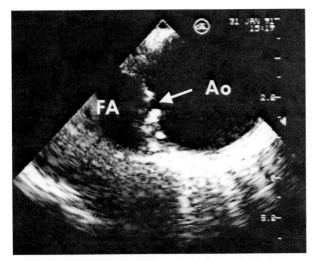

**Figure 11.7** Aortic rupture. In this descending aortic short axis view, a tear (arrow) in the aortic wall can be seen, connecting the aorta (Ao) and a false aneurysm (FA). There is haematoma (speckled appearance) around part of the false aneurysm. Image reproduced from Snow C et al. *Journal of the American Society of Echocardiography* 1992;5:101, courtesy of Mosby Inc.

# REFERENCES

1. Royse C, Royse A, Blake D, et al. Assessment of thoracic aortic atheroma by echocardiography: a new classification and estimation of risk of dislodging atheroma during three surgical techniques. *Annals of Thoracic and Cardiovascular Surgery* 1998;4:72–77.

2. The French Study of Aortic Plaques in Stroke Group. Atherosclerotic disease of the aortic arch as a risk factor for recurrent ischemic stroke. *New England Journal of Medicine* 1996;334:1216–1221.

3. Roach GW, Kanchuger M, Mangano CM, et al. Adverse cerebral outcomes after coronary bypass surgery. Multicenter Study of Perioperative Ischemia Research Group and the Ischemia Research and Education Foundation Investigators. *New England Journal of Medicine* 1996;335:1857–1863.

4. Hammon JW, Stump DA, Kon ND, et al. Risk factors and solutions for the development of neurobehavioural changes after coronary artery bypass grafting. *Annals of Thoracic Surgery* 1997;63:1613–1618.

5. Wareing TH, Davila-Roman VG, Daily BB, et al. Strategy for the reduction of stroke incidence in cardiac surgical patients. *Annals of Thoracic Surgery* 1993;55:1400–1408.

6. Katz ES, Tunick PA, Rusinek H, et al. Protruding aortic atheromas predict stroke in elderly patients undergoing cardiopulmonary bypass: experience with intraoperative transesophageal echocardiography. *Journal of the American College of Cardiology* 1992;20:70–77.

7. Hartman GS, Yao F-S, Bruefach M 3rd, et al. Severity of aortic atheromatous disease diagnosed by transesophageal echocardiography predicts stroke and other outcomes associated with coronary artery surgery: a prospective study. *Anesthesia and Analgesia* 1996;83:701–708.

8. Konstadt SN, Reich DL, Kahn R, et al. Transesophageal echocardiography can be used to screen for ascending aortic atherosclerosis. *Anesthesia and Analgesia* 1995;81:225–228.

9. Royse C, Royse A, Blake D, et al. Screening the thoracic aorta for atheroma: a comparison of manual palpation, transesophageal and epiaortic ultrasonography. *Annals of Thoracic and Cardiovascular Surgery* 1998;4:347–350.

10. Royse AG, Royse CF, Ajani AE, et al. Reduced neuropsychological dysfunction using epiaortic echocardiography and the exclusive Y graft. *Annals of Thoracic Surgery* 2000;69:1431–1438.

11. David TE, Armstrong S, Ivanov J, et al. Aortic valve sparing operations: an update. *Annals of Thoracic Surgery* 1999;67:1840–1842.

12. Burakovsky VI, Podsolkov VP, Sabirow BN, et al. Ruptured congenital aneurysm of the sinus of Valsalva. Clinical manifestations, diagnosis, and results of surgical corrections. *Journal of Thoracic and Cardiovascular Surgery* 1988;95:836–841.

13. Nienaber CA, von Kodolitsch Y, Nicolas V, et al. The diagnosis of thoracic aortic dissection by noninvasive imaging procedures. *New England Journal of Medicine* 1993;328:1–9.

# 12

# Prosthetic Valves

*Roman Kluger*
*Mario Kalpokas*

In the practice guidelines published in 1996 by the ASA/SCA, the assessment of valve replacement surgery is a category II indication for TOE (see Table 1.1). Since that time the evidence supporting the use of TOE during routine valve replacement surgery has been consolidated. For example, in patients undergoing AV replacement, routine intra-operative TOE changed the surgical plan in 13% of cases (which involved the addition of an unplanned MV replacement in 1.6%) in one study,[1] and the extension of a perioperative TOE service to include all valve replacement surgery actually resulted in an overall cost saving in another.[2] Situations in which complicated valve replacement surgery (involving a perivalvular abscess or haemodynamic instability) or valve repair is contemplated are a category I indication for perioperative TOE.

## APPROACH TO IMAGING PROSTHETIC VALVES

It is important to conduct a systematic TOE examination in all patients presenting for valve replacement surgery and to interpret the findings in light of the patient's clinical history. In the context of redo surgery, it can be helpful to know the type and size of valve, the year it was inserted, previously documented gradients and whether there were any problems at the time of the original operation.

All prosthetic valves produce a degree of acoustic shadowing and reverberation artifact due to material in the stents, sewing rings and discs. This can result in misdiagnosis, firstly because of over-interpretation of the reverberation artifact and secondly because pathology or abnormal flow may be hidden by acoustic shadowing, and therefore missed. This is a particular problem with mechanical valves as, in addition to the sewing ring and struts, the occluders (leaflets) are strongly echogenic. To avoid missing pathology in the far field it is important to examine the valve from multiple views (including non-standard image planes) so that, as far as possible, the entire structure is visualised. Decreasing the gain setting is helpful in minimising the intense echo reflections from mechanical surfaces. It is also useful to acquire short digital loops, and then toggle the colour map on and off while scrolling through each loop, to identify the origins of any jets.

### Mitral prosthetic valves

TOE is far superior to transthoracic imaging for the assessment of prosthetic MV function because the LA (where regurgitant jets and other complications such as thrombus and vegetations are most frequently seen) is not in the acoustic shadow of the prosthetic valve. As with native MV dysfunction, the mid oesophageal ventricular views (four-chamber, commissural, two-chamber and long axis) are the most useful. Rarely, prosthetic MV pathology occurs on the LV side of the valve (e.g. thrombus formation) and in these situations transthoracic imaging may be required.

## Aortic prosthetic valves

In general, prosthetic valves in the aortic position are not as well visualised as those in the mitral position. The mid oesophageal AV views (short axis and long axis) are the most useful for detecting regurgitant jets. However, with mechanical valves, echo dropout of the anterior elements of the valve (from the posterior sewing ring) makes leaflet motion difficult to visualise at the mid oesophageal level. Leaflet motion, transvalvular flow patterns and pressure gradients may be better assessed from the deep transgastric long-axis and transgastric long axis views. However, these views may be difficult to obtain, and poor alignment of the Doppler signal with flow may result in underestimation of transvalvular gradients. In cases of uncertainty the transvalvular gradient can be assessed by direct needle pressure measurements in the operating room, but these measurements may also be misleading.[3]

The adequate assessment of an aortic prosthesis (especially in relation to regurgitant jets) is made more difficult by the presence of an adjacent MV prosthesis.

## Specific points to address during the TOE examination

The following points should be emphasised during pre and postbypass echocardiographic examinations.

### Prebypass

- Confirm the indications for replacement (versus repair or no intervention) by an assessment of the aetiology and severity of the dysfunction.
- Look for associated pathology that may alter the surgical plan:
  - Dilatation of the aortic root that may necessitate a combined valve–root replacement.
  - Extensive calcification of valve annulus or aortic root that may complicate valve implantation – a particular problem with mitral annular calcification.
  - The presence of an atrial septal defect or small LA that may influence the surgical approach (e.g. a transseptal incision may be used instead of an incision directly into the LA for MV replacement).
  - The presence of thrombus, particularly in the LA appendage.
  - The presence of vegetations, abscesses or fistulas – particularly in redo valve surgery.
  - The presence of subvalvular obstruction rather than aortic stenosis (severe "aortic stenosis" in the absence of valvular calcification should raise this possibility).
  - Severe LV dysfunction that may increase the risk of procedures associated with a prolonged cardiopulmonary bypass time.
- Measure dimensions that have implications for specific surgical procedures:
  - In patients undergoing AV replacement, measurement of the annular diameter is highly predictive of the required prosthesis size.[4,5]
  - If a stentless AV prosthesis is planned it is also important to measure the diameter of the sinotubular junction as this may identify patients who require sinotubuloplasty.[5] The measurement technique is described on p.157.
  - If the annulus is small relative to the size of the patient and to the anticipated cardiac output, specific valves (e.g. stentless) or surgical techniques (e.g. supravalvular placement) may be required in order to avoid prosthesis–patient mismatch (p.198).

Postbypass
- Assess adequacy of replacement:
  - Proper seating of the prosthesis and the absence of paravalvular leaks.
  - Normal prosthetic valve function including leaflet motion, Doppler evaluation and characteristic regurgitant (signature) jets.
- Exclude complications involving other structures (p.197).
- Verify adequacy of de-airing.

# PROSTHETIC VALVES IN CURRENT USE

More than 80 models of prosthetic valves have been used since 1950. They vary in durability, thrombogenicity and haemodynamic profile. A basic knowledge of those in common use (Table 12.1), their echocardiographic features and their transvalvular blood flow patterns is important in order to differentiate normal from abnormal function.

The main advantage of **mechanical valves** is durability and therefore longevity. Their main disadvantage is thrombogenicity, necessitating lifelong anticoagulation.

**Bioprosthetic valves** do not require long-term anticoagulation, but are less durable.

Bileaflet valves and tilting disc valves make up the majority of mechanical valves currently in use. In general most stented bioprosthetic valves and all mechanical valves can be used in the aortic, mitral, tricuspid and pulmonary positions. The use of unstented bioprosthetic valves is restricted to the aortic or pulmonary position.

Available prosthetic valve sizes depend on the manufacturer and the specific model. Model-specific sizers are used intraoperatively to determine appropriate valve size. Most

| **Table 12.1** Commonly used prosthetic valves |
|---|
| **Mechanical valves** |
| Bileaflet (e.g. St Jude Medical, Carbomedics, ATS, Duromedics) |
| Tilting disc (e.g. Bjork–Shiley, Medtronic–Hall) |
| Ball and cage (e.g. Starr–Edwards) |
| Disc and cage (rare) |
| **Bioprosthetic (tissue)** |
| *Stented* |
| Porcine aortic valve (e.g. Carpentier–Edwards, Medtronic Mosaic) |
| Bovine pericardial valve (e.g. Carpentier–Edwards Perimount, Ionescu–Shiley) |
| *Stentless* |
| Porcine (e.g. Toronto SPV®, Freestyle®) |
| Homograft (human cadaveric) |
| Autograft (Ross procedure) |
| Valves of porcine and bovine origin are also known as **heterografts** or **xenografts**; homografts are sometimes referred to as **allografts**. |

adults receive a 19–23 mm valve in the aortic position; larger valves are used in the mitral position (usually 27–31 mm). However, sizes can vary from 19 to 31 mm for aortic prostheses and from 19 to 33 mm for mitral prostheses.

## Bileaflet valves

There are many different brands and models, but all have similar structural and echocardiographic characteristics (Figure 12.1a). Each valve consists of two semicircular rigid leaflets attached to a pyrolytic carbon ring. The leaflets pivot at two recessed hinges located slightly lateral to the central axis of the valve. The carbon ring is reinforced and enclosed by a sewing ring. Flow through the valve is symmetrical via two large lateral semicircular orifices and a narrow rectangular central orifice. Leaflets typically open to about 80°. The result is relatively unobstructed forward flow, a very small area of stagnation on the downstream side of the leaflets (which may reduce the risk of thromboembolism), and a relatively large regurgitant volume (because the leaflets must swing through a large arc to close). After the valve closes, characteristic regurgitant "signature" jets help "wash" the leaflet surfaces and reduce the formation of thrombus. Most current models allow the valve mechanism to be rotated within the sewing ring to minimise the risk of leaflets being caught up on perivalvular structures.

Bileaflet valves may be placed in an annular or supra-annular position. In the aortic position, supra-annular placement may allow the use of a larger valve than would otherwise be possible; in the mitral position, it may be used to separate the leaflets from the subvalvular apparatus in a chordal sparing operation. With double valve replacement, supra-annular placement provides a greater separation between the two valves, which facilitates implantation.

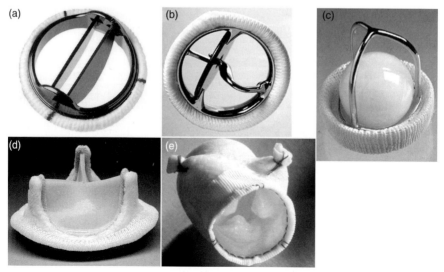

**Figure 12.1** Prosthetic valves in common usage: (a) bileaflet mechanical valve (St Jude Medical); (b) tilting disc valve (Medtronic–Hall); (c) ball and cage valve (Starr–Edwards aortic valve); (d) stented tissue valve (Carpentier–Edwards Perimount); (e) stentless tissue valve (Medtronic Freestyle). (a) Courtesy of St Jude Medical Ltd; (b, e) courtesy of Medtronic Ltd; (c, d) courtesy of Edwards Lifesciences.

Echocardiographic appearances

On 2-D imaging the echogenic sewing ring is seen at the level of the annulus. When supra-annular implantation is used in the mitral position, the valve is seen sitting in the LA more noticeably than when annular placement is used. In the aortic position it is difficult to differentiate between annular and supra-annular placement.

In the mitral position the leaflets can be clearly seen with mid oesophageal imaging. If the image plane is perpendicular to the central line of leaflet coaptation, the two leaflets should be seen opening and closing symmetrically and in synchrony (Figure 12.2). They should swing through the full opening arc to about 80°, then close at about 25°. Some imaging planes may give the false impression that the leaflet motion is unequal, so it is important to rotate the transducer through a range of views to obtain one in which the ultrasound beam is aligned perpendicularly to the central line of leaflet coaptation. The correct angle will vary depending on the orientation of the valve.

In the aortic position the leaflets are usually poorly seen in the mid oesophageal views, owing to shadowing from the sewing ring. Leaflet motion may be better appreciated in the deep transgastric long axis or transgastric long axis views.

Colour flow Doppler imaging usually displays two or more characteristic narrow signature jets, usually 2–5 cm in length. The direction of these jets will depend on the angle of the imaging plane relative to the valve. When the image plane is *parallel* to the central line of leaflet coaptation there will usually be two convergent jets, originating from within the sewing ring at the pivot points (Figure 12.3a). When the image plane is *perpendicular* to the central line of leaflet coaptation a central jet (originating from the central coaptation line) and a number of diverging peripheral jets of variable length (originating from the space between the valve leaflets and the ring) will be seen (Figure 12.3b). Although colour jets are usually well seen in long axis views, short axis imaging will often help to localise the origins of jets and to distinguish transvalvular from paravalvular regurgitation (pp.193–196).

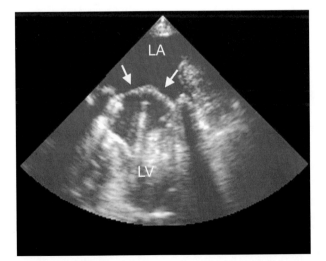

**Figure 12.2** Bileaflet mechanical valve in the mitral position (2-D imaging). The two leaflets (arrows) are shown in the closed position. This is a systolic frame in which the image plane is perpendicular to the central line of leaflet coaptation. Note the extensive far field shadowing, obscuring the LV.

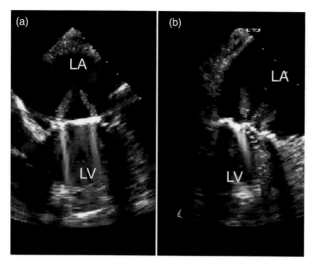

**Figure 12.3** Bileaflet mechanical valve in the mitral position (colour flow Doppler imaging). Both images are systolic frames. (a) The sector scan is parallel to the central line of leaflet coaptation, and two convergent jets can be seen. (b) The sector scan is perpendicular to the central line of leaflet coaptation, and a central jet, along with two small divergent jets, can be seen.

The pressure gradient across a prosthetic valve may be evaluated with CW Doppler (pp.196–197). With bileaflet valves, the following points are important:

- Avoid using the narrow central orifice as this may overestimate the transvalvular gradient because of pressure recovery (p.196).

- The mean gradient should be used rather than peak gradient as there may be transient high velocities within the valve.

## Tilting disc valves

A tilting disc valve consists of a single circular disc suspended from the supporting sewing ring by a single strut (Figure 12.1b). The strut attaches to the disc eccentrically so that the back pressure on the larger segment of the disc will tend to close the valve. The leaflet opens to 55–75° (compared with about 80° for a bileaflet valve). This results in a complex flow pattern (70% of flow passes through the major orifice and 30% through the minor orifice), greater impedance to forward flow, and a relatively large area of stagnation on the downstream surface of the disc (theoretically increasing the likelihood of thromboembolism).

### Echocardiographic appearances

The strut can be seen in a central position above the sewing ring (Figure 12.4). Motion of the leaflet is best visualised by imaging the valve in a scan plane through the hinge point and perpendicular to the axis of disc motion, and is much easier to see in the mitral position than in the aortic position. The correct sector scan angle will depend on the orientation of the valve.

In many planes small regurgitant jets can be seen with colour flow Doppler from the periphery of the valve (between the disc and the ring), and from the central strut attachment in some models. With the Medtronic–Hall valve the central jet is characteristically very long (up to 6 cm; Figure 12.4).

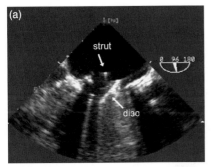 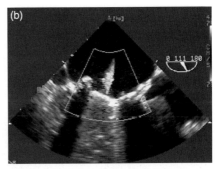

**Figure 12.4** Tilting disc valve in mitral position. (a) The valve in diastole with 2-D imaging. The supporting strut and disc (in the open position) can be seen. (b) The valve in systole with colour flow Doppler imaging. A central jet of regurgitation, characteristic of a Medtronic–Hall valve, can be seen.

On CW Doppler, velocities through the major and minor orifices are usually similar, but the gradient should ideally be measured across the major orifice.

## Ball and cage valves

A ball and cage valve consists of a sewing ring to which is attached a cage, usually made up of three struts for AVs and four for MVs. Within the cage is a Silastic ball. The most common brand is the Starr–Edwards, which over the past 20 years has proved to be very durable (Figure 12.1c). Flow through the valve passes between the ring and the ball, and is directed laterally from the midline of the valve and around the periphery of the ball to converge downstream from the valve. This creates a large area of stagnation behind the ball, resulting in a greater risk of thromboembolism than with other mechanical valves. Ball and cage valves are also associated with an increased risk of acute thrombotic occlusion and haemolysis.

A significant limitation of these valves is their high profile. This can cause intrusion of the valve into the LVOT (in the mitral position) and into the sinuses of Valsalva (in the aortic position).

### Echocardiographic appearances

Downstream from the echogenic sewing ring it is usually possible to see parts of the metallic cage, which are in the plane of the ultrasound beam. A partial outline of the leading edge of the ball may be seen moving within the cage (Figure 12.5).

Colour flow Doppler will display the laterally directed forward flow and the low-velocity closure backflow around the ball. Velocity should be assessed with the ultrasound beam aligned with the laterally directed forward flow.

## Stented bioprosthetic valves

A stented bioprosthetic valve will be either a porcine AV or a valve fashioned from bovine pericardium, suspended from a semiflexible frame (the stent) that provides support for the leaflets (Figure 12.1d). Three projections (stent posts) extend beyond the plane of the annulus to provide support for the leaflet commissures. The leaflets are stiffer than native valve leaflets (a result of the preservation technique). Stented porcine AVs are available in only a limited range of sizes. Some models (e.g. the Carpentier–Edwards supra-annular valve) are designed for supra-annular implantation. Pericardial valves are available in a wide range of sizes.

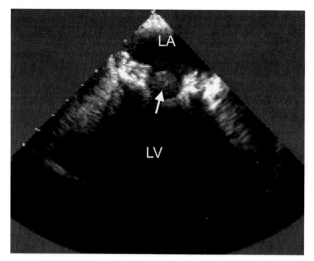

**Figure 12.5** Ball and cage (Starr–Edwards) valve in the mitral position (2-D imaging). The ball is clearly seen (arrow), but little detail of the cage can be identified. Often only the leading edge of the ball is visualised.

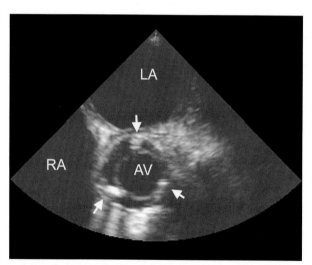

**Figure 12.6** Stented tissue valve in the aortic position (2-D imaging); mid oesophageal AV short axis view. The three echogenic stent posts of the valve can be seen (arrows), as well as the valve leaflets, which are in the open (systolic) position.

## Echocardiographic appearances

In all stented bioprosthetic valves, an echo-dense sewing ring can be seen. Parts of the stent posts may be seen within this ring.

In the aortic position, the three leaflets and stent posts can be seen in the mid-oesophageal AV short axis view (Figure 12.6). In the AV long axis view, dropout from the sewing ring may impair visualisation of the leaflets. Occasionally, when the valve is

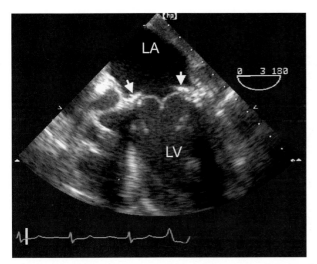

**Figure 12.7** Stented tissue valve in the mitral position (2-D imaging). Two leaflets and the echogenic sewing ring (arrows) can be identified. Some far field shadowing from the sewing ring can be seen, but compared with a mechanical valve, a reasonable view of the LV is obtained.

implanted into a dilated aortic root, a space will be seen between the sewing ring and the sinuses of Valsalva in the mid oesophageal AV short axis view. This is a normal finding and must be differentiated from a pathological paravalvular space (e.g. abscess) that may be associated with a paravalvular leak. This distinction is best made in the mid-oesophageal long axis AV view. Colour flow Doppler (or colour M-mode), with careful scrolling through a digital loop, should be used to assess and time the flows in the para-valvular space, the LVOT and the aortic root.

In the mitral position, the sewing ring and two of the three leaflets can usually be seen from the mid oesophageal ventricular views (Figure 12.7). One or two stent posts may be seen protruding into the LV. All three leaflets and stent posts can sometimes be seen in the transgastric basal short axis view.

Colour flow Doppler will often show a small central regurgitant jet (Figure 12.8). Immediately after separation of the patient from bypass, one to three small regurgitant jets may be seen, originating at the commissures and directed towards the centre of the valve. These will usually reduce in size over an hour or so, as the leaflets soften and remould.

### Stentless porcine valves

These are preserved porcine AVs, designed for use in the aortic position. The Toronto SPV® valve (St Jude Medical) is supported by Dacron cloth, has the sinuses trimmed down, and is designed for subcoronary implantation. The Freestyle® aortic root bio-prosthesis (Medtronic; Figure 12.1e) is a valve–root xenograft that can be used as a subcoronary valve or to replace the valve and root.

The main advantage of stentless valves is their increased orifice area and reduced trans-valvular pressure gradient, and therefore they are often used in people with relatively small aortic annuli. However, they are technically demanding to implant. When stentless valves are used as subcoronary implants the appropriate valve size is determined by the diameter of the *sinotubular junction* as this is the level at which the upper part of the

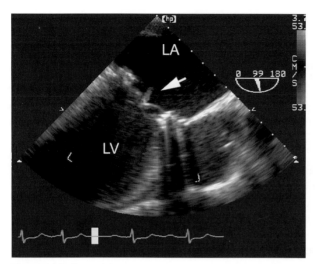

**Figure 12.8** Stented tissue valve in the mitral position (colour flow Doppler imaging). A small central jet of mitral regurgitation (arrow) can be seen.

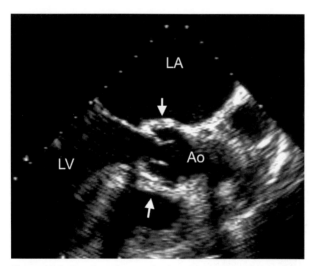

**Figure 12.9** Stentless tissue valve in aortic position (2-D imaging); mid oesophageal AV long axis view. Slight thickening of the aortic root is identified (arrows). This is usually the only clue to the presence of a stentless aortic prosthesis.

commissures sit. If a patient's sinotubular junction is more than 10% larger than his or her annular diameter, a sinotubuloplasty may be required to prevent postoperative aortic regurgitation.

## Echocardiographic appearances

These valves have similar echocardiographic appearances to those of a native AV. The only distinguishing feature may be an increase in tissue thickness in the region of the annulus and sinuses of Valsalva – best seen in the mid oesophageal AV long axis view (Figure 12.9). Trivial central regurgitation may be seen.

## Homograft aortic valve

These cryopreserved AVs come from human cadavers, or from patients receiving transplanted hearts. Like stentless porcine AVs, they have a favourable haemodynamic profile but are technically demanding to implant. They may be used as subcoronary or valve–root replacements. The correct size, based on aortic annular and sinotubular junction dimensions, must be obtained and prepared in advance. Availability of various sizes is often limited.

In the **Ross procedure** a pulmonary autograft is used to replace the diseased AV and a homograft is used to replace the PV. The native pulmonary and aortic valves must have similar annular dimensions for this procedure to be viable.

### Echocardiographic appearances
Homografts have echocardiographic appearances and pressure gradients similar to those of stentless AVs.

# EVALUATING REGURGITATION THROUGH A PROSTHETIC VALVE

Regurgitation may be **transvalvular** (within the sewing ring) or **paravalvular** (outside the sewing ring).

## Transvalvular regurgitation

Trivial transvalvular regurgitation is a normal finding for many prosthetic valves and often provides a "signature" for a particular model or type. Pathological transvalvular regurgitation may be associated with leaflet prolapse (bioprosthetic valve; Figure 12.10) or incomplete disc closure (mechanical valve) on 2-D imaging. The diagnosis of transvalvular regurgitation can be confirmed with colour flow Doppler (Figure 12.11).

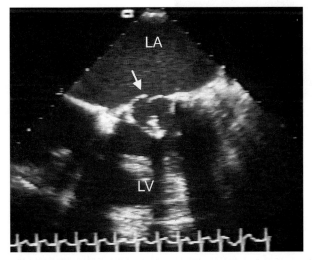

**Figure 12.10** Stented tissue valve in mitral position showing prolapse (arrow) of one of the leaflets. The far field shadowing is more extensive than normal (compare with Figure 12.7), suggesting prosthetic calcification.

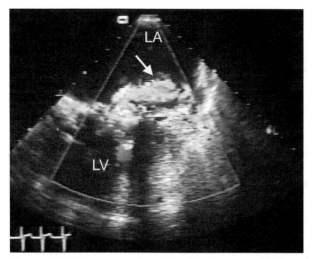

**Figure 12.11** Severe transvalvular regurgitation in the same valve as shown in Figure 12.10. Colour flow Doppler has been applied, and a large eccentric jet of mitral regurgitation can be seen (arrow).

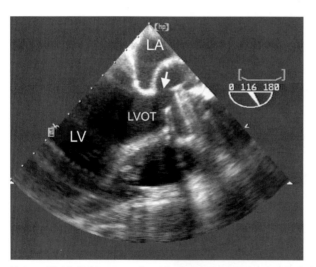

**Figure 12.12** Dehiscence of a bileaflet mechanical valve (2-D imaging). In this mid oesophageal long axis view, a bileaflet mechanical valve can be seen in the aortic position. The aortic root is dilated and the sewing ring has dehisced, creating a large paravalvular space (arrow). This resulted in severe paravalvular aortic regurgitation.

## Paravalvular regurgitation

Persistent paravalvular leaks are never normal. Trivial paravalvular jets seen immediately after surgery are common (possibly through stitch holes) and usually resolve following protamine administration or in the first few postoperative weeks as the sewing ring becomes covered with endothelium. More serious paravalvular regurgitation may be due to dehiscence of part of the sewing ring, usually by suture disruption or endocarditis (Figure 12.12). This situation produces a characteristic rocking motion of the prosthesis.

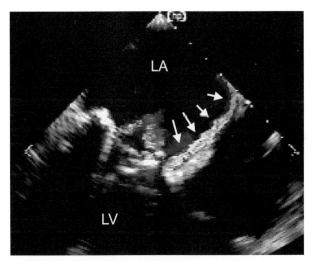

**Figure 12.13** Paravalvular regurgitation of a bileaflet valve in the mitral position (colour flow Doppler imaging); mid oesophageal view. A large eccentric paravalvular jet (arrows) can be seen originating from outside the sewing ring. Two washing jets are also visible.

On colour flow Doppler, the jet can usually be seen to originate outside the sewing ring and is typically eccentric (Figure 12.13). However, differentiating transvalvular from paravalvular regurgitation is not always straightforward, particularly if the sewing ring is not well visualised. It may be especially difficult if there is a peripheral transvalvular jet (which is common with degenerating bioprostheses), because tears and perforations of the cusps frequently occur near the point of their attachment to the stent. It is important to follow jets right back to the valve to identify their origin. Freezing an image and then adding and removing the colour map may help localise the regurgitant jet relative to the sewing ring. A markedly eccentric jet suggests a paravalvular origin.

## Aortic paravalvular regurgitation

Because of acoustic shadowing it can be difficult to visualise the origin of regurgitant jets in the mid oesophageal views, which may make it very difficult to distinguish trans-valvular from paravalvular leaks. It is important to use multiple views to visualise, and then to localise the origins of, any regurgitant jets. Localisation is particularly problematic if the patient has both mitral and aortic prostheses. The transgastric long axis and deep transgastric views may be helpful. Eccentric aortic jets that are directed across the LVOT may lead to *overestimation* of the degree of aortic regurgitation (as it is easy to confuse jet length with jet width).

## Mitral paravalvular regurgitation

This is usually well seen on TOE, but markedly eccentric jets that track along the wall of the LA may be overlooked. In this situation, the presence of significant proximal flow acceleration may be the only indication of severity. In contrast to the AV, eccentric mitral jets may result in *underestimation* of the degree of regurgitation.

As with native mitral regurgitation, it is possible to quantify the anatomical position and extent of the regurgitant jet. Foster and colleagues describe a technique whereby the cir-cumference of the sewing ring is overlaid with a clock face (Figure 12.14).[6] In the mid oesophageal ventricular views, the transducer can be rotated from 0° to 180° to visualise

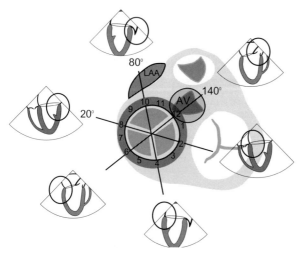

**Figure 12.14** Identification of the location and extent of paravalvular mitral regurgitation as described by Foster et al.[6] The face of a clock is superimposed on the valve. The AV is defined as the 12 o'clock position (which is its position from the surgeon's perspective). The LA appendage (LAA) lies in the 10 o'clock position. The valve is then imaged with colour flow Doppler from the standard mid-oesophageal ventricular views: four-chamber (2 and 8 o'clock), two-chamber (4 and 10 o'clock) and long axis (6 and 12 o'clock). The extent and location of a paravalvular leak is reported with respect to the clock face (e.g. from 2 to 6 o'clock).

the entire sewing ring. The location and extent of the paravalvular leak is then reported (e.g. a localised leak in the 12 o'clock position or an extensive leak from 9 to 12 o'clock).

## EVALUATING FLOWS, PRESSURE GRADIENTS AND ORIFICE AREAS IN PROSTHETIC VALVES

Standard quantitative Doppler techniques can be used to assess the function of prosthetic valves (see Chapter 16 ), but some specific points need to be taken into account.

All mechanical and stented bioprosthetic valves exhibit varying degrees of obstruction, and the **pressure gradients** across many prosthetic valves would be consistent with mild to moderate stenosis in a native valve. Measuring these gradients depends on the accurate interrogation of transvalvular flow using CW Doppler, so it is important to understand the normal flow patterns of the particular prosthesis and to use colour flow Doppler to guide the alignment and placement of the CW Doppler beam. Prosthetic valves (especially mechanical) have complicated velocity profiles and transient high velocities can occur. The maximum velocity will vary directly with cardiac output. As a rule of thumb, a maximum systolic velocity greater than 3.5 m/s in the aortic position, or a maximum diastolic velocity greater than 2.5 m/s in the mitral position, suggests haemodynamically significant stenosis and/or regurgitation.

Applying the **Bernoulli equation** to the high velocities seen at the narrowest part of the valve orifice may overestimate the true pressure gradient, because some of the kinetic energy at the orifice may be converted back to pressure (i.e. potential energy) distal to the valve – the phenomenon of **pressure recovery.** Therefore, the actual pressure drop across this orifice may be less than the calculated gradient. This may explain why velocities measured through the narrow central orifice of bileaflet valves are higher than those measured at the two lateral orifices.

Decisions to replace valves should never be made on velocities and pressure gradients alone. In many reported series of Doppler derived gradients, across clinically normal prosthetic valves, there are a few outliers with abnormally high measured gradients. These may represent problems in measurement or a patient-prosthesis mismatch (p.198). There is great inter-patient variability in "normal" measurements associated with prosthetic valves and it is difficult to specify values to differentiate abnormal from normal function. It is important to consider the measured gradients in the context of the normal Doppler patterns described for the particular valve size and type (the manufacturer's information should be consulted), the 2-D echo appearance of the valve, the gradient reported at the time of valve implantation, and the patient's cardiac output.

Assessment of prosthetic valve area may also be helpful since it does not vary significantly with changes in cardiac output; however a few points should be kept in mind. Measurement of the dimensions of the LVOT (which is required in the estimation of the orifice area of a prosthetic AV using the **continuity equation**; Examples 16.2 and 16.3) is often difficult because of poor image quality. The prosthetic valve size can be used in place of the measured LVOT diameter, or a value of 2.0 cm can be assumed (i.e. the average diameter of the LVOT). Alternatively, the **Doppler velocity index** can be used as an index of the severity of aortic stenosis and has been validated for St Jude Medical valves in the aortic position.[9] It is the ratio of peak velocity in the LVOT to the peak velocity through the AV and is proportional to the ratio of AV area to LVOT area. A value of $< 0.23$ suggests severe stenosis.

In the case of prosthetic valves in the mitral position, the **pressure half time** tends to overestimate the effective orifice area and is unreliable.[7,8] The flow convergence (**PISA**) method of calculating effective orifice area provides acceptable results.[7,10] A simple method for estimating the effective orifice area of mitral bioprosthetic valves is to measure the width of the forward colour flow jet (at the tips of the leaflets) in two orthogonal planes. The average of the two widths is taken as the diameter of the effective orifice area, which is assumed to be circular.[7]

# COMPLICATIONS ASSOCIATED WITH PROSTHETIC VALVES

Most complications of prosthetic valves result in stenosis, regurgitation or ventricular failure – or a combination of these. Complications can occur early, typically as manifestations of technical problems with the insertion of the valve, or late, as the valve ages and various pathological processes begin to influence its function.

## Early complications

At the time of implantation, **damage to leaflets** may occur because of a defective valve, or because poor technique results in a leaflet tear, or due to kinking of a stentless valve or homograft.

**Restriction of leaflet motion** by perivalvular tissues (e.g. retained MV apparatus) or by a suture looped around a stent post may result in the deformation of two associated leaflets.

Damage to other structures may occur. The **non-coronary leaflet of the AV** may be captured, or the **circumflex coronary artery** obstructed, by an annular suture during MV replacement. An **atrial septal defect** may be created during a transseptal approach to the MV or secondary to surgical trauma during MV replacement.

**Retained air** following separation of the patient from bypass frequently results in air embolism down the right (i.e. the most anterior) coronary artery, causing myocardial ischaemia. A **coronary ostium** may be obstructed by suture material or an incorrectly positioned prosthesis during AV replacement.

**Dynamic intracavity or LVOT obstruction** may occur after AV replacement. Decreased LV afterload can lead to reduced cavity and outflow tract diameters, and significant systolic intracavity gradients or systolic anterior motion of the anterior mitral leaflet (SAM; pp.149–150 and Figure 9.16). This is more likely in patients with marked LV hypertrophy.[11]

## Complications that typically occur later

A normal-looking prosthesis may have a gradient greater than would be expected from the valve type and size, simply because the effective orifice area is inadequate for the patient's required cardiac output. Such **patient–prosthesis mismatch** is most often seen in patients with small annular dimensions. The patient remains symptomatic following valve replacement. Diagnosis requires exclusion of prosthesis dysfunction with careful 2-D and colour imaging and may require stress echocardiography.

Bioprosthetic **valve failure** is usually progressive. It is uncommon before 7 years, but by 15 years 30–60% fail.[12] The mechanism of failure is usually calcification, with leaflet thickening and rigidity, which results in progressive stenosis with some regurgitation (transvalvular rather than paravalvular). Thrombus may occur, and cause stenosis. Occasionally, a rigid leaflet may fracture, resulting in acute severe regurgitation. Mechanical valves are extremely durable but, very occasionally, **structural failure** such as a strut fracture in a tilting disc valve can occur and cause acute severe regurgitation. Impairment of valve function by **pannus formation** (fibrous ingrowth from the sewing ring), **thrombus** or **vegetations** (any of which can limit leaflet movement and cause stenosis and/or regurgitation) is much more common as a reason for replacing a mechanical valve. Thrombus itself may be difficult to see with TOE as it may lie in the acoustic shadow of the valve apparatus or be very small; careful examination for limited leaflet excursion is therefore essential.

Between 3% and 6% of all patients with prosthetic valves will at some time develop **endocarditis**. This complication is less likely with homografts, but equally likely with bioprosthetic or mechanical valves.[13] **Vegetations** usually appear as irregular masses of echoes attached to valve components. Small vegetations may be difficult to see or to distinguish from suture material, valve strands, thrombi or the irregular surface of a degenerating bioprosthetic valve. Endocarditis on bioprosthetic valves usually results in leaflet destruction, which leads to regurgitation. With mechanical valves, vegetations may interfere with leaflet motion, and this may result in either stenosis or regurgitation. For both types of valve, endocarditis may cause dehiscence of the sewing ring from the valve annulus, resulting in severe paravalvular regurgitation and a rocking motion of the prosthesis on 2-D imaging. Endocarditis may also result in a **paravalvular abscess** (p.168; Figure 10.8).

**Thrombus** formation may result in valvular stenosis, regurgitation or systemic embolisation. The risk of thrombus formation is similar for bioprosthetic (not anticoagulated) and mechanical valves (adequately anticoagulated) and is 1–4% per patient. **Valvular strands** are mobile, linear echodensities attached to the sewing ring, stents or hinge points of prosthetic valves (p.78; Figure 5.11). Subclinical **haemolysis** occurs with all mechanical prostheses. Severe haemolysis is usually associated with a paravalvular leak.

## REFERENCES

1. Nowrangi SK, Connolly HM, Freeman WK, et al. Impact of intraoperative transesophageal echocardiography among patients undergoing aortic valve replacement for aortic stenosis. *Journal of the American Society of Echocardiography* 2001;14: 863–866.

2. Ionescu AA, West RR, Proudman C, et al. Prospective study of routine perioperative transesophageal echocardiography for elective valve replacement: clinical impact and cost-saving implications. *Journal of the American Society of Echocardiography* 2001;14:659–667.

3. Rehfeldt KH, Click RL. Prosthetic valve malfunction masked by intraoperative pressure measurements. *Anesthesia and Analgesia* 2002;94:857–858.

4. Abraham TP, Kon ND, Nomeir AM, et al. Accuracy of transesophageal echocardiography in preoperative determination of aortic anulus size during valve replacement. *Journal of the American Society of Echocardiography* 1997;10:149–154.

5. Bridgman PG, Bloomfield P, Reid JH, et al. Prediction of stentless aortic bioprosthesis size with transesophageal echocardiography and magnetic resonance imaging. *Journal of Heart Valve Disease* 1997;6:487–489.

6. Foster GP, Isselbacher EM, Rose GA, et al. Accurate localization of mitral regurgitant defects using multiplane transesophageal echocardiography. *Annals of Thoracic Surgery* 1998;65:1025–1031.

7. Degertekin M, Gençbay M, Başaran Y, et al. Application of proximal isovelocity surface area method to determine prosthetic mitral valve area. *Journal of the American Society of Echocardiography* 1998;11:1056–1063.

8. Dumesnil JG, Honos GN, Lemieux M, et al. Validation and applications of mitral prosthetic valvular areas calculated by Doppler echocardiography.

*American Journal of Cardiology* 1990;65:1443–1448.

9. Chafizadeh ER, Zoghbi WA. Doppler echocardiographic assessment of the St Jude Medical prosthetic valve in the aortic position using the continuity equation. *Circulation* 1991;83:213–223.

10. Leung DY, Wong J, Rodriguez L, et al. Application of color Doppler flow mapping to calculate orifice area of St Jude mitral valve. *Circulation* 1998;98:1205–1211.

11. Laurent M, Leborgne O, Clement C, et al. Systolic intra-cavitary gradients following aortic valve replacement: an echo-Doppler study. *European Heart Journal* 1991;12:1098–1106.

12. Fann JI, Burdon TA. Are the indications for tissue valves different in 2001 and how do we communicate these changes to our cardiology colleagues? *Current Opinion in Cardiology* 2001;16:126–135.

13. Bloomfield P, Wheatley DJ, Prescott RJ, et al. Twelve-year comparison of a Bjork–Shiley mechanical heart valve with porcine bioprostheses. *New England Journal of Medicine* 1991;324:573–579.

# 13

# The Right Ventricle, Tricuspid Valve and Pulmonary Valve

*Selwyn Wong*

The importance of the RV as a cause of perioperative morbidity is being increasingly recognised. RV failure is responsible for approximately one-fifth of cases of circulatory failure after cardiac surgery[1] and has a higher mortality rate than failure associated with LV dysfunction.[2]

Although the right heart structures are anterior in location and therefore less well visualised by the posteriorly placed oesophageal probe than the LV, TOE can provide valuable information regarding their function.

## ANATOMY

Normal values for the dimensions and flow patterns of right heart structures are provided in Appendix 2.

### Right ventricle and atrium

The geometry of the RV is complex and does not conform to any regular shape. It is separated into an **inflow tract,** consisting of the TV, papillary muscles, chordae tendinae and chamber walls, and an **outflow tract** consisting of the **infundibulum.** The inflow portion of the RV forms the base of a pyramid, with the three walls formed by the interventricular septum and the anterior and posterior aspects of the RV free wall. A small muscle bundle (the **crista supraventricularis**) separates the inflow (with trabeculated myocardium) and outflow (with non-trabeculated myocardium) regions of the RV. The **moderator band** is a large muscle bundle that runs from the septum to the free wall. The interventricular septum bulges into the RV cavity, imparting a crescent shape to the chamber when viewed in short axis. RV wall thickness is approximately half that of the LV.

In most patients the RV myocardium is predominantly supplied by branches of the **right coronary artery.** A small area, notably the anteroseptal wall, and part of the mid and distal anterior free wall, are supplied by branches of the **left anterior descending coronary artery** (see Figure 7.6). In patients with a left-dominant coronary system, the entire ventricular septum is supplied by branches of the left main coronary artery (p.109).

The RA lies superior and medial to the RV. It has a triangular appendage that is broad based and trabeculated. The anatomy of the **crista terminalis, eustachian valve** (or **Chiari network**) and **thebesian valve** is described in Chapter 5. The **coronary sinus** runs along the posterior atrioventricular groove behind the LA, and drains into the inferior aspect of the RA between the septal leaflet of the TV and the eustachian valve.

### Tricuspid valve

The TV consists of three leaflets (the **anterior, posterior** and **septal**). The leaflets are thinner and less individually distinct than those of the MV. The largest is the septal leaflet (see Figure 9.6), which attaches to the fibrous skeleton of the heart in a slightly more apical position than the anterior mitral leaflet. The anterior leaflet is usually larger than the posterior leaflet.

There are three **papillary muscles**, each associated with a tricuspid leaflet. The septal papillary muscle is usually small and may be absent. The RV papillary muscles are more variable than those of the LV and therefore less useful as an echocardiographic reference point. **Chordae tendinae** attach the papillary muscles to the leaflets.

### Pulmonary valve and artery

The PV is a trileaflet (anterior, left and right; see Figure 9.6) semilunar valve, similar in appearance, but oriented perpendicularly to, the AV. The pulmonary leaflets are thinner and the sinuses of Valsalva less prominent than in the AV.

The pulmonary artery is a short wide vessel, approximately 5 cm in length. It follows an oblique course, arising superiorly from the PV and then curving posteriorly underneath the aortic arch, as it divides into left and right branch pulmonary arteries.

## PHYSIOLOGY AND PATHOPHYSIOLOGY[3]

The function of the RV is to propel deoxygenated blood through the low-impedance pulmonary circulation. The resistance of this circulation is one-tenth that of the systemic circulation and requires a perfusion gradient of just 5 mmHg.

Under normal circumstances the interventricular septum can be considered functionally as part of the LV; consequently the RV free wall contributes most to systolic ejection. The thin wall and crescent shape make the RV highly compliant, and therefore able to accommodate a large increase in preload with minimal change in end diastolic pressure. Thus, the primary compensatory mechanism of the RV is dilatation. For this reason acute (e.g. with exercise) and chronic (e.g. with an atrial septal defect) RV volume overload is relatively well tolerated. However, with severe volume overload functional tricuspid regurgitation develops and the RV loses its crescent shape, becoming ellipsoid like the LV.

The RV is less tolerant of increases in afterload (pressure overload). An acute rise in pulmonary vascular resistance (e.g. due to pulmonary embolus), requiring a mean pulmonary artery pressure of 40 mmHg to perfuse the pulmonary bed, is beyond the capacity of the RV and will result in rapid RV dilatation, failure and circulatory collapse.[4] Chronic pressure overload (e.g. due to emphysema) is, however, somewhat better tolerated through a combination of ventricular dilatation and hypertrophy.

RV dysfunction can also occur as a consequence of direct myocardial injury, most commonly due to ischaemia, infarction, stunning or contusion.

## ECHOCARDIOGRAPHIC EXAMINATION

The anterior location of the right heart structures creates difficulties for imaging with TOE. The RV lies in the far field and image resolution is reduced compared with that of the LV (particularly when colour flow Doppler is used). The presence of strong reflectors within the left heart (e.g. prosthetic aortic or mitral valves) can lead to echo dropout of the right heart structures. In addition, the RV is commonly imaged in an oblique plane, making assessment of chamber size and wall thickness unreliable. This is a particular problem in the transgastric mid short axis view. Despite these limitations, careful imaging using a systematic approach and multiple views can yield important information.

To examine the right heart, five standard views must be obtained:

1. mid oesophageal four-chamber;
2. mid oesophageal RV inflow–outflow;
3. mid oesophageal bicaval;

4. transgastric mid short axis;

5. transgastric RV inflow.

Additional views can also be helpful (Table 13.1, and see Chapter 4).

There is no standardised nomenclature for the RV free wall but the terms basal, apical, inferior, anterior and lateral are used in the ASA/ASE guidelines.[5]

## The mid oesophageal views

Starting with the **four-chamber view**, with the image centred on the RV (Figure 13.1), the basal and apical segments of the RV free wall, the interatrial and interventricular septa, and the anterior and septal leaflets of the TV can be seen. Advancing the probe slightly shows the posterior TV leaflet (identified as the coronary sinus comes into view).

The **RV inflow–outflow view** (see Figure 4.8) is used to visualise the inferior free wall, the RVOT, the posterior and anterior TV leaflets, and the PV. In this view it is usually

| Table 13.1 Optimal views for visualisation of the right heart and pulmonary structures with TOE | |
|---|---|
| **Probe position** | **Structures** |
| **Mid oesophageal** | |
| Four-chamber view (15°) with the probe turned to the right to centre on the right heart | RV free wall, interventricular septum, TV (anterior and septal leaflets), interatrial septum |
| Coronary sinus view (0°) | TV (posterior and septal leaflets), coronary sinus |
| RV inflow–outflow view (80°) | RV, TV (posterior and anterior leaflets), RVOT, PV |
| Bicaval view (110°) | RA and appendage, interatrial septum, vena cavae |
| AV short axis view (40°) | PV (long axis) |
| AV long axis view (130°) | PV (short axis) |
| **Transgastric** | |
| Short axis (0°) with the probe turned to the right to centre on the RV | RV, TV (*en face* view) |
| RV inflow (90°) | RA, TV (anterior and posterior leaflets), RV |

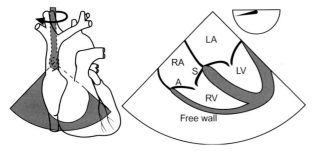

**Figure 13.1** Mid oesophageal four-chamber view with the probe turned to the right, to centre on the right heart structures.

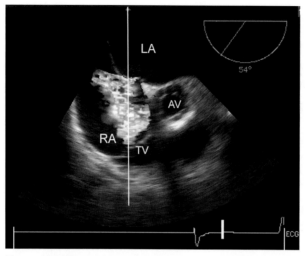

**Figure 13.2** Tricuspid regurgitation seen in a modified mid oesophageal RV inflow–outflow view. The transducer has been rotated backwards from the standard position to improve alignment with a Doppler signal.

possible to align a CW Doppler signal through the TV, although it may be necessary to rotate the transducer backwards 10–20° (Figure 13.2). Improved visualisation of the PV leaflets may be obtained in the AV short or long axis views, but identification of individual leaflets may still be difficult – fortunately this is rarely required.

The **bicaval view** (see Figure 4.9) is useful for examination of the vena cavae and the interatrial septum. The eustachian valve or a Chiari network may be seen adjacent to the IVC (see Figure 5.2) and the crista terminalis may be seen adjacent to the SVC (see Figure 5.1). Turning the probe to the left (anticlockwise) often brings the TV into view at the bottom of the image. This manoeuvre is useful if adequate alignment of a CW Doppler signal with a jet of tricuspid regurgitation cannot be obtained in other views. Advancing the probe allows inspection of more of the IVC; withdrawing the probe allows inspection of more of the SVC.

To examine the main pulmonary artery it is necessary to obtain the **ascending aortic short axis view** (see Figure 4.6). Turning the probe to the right (clockwise) may improve visualisation of the distal segments of the right pulmonary artery. The left pulmonary artery is rarely seen due to interposition of the large airways.

## Transgastric short axis views

In the **transgastric mid short axis view**, with the image centred on the RV (Figure 13.3), all segments of the free wall can be seen (anterior, lateral and inferior). The probe may be advanced or withdrawn to inspect the apical or basal segments respectively. Withdrawing the probe may also provide an *en face* view of the TV, with the anterior leaflet to the left (in the far field), the posterior leaflet to the left (in the near field), and the septal leaflet to the right of the display. Rotating the transducer forward to approximately 35° may improve alignment with the tricuspid annulus.

The **transgastric RV inflow view** (see Figure 4.20) is useful for evaluation of the TV subvalvular apparatus.

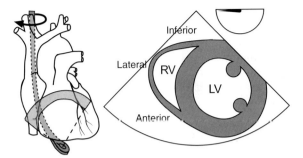

**Figure 13.3** Transgastric mid short axis view with the probe turned to the right, to centre on the RV.

# ECHOCARDIOGRAPHIC ASSESSMENT OF RIGHT VENTRICULAR FUNCTION

## Global function

The complex non-geometric shape of the RV makes echocardiographic assessment of RV volume difficult. Furthermore, RV volume can change substantially with changes in pre-load. A simple method to grade RV volume is to compare the relative sizes of the RV and LV in the mid oesophageal four-chamber view. The RV can be classified as mildly dilated (enlarged but RV area less than LV area), moderately dilated (RV area equals LV area), or severely dilated (RV area greater than LV area). Oblique imaging can sometimes render this comparative technique misleading. As an alternative, the apex of the heart can be inspected. Normally, the RV extends two-thirds of the way to the apex. If the apex includes both the RV and LV, dilatation is moderate; if the RV extends beyond the LV at the apex, dilatation is severe.

The use of ejection fraction to quantify RV systolic function by TOE is limited by the problems inherent in measuring RV volume. Tracing the RV endocardial border at end systole is difficult because of extensive trabeculations and because the RV lies in the far field. While RV fractional area change (using automated border detection in the mid oesophageal four-chamber view) has been described with TOE, and has shown good agreement with stroke volume,[6] it is rarely used in clinical practice.

## Tricuspid annular plane systolic excursion

As the RV contracts during systole, it decreases in both its short and long axis dimensions. The magnitude of long axis shortening provides a useful measure of global RV systolic function. This can be evaluated by calculation of the end diastolic to end systolic fractional shortening of RV length (Figure 13.4) and is normally about 35%.[7] In most patients the systolic excursion is >25 mm. While formal measurement is rarely done, subjective assessment of the descent of the tricuspid annulus provides a useful qualitative guide to global RV systolic function.

## Right ventricular wall motion

Assessment of systolic RV function should include a description of myocardial thickening and wall movement (see Table 7.1). However, evaluation of RV wall motion is limited by a number of factors:

- Difficulties related to image quality, oblique views and the complex shape of the RV, as described above.

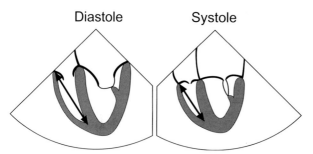

**Figure 13.4** Reduction in long axis dimension of the RV. During systole the long axis of the RV decreases and can be used as a measure of RV systolic function. In the mid oesophageal four-chamber view long axis shortening is normally more than 25 mm. Clinically this is seen as descent of the tricuspid annulus (or tricuspid annular plane excursion).

- It can be difficult to be absolutely sure which RV segments (and which coronary territories) are being visualised in a particular view.
- Systolic excursion is less than with the LV because of the smaller muscle mass of the RV.

In addition, the character of RV wall motion is different from that seen with the LV (RV motion has a sliding quality rather than the piston-like inward movement seen with the LV). It follows that the diagnosis of subtle regional disturbances of RV function should be made with caution. The SCA/ASE guidelines recommend limiting the categorisation of RV regional function to akinetic or dyskinetic segments.[5]

## Volume and pressure overload

Abnormalities of the **shape** and **motion** of the **interventricular septum** occur with both pressure and volume overload of the RV (Figure 13.5). The nature and timing of the abnormalities help to differentiate the two conditions. Timing may be facilitated by placing an M-mode cursor across the interventricular septum, or by replaying the loop of a single cardiac cycle in slow motion. Normally the interventricular septum is *curved* towards the RV in both systole and diastole; it *moves* towards the RV in diastole and towards the LV in systole.

### Volume overload

Chronic RV volume overload causes RV dilatation and, to a lesser extent, hypertrophy. The interventricular septum shows *diastolic* septal flattening (during ventricular filling), with the LV appearing D-shaped in cross-section.

With severe volume overload the RV may appear circular in cross-section (i.e. the septum is curved towards the LV in diastole), and the interventricular septum may show paradoxical motion (it moves towards the LV in diastole).

Causes of RV volume overload include left-to-right shunts (e.g. atrial septal defect, ruptured sinus of Valsalva aneurysm), and severe pulmonary or tricuspid regurgitation.

### Pressure overload

The cardinal features of RV pressure overload are ventricular hypertrophy and paradoxical septal motion in *systole*. Wall thickness can be measured in the mid oesophageal four-chamber view with the image centred on the RV using M-mode imaging; the RV is normally half as thick as the LV. An end diastolic RV wall thickness greater than 5 mm is indicative of hypertrophy. Note that oblique imaging can overestimate wall thickness.

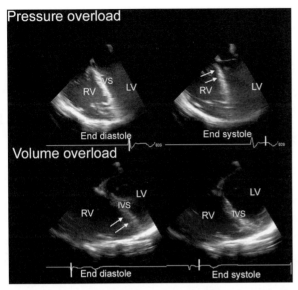

**Figure 13.5** Shape of the interventricular septum (IVS) with RV pressure and volume overload. In pressure overload, at end systole the IVS is curved towards the LV and away from the RV. In the presence of volume overload the IVS appears to curve towards the LV at end diastole. Normally the septum is curved towards the RV in both systole and diastole.

Initially RV pressure overload decreases the motion of the interventricular septum and leads to septal flattening throughout the cardiac cycle. Chronic RV pressure elevation eventually leads to hypertrophy and progressively shifts the centre of mass of the heart towards the RV. This causes the septum to be curved towards the LV in systole and to show paradoxical motion (i.e. the septum moves towards the RV in systole).

RV pressure overload may occur as a consequence of PV stenosis or pulmonary artery hypertension.

## Movement of the interatrial septum
Normally the interatrial septum bows towards the RA throughout most of the cardiac cycle (with mid systolic reversal in both inspiration and expiration in the ventilated patient), but if RA pressure is greater than LA pressure abnormal right-to-left bowing may be seen (Figure 13.6).

## Doppler assessment of right ventricular function
The normal values for tricuspid and SVC filling velocities are given in Appendix 2. The tricuspid inflow pattern is similar to that of the MV, although absolute velocities are lower as the tricuspid annulus is larger than the mitral annulus.

### Estimation of pulmonary artery pressures
There are several echocardiographic techniques for the estimation of pulmonary pressures. With TOE, the most clinically useful is the estimation of **systolic pulmonary artery pressure** from the peak velocity of a jet of tricuspid regurgitation, and the RA pressure (see Example 16.7 and related equations). Over 90% of subjects have a jet of tricuspid regurgitation suitable for measurement even if the degree of regurgitation is modest.[8]

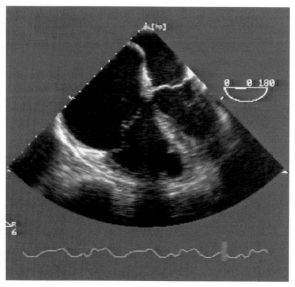

**Figure 13.6** Abnormal right-to-left bowing of the interatrial septum. The RA and RV are markedly dilated. These findings are consistent with pulmonary hypertension secondary to emphysema.

The peak velocity of the regurgitant jet is normally below 2.5 m/s. It is important to ensure that the directions of the Doppler beam and the regurgitant jet are similar to avoid underestimation of the velocity. Inspection of the jet from multiple windows should be undertaken and the highest velocity used.

In the presence of pulmonary regurgitation, the diastolic gradient between the pulmonary artery and RV can be added to the RA pressure to give an estimate of **diastolic pulmonary artery pressure** (p.240). Some degree of pulmonary regurgitation is often found in normal patients but satisfactory alignment of the regurgitant jet with a CW Doppler signal is frequently not possible with TOE.

With transthoracic echocardiography, the **mean pulmonary artery pressure** has been estimated from the time to peak velocity of systolic ejection in the pulmonary outflow tract (also referred to as the **pulmonary acceleration time**). A value shorter than 80–100 ms indicates an elevated mean pulmonary pressure (>20 mmHg).[9,10] Given the difficulties in obtaining adequate views (i.e. the ascending aortic short axis view), this technique is rarely used with TOE.

## PERIOPERATIVE RIGHT VENTRICULAR DYSFUNCTION

RV dysfunction is common during the perioperative period and is an important contributor to haemodynamic instability following cardiopulmonary bypass. Causes include:

- Direct compression of the RV from the retractors that may be used during dissection of the internal mammary artery.
- Prolonged cardiopulmonary bypass.
- Poor myocardial protection. RV protection is less effective if only retrograde cardioplegia is given (the thebesian veins drain directly to the RV cavity rather than into the coronary sinus), and antegrade cardioplegia is less effective in the presence of severe right coronary artery stenosis. These problems are worse in the presence of RV hypertrophy.

- Air embolism down the right coronary artery during separation of the patient from cardiopulmonary bypass. The consequences of this are usually transient.
- The effects of positive pressure ventilation and PEEP, which act to reduce RV preload and increase RV afterload. Lung hyperinflation, particularly in the presence of PEEP, can cause RV compression on sternal closure.
- Occlusion or kinking of a right coronary graft.
- Incipient RV failure due to pre-existing pulmonary hypertension (e.g. as a result of MV or pulmonary disease).

In addition, specific procedures are associated with an increased likelihood of RV dysfunction. These include:

- Heart transplantation and lung transplantation (Chapter 14).
- The surgical correction of lesions causing RV volume overload (e.g. atrial septal defect or repair of a ruptured sinus of Valsalva aneurysm).
- The repair or replacement of diseased TVs (e.g. carcinoid heart disease).

### Pulmonary embolus

In the ICU, particularly in postoperative patients, pulmonary embolus should always be considered in the context of acute cardiorespiratory deterioration. A large pulmonary embolus results in a sudden increase in RV afterload. On TOE this is seen as RV dilatation and hypokinesis, diastolic septal flattening, functional tricuspid regurgitation and pulmonary hypertension. In addition, inspection of the IVC, RA, RV and pulmonary arteries may show thrombus or thrombus in transit. For patients with proven major pulmonary embolus, TOE can be used to visualise central emboli with a high sensitivity (97%) and specificity (86%).[11] It may be possible to differentiate fresh thrombus (which has a floating, protruding or elongated appearance) from old thrombus. Small emboli may not produce any echocardiographic abnormalities.

## TRICUSPID VALVE PATHOLOGY

The TV leaflets are thinner and anatomically less distinct than the MV leaflets. This, combined with the fact that the TV lies some distance from the oesophagus, means that the fine detail of leaflet morphology can be difficult to define clearly with TOE. Compared with the obvious opening and closing of the MV, the TV displays a fluttering motion and may even be mistaken for a Chiari network.

## TRICUSPID REGURGITATION

RV dilatation can cause tricuspid regurgitation despite normal leaflet morphology (**functional tricuspid regurgitation**). The mechanisms involve:

1. annular dilatation, which leads to incomplete leaflet closure and a (typically) central jet of regurgitation;
2. papillary muscle dysfunction and ventricular dilatation, which can result in leaflet tethering and restriction.

Asymmetrical leaflet restriction typically results in an eccentric regurgitant jet directed towards the affected leaflet.

If tricuspid regurgitation is identified but leaflet morphology appears normal, a careful search for underlying RV dysfunction should be made, looking in particular for evidence of pressure or volume overload and systolic dysfunction. The development of new or worsened tricuspid regurgitation should raise the question of RV dysfunction and possible pulmonary hypertension.

**Structural tricuspid regurgitation** is far less common than functional tricuspid regurgitation. Causes include:

- Rheumatic heart disease, usually in association with aortic and mitral disease. Leaflet thickening and restriction may be evident.

- TV prolapse (myxomatous degeneration) – This usually occurs in association with MV prolapse, especially in patients with floppy valve syndromes such as Marfan or Ehlers–Danlos. The septal and anterior leaflets are most often involved.

- Ebstein's anomaly – In this condition, one or more of the tricuspid leaflets (usually the septal alone, or in association with a second leaflet) are displaced toward the RV apex causing "atrialisation" of a portion of the RV. Apical displacement of the TV leads to a separation of the mitral and tricuspid planes by more than 11 mm.

- Carcinoid heart disease – This causes thickening, shortening and immobility of the leaflets, usually resulting in regurgitation. The presence of pathology involving both the tricuspid and pulmonary valves should always raise the possibility of carcinoid heart disease.

- Endocarditis – See below.

- Chest trauma – This can lead to tricuspid regurgitation due to ruptured chordae or papillary muscles, leading to leaflet flail.

- In addition to the causes of tricuspid regurgitation listed above, a ventricular pacing wire or a pulmonary artery catheter that crosses the TV will prevent normal leaflet coaptation, resulting in mild regurgitation.

### Tricuspid endocarditis

Endocarditis leads to regurgitation due to leaflet destruction and perforation, or a failure of coaptation due to the presence of vegetations.

Vegetations appear as oscillating masses, usually on the upstream (RA) surface of the valve, and commonly occur within a regurgitant jet pathway (p.83). Small lesions are easily missed on TOE. The presence of vegetations on the mitral or aortic valve should prompt the echocardiographer to examine the TV carefully, from multiple views. Endocarditis is the most common cause of tricuspid regurgitation in intravenous drug users. Typically such patients are infected with virulent organisms that cause bulky friable lesions with extensive leaflet damage and severe regurgitation.

### Grading tricuspid regurgitation

Tricuspid regurgitation can be evaluated with semiquantitative Doppler techniques in a manner similar to that described for mitral regurgitation (see Chapter 9). The overall grading of the regurgitation as mild, moderate or severe should be based on a combination of techniques.

### Colour flow Doppler

Colour flow Doppler provides a visual representation of the regurgitant jet and is a practical and simple method for the assessment of severity. However, the use of colour flow Doppler to interrogate the TV is limited by the fact that the colour sample must be placed in the far field, which reduces the detail of the flow abnormality. Image quality is maximised by reducing the size of the 2–D sector scan and of the colour sample.

## Jet area

Given the issue of image quality, most practitioners rely on a subjective assessment of jet area to grade the severity of tricuspid regurgitation. A jet area of less than one-third of the RA area is consistent with mild regurgitation. One-third to two-thirds is consistent with moderate regurgitation and greater than two-thirds with severe regurgitation. However, jet area is also influenced by changes in machine gain and scale settings and ventricular loading conditions (see Table 9.5). Furthermore, use of jet area tends to underestimate the severity of eccentric jets because of the Coanda effect (p.230). To assess asymmetrical or eccentric jets more accurately, the TV should be examined from multiple views.

## Vena contracta width

This is the narrowest neck of regurgitant flow just distal to the flow convergence region (see Figure 16.1). Assessment of the width of the vena contracta has been validated for the quantification of aortic and mitral regurgitation, and for tricuspid regurgitation with transthoracic echocardiography. With transthoracic echocardiography, a vena contracta width of the tricuspid regurgitant jet ≥ 6.5 mm, measured from the apical four-chamber view, indicates severe regurgitation.[12]

## Proximal isovelocity surface area

This is a well described method for quantification of mitral regurgitant severity (pp.236 and 237). The use of PISA for grading tricuspid regurgitation has been validated only for transthoracic echocardiography. As a simple qualitative guide, the presence of a proximal flow convergence zone on the RV side of the valve in systole suggests significant tricuspid regurgitation. For a given Nyquist limit, the PISA radius increases as the regurgitant volume increases.

## Hepatic venous PW Doppler

Severe tricuspid regurgitation alters flow in the vena cavae. IVC flow can be recorded by PW Doppler inspection of a hepatic vein (Figure 13.7) – no valves are present between the hepatic veins and the heart. The hepatic veins are visualised by turning the probe to the right at the level of the transgastric mid short axis view until the liver is seen. It may be necessary to rotate the transducer forward and to turn the shaft of the probe further to the right to align the vein adequately with the Doppler beam.

Severe tricuspid regurgitation causes reversal of the normal systolic forward flow in the hepatic vein. Blunting of the hepatic venous systolic flow implies moderate regurgitation. However, in the presence of marked RA dilatation, systolic flow may be antegrade despite severe regurgitation.

## Transtricuspid CW Doppler

With CW Doppler, the *intensity* of the regurgitant signal is determined by the volume of blood traversing the valve and the Doppler gain setting. Comparison of the intensity of the regurgitant (systolic) signal with the intensity of the diastolic inflow signal provides a guide to the severity of the regurgitation that is independent of the Doppler gain setting (p.145). As with mitral regurgitation severe, or acute-onset, tricuspid regurgitation may be associated with a V wave cutoff sign (p.145). Severe tricuspid regurgitation may be associated with pulmonary hypertension; if this is the case, the *velocity* of the regurgitant jet will be increased (p. 207).

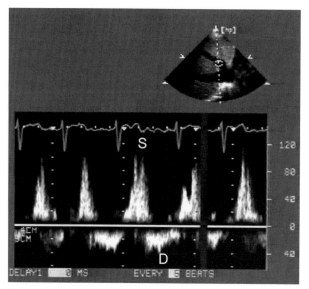

**Figure 13.7** Systolic flow reversal in a patient with severe tricuspid regurgitation. The Doppler signal was obtained from a transthoracic window, so the direction of flow is reversed compared with that seen with TOE. Flow in systole (S) is directed towards the transducer and away from the heart. Flow in diastole (D) is directed away from the transducer and towards the heart. No A wave is seen because the patient is in atrial fibrillation.

### Tricuspid valve repair

As the TV is subjected to relatively low pressures and the leaflets are usually morphologically normal, the valve is often amenable to successful repair, despite the presence of severe regurgitation.[13]

In the perioperative setting, the issue that arises most frequently is whether a tricuspid annuloplasty ring is required for functional tricuspid regurgitation in a patient undergoing surgery for left-sided heart disease (usually mitral regurgitation). When tricuspid regurgitation is mild, correction of the left-sided disease invariably eliminates the regurgitation. However, if the regurgitation is more severe, a tricuspid annuloplasty is usually warranted.[13]

## TRICUSPID STENOSIS

Tricuspid stenosis is rare. Causes include rheumatic heart disease (the most common cause), carcinoid heart disease and congenital abnormalities. Mass lesions in the RA (myxoma, thrombus and vegetations) may cause RV inflow obstruction leading to functional tricuspid stenosis.

Transthoracic imaging is better for assessing the aetiology and severity of tricuspid stenosis, but in the intraoperative setting examination with TOE is useful to rule out significant stenosis following TV repair.

Rheumatic disease causes leaflet thickening (usually starting at the leaflet tips) and diastolic doming. There may be accompanying thickening of the subvalvular structures and calcification of the leaflets. In the transgastric basal short axis view (with the image centred on the TV) commissural fusion may be evident.

Carcinoid heart disease causes characteristic thickening, shortening and immobility of the tricuspid leaflets and may result in stenosis. A search should also be made for thrombus in the RA.

### Grading tricuspid stenosis

With 2–D imaging, assessment should be made of the degree of leaflet immobility, thickening, diastolic doming and commissural fusion.

The severity of the stenosis can be graded by evaluating the transvalvular velocity profile using CW Doppler. This allows the peak and mean transvalvular velocity and pressure gradients to be estimated (pp.237–240). To assess stenosis accurately, it is important that the Doppler signal is aligned with diastolic flow; the valve should be examined from multiple views and the highest velocity used. Normal values are less than those for the MV: the normal peak E wave velocity is 0.5 m/s (range 0.3–0.7 m/s) and a mean pressure gradient of ≥5 mmHg is consistent with severe stenosis.[14] Peak transtricuspid velocity is also elevated in the presence of increased cardiac output and tricuspid regurgitation.

# PULMONARY VALVE PATHOLOGY

The PV is an anterior structure and is often poorly visualised with TOE. Unfortunately the substernal location of the PV also prevents optimal imaging by transthoracic echocardiography.

# PULMONARY REGURGITATION

Acquired pulmonary regurgitation is rare. Causes include pulmonary hypertension, endocarditis and carcinoid heart disease.

Mild pulmonary regurgitation is a normal variant. This can usually be assessed in the mid oesophageal AV short axis view. Congenital disease or carcinoid involvement may result in thickening and deformity of the leaflets. Pulmonary regurgitation may be assessed by the use of colour flow Doppler to estimate jet area and width, and CW Doppler to assess the intensity of the regurgitant signal. Holodiastolic flow reversal detected by PW Doppler in the main pulmonary artery indicates significant regurgitation. Severe pulmonary regurgitation leads to RV volume overload and functional tricuspid regurgitation.

# PULMONARY STENOSIS

Pulmonary stenosis is usually secondary to congenital obstruction, which may be subvalvular, valvular or supravalvular. Poststenotic pulmonary artery dilatation may be present.

Quantification of pulmonary stenosis requires estimation of the peak or mean transvalvular pressure gradient with CW Doppler. However, with TOE optimal alignment of the Doppler signal with valvular flow is frequently not possible.

# REFERENCES

1. Reichert CLA, Visser CA, Koolen JJ, et al. Transesophageal echocardiography in hypotensive patients after cardiac operations. *Journal of Thoracic and Cardiovascular Surgery* 1992;104:321–326.
2. Reichert CLA, Visser CA, van den Brink RBA, et al. Prognostic value of biventricular function in hypotensive patients after cardiac surgery as assessed by transesophageal echocardiography. *Journal of Cardiothoracic and Vascular Anesthesia* 1992;6: 429–432.
3. Dell'Italia LJ. The right ventricle: anatomy, physiology, and clinical importance. *Current Problems in Cardiology* 1991;16:653–720.
4. Barnard D, Alpert JS. Right ventricular function in health and disease. *Current Problems in Cardiology* 1987;12:417–449.

5.  Shanewise JS, Cheung AT, Aronson S, et al. ASE/SCA guidelines for performing a comprehensive intraoperative multiplane transesophageal echocardiography examination: recommendations of the American Society of Echocardiography Council for Intraoperative Echocardiography and the Society of Cardiovascular Anesthesiologists Task Force for Certification in Perioperative Transesophageal Echocardiography. *Anesthesia and Analgesia* 1999;89: 870–884.

6.  Ochiai Y, Morita S, Tanoue Y, et al. Use of transesophageal echocardiography for postoperative evaluation of right ventricular function. *Annals of Thoracic Surgery* 1999;67:146–153.

7.  Rafferty T, Durkin M, Harris S, et al. Transesophageal two-dimensional echocardiographic analysis of right ventricular systolic performance indices during coronary artery bypass grafting. *Journal of Cardiothoracic and Vascular Anesthesia* 1993;7: 160–166.

8.  Yock PG, Popp RL. Noninvasive estimation of right ventricular systolic pressure by Doppler ultrasound in patients with tricuspid regurgitation. *Circulation* 1984;70:657–662.

9.  Kitabatake A, Inoue M, Asao M, et al. Noninvasive evaluation of pulmonary hypertension by a pulsed Doppler technique. *Circulation* 1983;68:302–309.

10. Stevenson JG. Comparison of several noninvasive methods for estimation of pulmonary artery pressure. *Journal of the American Society of Echocardiography* 1989;2:157–171.

11. Wittlich N, Erbel R, Eichler A, et al. Detection of central pulmonary artery thromboemboli by transesophageal echocardiography in patients with severe pulmonary embolism. *Journal of the American Society of Echocardiography* 1992;5:515–524.

12. Tribouilloy CM, Enriquez-Sarano M, Bailey KR, et al. Quantification of tricuspid regurgitation by measuring the width of the vena contracta with Doppler color flow imaging: a clinical study. *Journal of the American College of Cardiology* 2000;36:472–478.

13. Hammond GL, Franco KL. Mitral, tricuspid, and aortic valve repair or reconstruction. *Current Opinion in Cardiology* 1997;12:100–107.

14. Grossman W. Profiles in valvular heart disease. In: Grossman W, Baim DS (eds). *Cardiac Catheterization, Angiography and Interventions*, 5th Edition. Baltimore: Williams and Wilkins, 1996:735–756.

# 14.

# Transplantation and Mechanical Cardiac Support

*Andrew McKee*

The management of patients undergoing transplantation or the placement of mechanical cardiac assist devices presents some of the greatest challenges in cardiac surgery and cardiac anaesthesia. Given the value of TOE in the management of complex cardiac surgical procedures generally, it is not difficult to appreciate its utility in this particular subset of patients. Furthermore, there are also a number of problems that can develop during these operations that can only be detected using TOE.

## HEART TRANSPLANTATION

End-stage ischaemic heart disease and dilated cardiomyopathy are the most common indications for heart transplantation. Patients with these conditions frequently have a degree of mitral and tricuspid regurgitation and pulmonary hypertension.

### Prebypass
The extent of pulmonary hypertension should be evaluated (p.207) as this may have deteriorated since the patient underwent a preoperative right heart catheter study. In addition, it is useful to search for the presence of aortic atheroma (important if an intra-aortic balloon pump is required) and for the presence of pleural effusions (as these can be drained by the surgeon).

More detailed examination of the native heart is not warranted.

### Postbypass
TOE allows assessment of preload and systolic function, detection of any valvular abnormalities, evaluation of the surgical anastomoses, and monitoring of the effectiveness of de-airing. Transplanted hearts all show some degree of impaired contractility, and the RV in particular is vulnerable to air emboli and to the effects of poor myocardial protection during harvesting. Acute RV failure is one of the most serious short-term complications following cardiac transplantation and is usually due to elevated pulmonary vascular resistance in combination with the factors mentioned above. The RV usually recovers with time, but a period of inotropic support may be required.

The donor heart is smaller than the native heart, more medial and rotated clockwise. Placing a small heart in a larger pericardial space creates room for fluid to accumulate and makes haemodynamically significant tamponade somewhat less likely.

A small degree of mitral and tricuspid regurgitation is common after heart transplantation; this usually resolves, but occasionally persists and even worsens over a number of years.[1]

Assessment of the pulmonary, aortic and LA suture lines is important. A small ridge is commonly seen at the site of the anastomosis in the pulmonary artery but there should not be a measurable gradient across this. The aortic anastomosis is not normally visible. The LA suture line usually appears as an echodense ridge within the atrium (Figure 14.1).

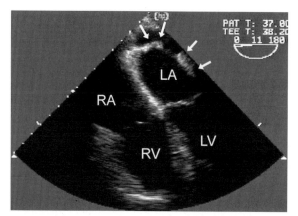

**Figure 14.1** LA suture line following heart transplantation: mid oesophageal four-chamber view. A prominent ridge can be seen straddling the LA (arrows). This is due to the LA suture line and gives the appearances of a partial cor triatriatum (see Chapter 5).

Residual native atrial tissue can create the appearance of an unusual echo-free space behind the heart (p.75) or give the appearance of an inverted LA appendage (pp.74–75; Figure 5.6). If the atrial suture line is too tight it can result in acquired cor triatriatum an a mid atrial stenosis.[2] New atrial septal defects have been reported following heart transplantation.[3]

# LUNG TRANSPLANTATION

Patients undergoing lung transplantation usually have minimal cardiorespiratory reserve. The procedure requires one-lung ventilation and manipulation of the heart, and these interventions are often poorly tolerated. Most patients have pre-existing pulmonary hypertension and RV dysfunction. Any further increase in pulmonary vascular resistance in this situation can precipitate acute RV failure and the need for urgent cardiopulmonary bypass; monitoring of RV function is therefore essential. It is also useful to assess the pulmonary and tricuspid valves, LV function and filling, and the pulmonary venous anastomoses.

## Right ventricular function

Quantitative assessment of RV contractility is difficult, but careful qualitative evaluation of filling and global RV function may provide important information on impending haemodynamic collapse that may not be apparent from a pulmonary artery catheter. It is useful to position the sector scan in the mid oesophageal four-chamber view centred on the RV, so that RV function can be continuously monitored in a "hands-off" manner.

Acute RVOT obstruction has been reported after transplantation in patients with severe RV hypertrophy when faced with sudden increases in pulmonary vascular resistance.[4] In most lung transplant patients who develop early acute RV failure, the cause is elevated pulmonary vascular resistance. This may arise from pulmonary oedema (secondary to reperfusion injury or acute rejection) or from pulmonary venous obstruction related to the surgical anastomoses. Tricuspid incompetence may be a manifestation of RV failure and may aggravate its haemodynamic consequences.

## Assessment of the interatrial septum and pulmonary veins

Two anatomical structures that specifically need to be examined in these patients are the interatrial septum and the pulmonary veins. Obstruction to normal pulmonary venous blood flow and right-to-left shunting through a patent foramen ovale (p.222) are the most common structural causes of hypoxia following lung transplantation. Abnormal right-to-left bowing of the interatrial septum is indicative of elevated RA pressure (p.207).

The pulmonary veins should be evaluated carefully for any signs of obstruction. Because of their posterior position the anastomoses are poorly seen through the surgical incision (particularly when the lungs are inflated) but are usually well visualised with TOE.[5] A region of narrowing may be seen on 2-D imaging, but pulmonary vein stenosis is best evaluated with colour Doppler, where a region of flow narrowing or aliasing may be identified. On PW Doppler, pulmonary vein stenosis results in loss of the phasic S, D and A waves and an overall increase in velocity. Pulmonary vein stenosis is an important cause of resistant pulmonary oedema and hypoxia following lung transplantation.[6]

The anterior location of the pulmonary artery anastomoses renders them difficult to visualise with TOE, but easy to inspect by the surgeon.

# MECHANICAL CARDIAC SUPPORT

## Positioning an intra-aortic balloon pump

The tip of the balloon catheter should be positioned just distal to the origin of the left subclavian artery. First, locate the left subclavian artery in the upper oesophageal aortic arch short axis view, then rotate back to 0° and advance the probe 1–2 cm; the aorta should now appear as a circle. Both the Seldinger wire and the balloon catheter can be seen as they are advanced in the aorta. When the tip of the balloon catheter is seen, the position is correct. Intra-aortic balloon pumps should be used with caution in patients with descending aortic aneurysms, moderate-to-severe aortic incompetence or severe atheroma (especially mobile plaque), and these conditions should be evaluated with TOE before insertion.

## Placing a left ventricular assist device

Left ventricular assist devices (LVADs) can be divided into two types – those for long-term use and those for short-term use.

The former are used as a bridge to transplantation in patients with end-stage LV dysfunction. Two examples are the Heartmate (Thoratec Inc.) and Novacor (Worldheart Inc.). Both devices drain blood from the LV apex and return blood to the proximal ascending aorta.

Devices for short-term use are usually used in an attempt to provide a bridge to recovery in patients who cannot be weaned from cardiopulmonary bypass. Blood is drained from the LA and returned to the proximal ascending aorta. The Thoratec (Thoratec Inc.) and Abiomed BVS 5000 (Abiomed Inc.) systems are examples, which can also be used as RV or biventricular assist devices. The comments below refer specifically to the bridge to transplantation devices implanted into the LV apex.

### Assessment preinsertion

Before placing an LVAD, it is important to look for the following specific abnormalities.

*Patent foramen ovale*

Patients with end-stage LV dysfunction often have elevated RA pressure. When the LVAD starts functioning, the LA pressure falls almost to zero. This can lead to right-to-left shunting across a patent foramen ovale (or other atrial septal defect), causing systemic desaturation and the risk of paradoxical embolisation. If such a defect is identified, then bicaval cannulation will be required, and the lesion should be repaired before the LVAD is activated.

### Aortic regurgitation

The LVAD withdraws blood from the LV and ejects it into the aorta. If significant aortic regurgitation exists then blood ejected into the aorta at high pressure will leak back into the decompressed LV, causing the pump to cycle faster without increasing systemic output. The LV may distend, with consequent reduction in coronary perfusion. Repair or replacement of the AV at the time of implantation is advocated by some authors if the regurgitation is more than mild.[7]

### Mitral stenosis

As LVAD inflow depends on passive flow through the MV, significant mitral stenosis will limit maximal pump flow.

### Intracavity thrombus

Patients with ventricular or atrial dilatation are at risk of developing thrombus (pp.82–83), which may be dislodged during LVAD insertion. The LA appendage and the LV apex are the most common sites for thrombus to develop (the LV apex is difficult to visualise reliably with TOE).

### Aortic atheroma

See pp.173–176.

### RV dysfunction

RV function is critical for the postoperative management and outcome of these patients.[8,9] Evaluation of the RV, and of the degree of tricuspid regurgitation (a marker of RV function), before insertion of the device is useful for comparative purposes later, when the LVAD is functioning.

## Assessment during insertion

### Positioning of inlet cannula

The inlet cannula for these devices sits in the apex of the LV. It is important that the cannula is central, does not lie against the ventricular wall, and is free of the mitral apparatus. These points can be checked in the mid oesophageal ventricular views (four-chamber or two-chamber). The position of the cannula should also allow the LV to drain completely, to maximise device stroke volume. Evidence of aliasing on colour flow Doppler or increased velocity on PW Doppler in the cannula orifice indicates obstruction to blood flow. The obstruction can usually be corrected by surgical repositioning of the inflow conduit.[7]

### De-airing

The adequacy of de-airing before activation of the device should be assessed by looking for "fireflies" in the descending thoracic aorta (the ascending aorta can be difficult to visualise). Aortic venting may be required.

## Activation of the device

The LVAD should be activated slowly. At this stage it is important to assess RV function and to check again for a patent foramen ovale. The AV should also be checked for regurgitation, and LA and LV decompression observed as the device begins to function. In fixed-rate mode the device can entrain air from around the sewing ring (and other sites) if poor ventricular filling leads to LV collapse around the cannula.

## Postbypass

The differential diagnosis of low pump flows includes hypovolaemia, tamponade, RV failure, inflow or outflow cannula obstruction and pulmonary embolism. Unexpectedly high flow rates, particularly in the later postoperative period, suggest sepsis, but aortic regurgitation needs to be excluded. Regurgitation through the inflow and outflow cannula valves has also been reported,[7] and can produce a clinical picture similar to that of volume overload.

## Establishing extracorporeal membrane oxygenation

Extracorporeal membrane oxygenation (ECMO) is predominantly used in neonates with persistent fetal circulation (usually due to meconium aspiration), but is sometimes used in adults with conditions such as myocarditis and pulmonary embolism (venoarterial: V–A) or pneumonia and adult respiratory distress syndrome (venoveno: V–V). V–A ECMO provides biventricular and respiratory support while V–V ECMO provides respiratory support only.

TOE is useful for ensuring the correct position of the venous drainage cannula within the RA. From the mid oesophageal bicaval view, the echocardiographer can follow a cannula as it is advanced into the RA from either the femoral or jugular vein (the venous drainage catheter is typically placed in the jugular vein for V–V ECMO but may be placed in either position for V–A ECMO).

Some patients placed on V–A ECMO who have minimal or no LV ejection (e.g. ventricular fibrillation) are at risk of LV distension and acute pulmonary oedema. TOE is useful for confirming this diagnosis and monitoring the response to treatment, such as percutaneous atrial septostomy or surgical septectomy. Unlike LVAD placement, a patent foramen ovale is not of major concern as, assuming correct function of the circuit, RA pressure will be low.

TOE is also useful in confirming the diagnosis of tamponade (a particular problem in postcardiopulmonary bypass ECMO), and in monitoring ventricular function and filling during weaning from ECMO.

# REFERENCES

1. Cladellas M, Abadal ML, Pons-Lladó G, et al. Early transient multivalvular regurgitation detected by pulsed Doppler in cardiac transplantation. American Journal of Cardiology 1986;58:1122–1124.

2. Oaks TE, Rayburn BK, Brown ME, et al. Acquired cor triatriatum after orthotopic cardiac transplantation. Annals of Thoracic Surgery 1995;59:751–753.

3. Voci P, Chiera A, Caretta Q, et al. Acquired atrial septal defect after heart transplantation. Journal of Heart and Lung Transplantation 1999;18:921–923.

4. Suriani RJ. Transesophageal echocardiography during organ transplantation. Journal of Cardiothoracic and Vascular Anesthesia 1998;12:686–694.

5. Hausmann D, Daniel WG, Mügge A, et al. Imaging of pulmonary artery and vein anastomoses by transesophageal echocardiography after lung transplantation. Circulation 1992;86:II251–II258.

6. Schulman LL, Anandarangam T, Leibowitz DW, et al. Four-year prospective study of pulmonary venous thrombosis after lung transplantation. Journal of the American Society of Echocardiography 2001;14: 806–812.

7. Scalia GM, McCarthy PM, Savage RM, et al. Clinical utility of echocardiography in the management of implantable ventricular assist devices. Journal of the American Society of Echocardiography 2000;13: 754–763.

8. Henry D, Lim LL-Y, García Rodríguez LA, et al. Variability in risk of gastrointestinal complications with individual non-steroidal anti-inflammatory drugs: results of a collaborative meta-analysis. British Medical Journal 1996;312:1563–1566.

9. Savage RM, Scalia G, Smidera N, et al. Intraoperative echocardiography is indicated in implantable left ventricular assist device placement [abstract]. Journal of the American Society of Echocardiography 1996; 9:375.

# 15

# Adult Congenital Heart Disease

*Roger Hall*
*Thomas Gentles*

Congenital heart disease is common, occurring in approximately 1% of all live births, and includes a diverse range of conditions from the innocuous to the lethal. The population seen in adulthood is different from that seen in childhood. Reasons for this include the effects of cumulative mortality and the fact that most surgery for congenital heart disease is carried out in children (often in the neonatal period). In addition, some conditions that are present at birth may disappear over time (e.g. patent ductus arteriosus and some ventricular septal defects – VSDs). Thus many adults with congenital heart disease have already undergone either an anatomical correction or a palliative procedure.

The role of intraoperative TOE in this group of patients is similar to that in other adults undergoing cardiac surgery, namely:

- Assessment of ventricular function.
- Assessment of valvular function and the adequacy of valve repair.
- Troubleshooting difficulties in separating patients from cardiopulmonary bypass.
- In addition, operation-specific assessment of intracardiac repairs and connections may also be required.

Patients with congenital heart disease present to the adult TOE practitioner under three circumstances:

- When patients with known congenital heart disease require "routine" adult surgery (e.g. coronary artery bypass grafting).
- When a congenital lesion presents as an unexpected intraoperative finding.
- When the congenital lesion is the primary reason for surgery.

This last group of patients will most commonly have either a simple lesion (e.g. an atrial septal defect – ASD) or a lesion requiring a "standard" adult operation (e.g. replacement of a congenitally bicuspid valve or repair of a cleft mitral leaflet). The lesions commonly seen in these three groups fall within the scope of standard adult TOE, and are the subject of this chapter. In contrast, the echocardiographic assessment of complex congenital heart lesions is highly specialised and should be be undertaken only by an appropriately trained and experienced practitioner. In most centres this will be a cardiologist with training in congenital heart disease.

## ATRIAL SEPTAL DEFECTS

ASDs are associated with RV volume overload that is usually well tolerated and frequently results in only minor limitation in exercise tolerance. However, with each passing decade the risks increase of developing atrial arrhythmias (as a consequence of atrial dilatation), RV dysfunction and, less commonly, pulmonary hypertension. In addition, the presence of an ASD or patent foramen ovale is associated with an increased risk of cerebral events related to paradoxical embolism. Consequently the chance finding of an ASD always warrants further investigation.

ASDs may be further classified into the following subtypes: primum, secundum, sinus venosus or coronary sinus. Irrespective of the type of ASD, echocardiographic features of RA and RV volume overload, paradoxical septal motion and pulmonary hypertension may be present.

## Secundum atrial septal defect

Over 80% of ASDs are of the secundum subtype. The defect is confined to the fossa ovalis. When there is no deficiency in septal tissue but an interatrial communication exists, the defect is more correctly termed a **patent foramen ovale** (PFO). A secundum ASD may be seen in the mid oesophageal four-chamber and bicaval views (Figures 15.1a and 15.2). Colour flow Doppler should be used to confirm shunt direction, which in most cases will be left-to-right. Shunting occurs predominantly during *diastole*. The Nyquist limit should be set at a low level (<30 cm/s) to highlight low-velocity transseptal flow.

Detection of a PFO may be difficult. The foramen ovale acts as a trapdoor that opens from the RA to the LA (Figure 15.3). Sometimes an edge of the septum primum may prolapse, allowing a small left-to-right shunt. The foramen will usually be closed, except when RA pressure is higher than LA pressure.

One method of demonstrating a right-to-left shunt across a PFO is to inject 10 ml of agitated saline into a systemic vein; in the presence of such a shunt this rapidly results in a contrast effect ("fireflies") within the LA. The detection rate is substantially improved by transiently raising RA pressure. In a ventilated patient this can be achieved by the

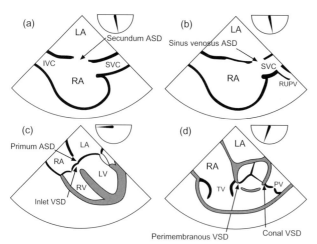

**Figure 15.1** Common types of ASD and VSD. (a, b) Secundum and sinus venosus ASDs in the mid-oesophageal bicaval view; (b) also demonstrates partial anomalous pulmonary venous return, which is commonly associated with a sinus venosus ASD. (c) A primum ASD and inlet VSD from the mid oesophageal four-chamber view. These defects may occur together as part of an atrioventricular canal defect. (d) Mid oesophageal RV inflow–outflow view with perimembranous and conal VSDs. These defects do not usually occur together, but both can lead to AV cusp prolapse and aortic incompetence.

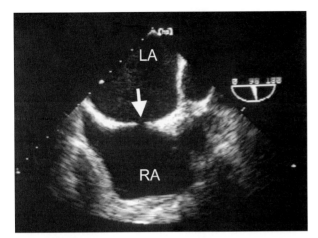

**Figure 15.2** Secundum ASD (arrow) from the mid oesophageal bicaval view.

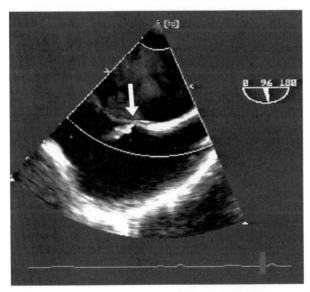

**Figure 15.3** In this modified mid oesophageal bicaval view a patent foramen ovale (arrow) has been identified with colour flow Doppler.

release of a large positive pressure breath. This manoeuvre should be routinely performed in conjunction with the injection of agitated saline.

MV prolapse is associated with secundum ASDs and should be actively sought. A small number of secundum ASDs are associated with anomalous pulmonary venous drainage, most commonly of the right pulmonary veins.

TOE has an important role in guiding transcatheter closure of secundum ASDs. It is important to determine whether there is a sufficient rim of normal atrial tissue between the defect and adjacent structures, including the mitral and tricuspid valves, the pulmonary veins and the cavae, before deploying the device. TOE also allows assessment of any residual defect following device deployment.

## Primum atrial septal defect

A primum ASD is part of a constellation of conditions known as endocardial cushion defects. These defects range from a simple ASD to a complete atrioventricular canal defect, and include atrial and ventricular septal defects and varying degrees of tricuspid and mitral valve abnormality.

With TOE, a primum ASD is best seen in the modified mid oesophageal four-chamber view with the probe turned to the right to centre on the interatrial septum (Figures 15.1c and 15.4). The defect occurs adjacent to the mitral and tricuspid valves, which appear to arise at the same level (rather than from different levels with slight ventricular displacement of the TV as is normally seen). A cleft anterior mitral leaflet (which may be regurgitant) is commonly associated with a primum ASD. In addition, a VSD may be seen just below the atrioventricular valves.

## Sinus venosus and coronary sinus atrial septal defects

Sinus venosus defects occur in the region of the superior or inferior vena cavae, most frequently at the junction of the RA and SVC. A superior defect is usually visible in a modified mid-oesophageal bicaval view, obtained by turning the shaft of the probe to the right (clockwise) from the standard position (Figures 15.1b and 15.5).

Superior defects are associated with anomalous drainage of the right upper pulmonary vein (Figure 15.1b). If the defect extends inferiorly there may also be anomalous drainage of the right lower pulmonary vein.

A coronary sinus ASD is rare, and is a defect in the roof of the coronary sinus that allows communication between the right and left atria via the coronary sinus ostium. This type of defect may be associated with a persistent left SVC that may appear to drain directly into the LA.

An isolated left SVC that drains to the coronary sinus is a normal variant. It may be easily identified by the injection of agitated saline into a left arm vein, which will rapidly produce opacification of the coronary sinus. A left SVC may be associated with other congenital anomalies, including anomalous drainage of the left pulmonary veins,

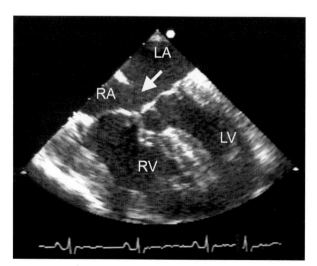

**Figure 15.4** Primum ASD (arrow): mid-oesophageal four-chamber view.

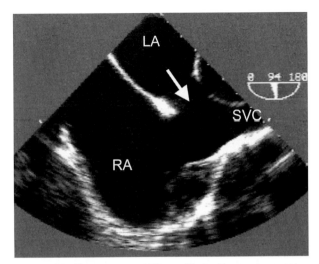

**Figure 15.5** Sinus venosus ASD: modified mid oesophageal bicaval view.

hypoplasia of left-sided structures (e.g. mitral stenosis or coarctation), and other complex congenital heart disease. When the left SVC drains to the coronary sinus the latter structure will be large (see Figure 5.3) and the left SVC may be visualised anterior to the left upper pulmonary vein (see Figure 5.14).

## VENTRICULAR SEPTAL DEFECTS

Nearly all VSDs have either closed spontaneously or have been surgically corrected by adulthood. Thus, adult patients with a VSD usually have either a small defect of no haemodynamic significance or a large defect with severe pulmonary vascular obstructive disease to an extent that repair is contraindicated.

The anatomy of the ventricular septum is complex and the nomenclature confusing. When viewed from the RV, the septum can be divided into **muscular** and **subaortic** components. The muscular septum can be divided into **inlet**, **mid**, **apical** and **anterior** regions, while the subaortic septum can be divided into the **membranous** septum and **conal** septum. The membranous septum is a small oval-shaped area adjacent to the TV (in the region of the junction of the septal and anterior leaflets), which lies below the ridge of the crista supraventricularis. VSDs in this region are known as **membranous** or **perimembranous**.

The RVOT lies above the crista supraventricularis. VSDs in this region are termed **conal** or **subpulmonary**. Both perimembranous and conal defects communicate with the LVOT and can be visualised in the mid oesophageal RV inflow–outflow view; a perimembranous defect can be seen adjacent to the TV and a conal defect can be seen adjacent to the PV (Figure 15.1d). Each of these defects (particularly conal) can lead to prolapse of the adjacent AV cusp and aortic incompetence.

Inlet and mid-muscular defects may be visible in the mid oesophageal four-chamber or transgastric short-axis views, but apical VSDs are frequently difficult to visualise with TOE because of the distance of the apical septum from the transducer. In a complete atrioventricular canal defect there is a deficiency of the atrioventricular septum resulting in an inlet VSD. This is best visualised in the mid oesophageal four-chamber view, where the VSD is seen immediately below the septal leaflet of the TV (Figure 15.1c).

Large VSDs produce predominantly LA and LV volume overload and pulmonary hypertension. Compared to ASDs, RV overload is less pronounced. Colour flow Doppler is useful to determine both the site of the defect (which may not be apparent on 2-D imaging) and the direction of flow. In contrast to ASDs, shunting occurs predominantly in *systole*. If possible, interrogation of the defect with CW Doppler is useful to determine the physiological significance of the lesion. The RV systolic pressure, and therefore the pulmonary artery systolic pressure, can be estimated as the difference between the systemic systolic blood pressure and the calculated systolic pressure difference between the two ventricles (p.241). In general, large VSDs that are unrestrictive to flow are associated with low velocities and small VSDs that are restrictive to flow are associated with high velocities.

## TETRALOGY OF FALLOT

Tetralogy of Fallot consists of a VSD, an aorta that overrides the VSD, RV hypertrophy and pulmonary stenosis that is usually subvalvular and often also valvular. There may also be hypoplasia of the branch pulmonary arteries.

In developed countries, virtually all patients with this condition undergo correction in early childhood, but late sequelae may present in adulthood. In particular, repair of the RVOT and PV frequently results in significant pulmonary regurgitation, which is initially well tolerated; however, in later life the chronic volume overload may cause progressive RV dilatation and dysfunction. Under these circumstances PV replacement may be beneficial.

The echocardiographic features are those of pulmonary regurgitation, and RV dilatation and dysfunction. Pulmonary regurgitation is best seen in the mid oesophageal RV inflow–outflow view.

Some patients with tetralogy of Fallot also have pulmonary atresia and require a valved conduit from the RV to the pulmonary artery. These conduits may be of homograft, xenograft or prosthetic material and are prone to calcification, stenosis and regurgitation. They are anterior structures and therefore are often poorly visualised with TOE.

## PALLIATION FOR SINGLE-VENTRICLE LESIONS

Patients with single right (e.g. tricuspid atresia) or left (e.g. double-inlet LV) ventricle lesions usually undergo a staged palliation in which the end result is a Fontan-type circulation. There are a number of variations, but all have the common feature of SVC and IVC return passing directly to the pulmonary artery:

- The SVC is usually connected directly to the pulmonary artery.
- The IVC connection may be more complicated, involving an intra-atrial baffle or extra cardiac conduit. With this arrangement, pulmonary blood flow is dependent on an unobstructed cavopulmonary connection, low pulmonary vascular resistance and a low LA pressure. Failure to meet any of these conditions may result in low cardiac output and elevated systemic venous pressure. To minimise this problem a small (4–5 mm) connection or fenestration is frequently created between the systemic venous pathway and the pulmonary venous atrium. This allows cardiac output to be maintained at the cost of oxygen saturation.

Formal assessment of the Fontan-type circulation remains within the realm of the specialist congenital echocardiographer. However, patients with this anatomy may present for other reasons to the adult TOE practitioner. In such situations the examination should focus on ventricular function and filling, and on the atroventricular valve. In the poorly functioning Fontan circulation, systemic venous pressure is likely to be markedly elevated and there may be significant enlargement of the systemic venous pathway, particularly if it incorporates the RA. Spontaneous echo contrast may be present and thrombosis within the cavopulmonary pathway should be excluded. The systemic ventricle may be dilated and there may be significant ventricular dysfunction and bilateral pleural effusions.

# 16

# Aspects of Quantitative and Semiquantitative Echocardiography

*Alan Merry*

The aim in this chapter is to explain the theory underlying some of the quantitative and semi-quantitative methods used in perioperative TOE to estimate cardiac output, to evaluate the orifice size in valve lesions and to estimate pressures and pressure gradients. Most of the quantitative methods involve simple algebra, geometry and physics. However, it is often difficult to obtain accurate data for the calculations, so their results should always be interpreted in the light of other echocardiographic and clinical information. The application of the theory presented in this chapter to particular clinical situations is discussed elsewhere in the book.

## BASIC CONCEPTS

Blood is a fluid. The defining characteristic of a fluid is that it is capable of flowing from one place to another under the influence of force. Force per unit area is pressure. Pressure and flow are integrally related, because fluids flow down pressure gradients.

Neither flow nor pressure can be measured directly with echocardiography but the **Doppler effect** allows the velocity of blood to be estimated (Chapter 3), and the dimensions of cardiac structures can be obtained with 2-D imaging. From this information volumes and flows can be derived. The pressure gradient across a restrictive orifice can also be estimated from velocity (using the simplified Bernoulli equation). This provides a means of grading the severity of valvular stenoses and of estimating an unknown pressure on one side of a restrictive orifice from a known pressure on the other side. The rate of change of a pressure gradient provides an alternative approach to the estimation of orifice size in mitral stenosis and aortic incompetence – the pressure half-time method.

## JETS

As blood flowing down a pressure gradient approaches a narrow orifice it speeds up. This results in characteristic appearances proximal to, at and distal to the orifice (Figure 16.1). The semiquantitative interpretation of these appearances is an integral part of the evaluation of valvular lesions with echocardiography (Chapters 9, 10 and 13).

Proximal to the orifice, depending on its size, the pressure gradient and the settings of the machine, more than one PISA (p.235) may become visible with colour flow Doppler. The dimensions of the PISA can be used to assess the size of the valvular orifice.

The narrowest point of flow occurs just distal to the orifice and is called the **vena contracta.** The width of the vena contracta (seen with colour flow Doppler) is used in grading the severity of valvular regurgitation (pp.144, 166 and 211).

Distal to the vena contracta a **jet** is formed. Blood flow velocity decreases but, in accordance with the principle of conservation of momentum, the **jet** entrains mass and its volume increases. The volume of the fully developed jet is a function of its kinetic energy. The area of a jet, seen with colour flow Doppler, is usually assumed to be

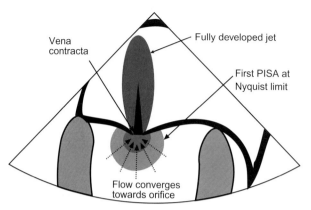

**Figure 16.1** Appearances on colour Doppler as blood converges towards a regurgitant MV orifice (see text).

proportional to its volume. In theory, therefore, jet area may be an index of lesion severity; however, a jet is three dimensional and its cross-sectional area may vary from plane to plane. Furthermore the dimensions of the jet may be affected by the geometry of the orifice, and by many other physiological, physical and machine-related factors.

Jets may be defined as **free** or **confined**:

- A free jet flows into the centre of a relatively stagnant chamber (such as the LA) whose cross-sectional area is large in comparison with that of the jet (see Figure 12.4). The geometry of a free jet is unaffected by the boundaries of the chamber.

- In contrast, solid boundaries close to the jet (e.g. in aortic stenosis or eccentric mitral regurgitation) will modify its geometry and confine its volume (the **Coanda effect** is the tendency of a jet to follow a surface, especially a convex surface). Reliance on jet size may then lead to an underestimation of lesion severity.

Jets may also be affected by interaction with other jets. Dual jet interaction will attenuate the size of the jet of interest if the second jet is in the opposite direction, and accentuate it if the second jet is in the same direction.

The intensities of the flow signals obtained with CW Doppler for jets and normal flows, at a particular gain setting, depend on the number of blood cells from which the echo beam has been reflected in each case and their comparison provides an alternative index of jet volume (see Figure 9.14).

## USING VELOCITY TO ESTIMATE FLOW AND VALVE AREAS

### Flow as a function of velocity and cross-sectional area

Consider a rigid uniform cylinder of radius $r$, through which flows blood containing cells from which the echo signal is reflected (Figure 16.2). Assume flow is constant, laminar (i.e. the blood is moving along parallel streams with uniform flow velocities, with the cells all moving in the same direction) and has a flat flow–velocity profile (i.e. cells in the parallel streams at the centre of the structure flow at the same speed as cells in the streams near its sides). If the blood moves a distance $s$ over time $t$, then velocity ($V$) will equal $s/t$. Flow ($Q$) will equal the product of $V$ (the distance travelled by blood in a given direction per unit time) and the cylinder's cross-sectional area (CSA). Flow is the volume of blood passing a given point per unit time. Units of measurement are very important

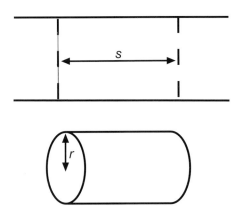

**Figure 16.2** The volume of a section of a cylinder of radius $r$ cm and length $s$ cm is given by cross-sectional area $\times s$ cm$^3$ (cross-sectional area = $\pi r^2$).

and should be included in each step of any haemodynamic calculation. Typically $V$ is in cm/s or m/s, $s$ is in cm or m, CSA is in cm$^2$ and Q is in ml/s or l/min. Thus:

$$V = \frac{s}{t}$$

(Equation 16.1)

and

$$Q = CSA \times V$$

(Equation 16.2)

## Calculation of cross-sectional area

Because there are often difficulties in obtaining the CSA of a cardiac structure using planimetry, certain shapes have been attributed empirically to particular structures for the (approximate) calculation of CSA by standard formulae using dimensions obtained with 2-D imaging (Table 16.1).

## Accounting for varying flow

The assumption that flow is laminar and has a flat profile is reasonable in great vessels and across normal cardiac valves (although it may not always be true when pathological valve lesions are involved). However, cardiac structures are not usually uniform cylinders and the velocity of blood flow varies as CSA changes during the progression of the blood through the heart and great vessels. Furthermore, blood flow is pulsatile, starting from approximately zero velocity, accelerating to a maximum velocity, and then decelerating back to zero velocity. This is represented as a velocity–time curve on the spectral Doppler display (see, for example, Figures 4.25–4.28). Mean velocity is distance over time: $V_{mean} = \frac{s}{t}$ (typical units: cm/s or m/s) as in Equation 16.1, but in echocardiography the time used to calculate mean velocities is always one pulse period. Velocity at any instant is the differential of distance with respect to time: $V = \frac{ds}{dt}$. Conversely, the distance travelled by blood over any particular period is the product of mean velocity and time: $s = V_{mean} \times t$. It is also the integral of instantaneous velocity with respect to time: $s = \int v.dt$ (typical units: cm or m; note that cm/s $\times$ s = cm). This distance is the area under the velocity–time curve, and is known as the **velocity–time integral** (VTI). Most ultrasound machines calculate VTI automatically once the outline of a flow pattern (its velocity–time curve) has been traced.

**Table 16.1** Cross-sectional shapes attributed to various intracardiac structures, and the formula for calculating area in each case; $r$ is the radius and $d$ the diameter of a circle or ellipse. Formulae are often quoted for $d$ instead of $r$ ($\pi r^2 = \pi(d/2)^2 = \pi/4 \times d^2$ and $\pi/4 = 0.785$). For the AV, $s$ is the length of a side of an equilateral triangle, measured in the mid oesophageal AV short axis view from commissure to commissure. If the formula for an ellipse is used, the MV annulus should be measured in its long (see Figure 9.7) and short (see Figure 9.9) axes, but a recent report from the American Society of Echocardiography recommends the application of circular geometry to the MV annulus[1]

| Structure | Assumed cross-sectional shape | Formula for area |
|---|---|---|
| LVOT | Circle | $\pi r^2$ or $0.785\,d^2$ |
| PISA | Hemisphere | $2\pi r^2$ |
| MV annulus | Ellipse (or circle) | $\pi r_1 \times r_2$ or $0.785\,d_1 \times d_2$ |
| AV | Equilateral triangle | $0.433\,s^2$ |

## Stroke volume and cardiac output

In the absence of regurgitation, the total volume passing through a structure such as the MV or AV during diastole or systole represents stroke volume (SV, usually in ml). From Equation 16.2 the maximum instantaneous flow ($Q_{max} = CSA \times V_{max}$) can be calculated. The mean flow ($Q_{mean} = CSA \times V_{mean}$) could also be calculated in this way and used to derive the volume of blood passing through a structure during one pulse period (SV = $Q_{mean} \times t = CSA \times V_{mean} \times t$) but this volume is usually calculated as:

$$SV = CSA \times VTI \qquad \text{(Equation 16.3)}$$

Note that VTI is equivalent to $s$ in Figure 16.2, and equals $V_{mean} \times t$.

Stroke volume can be calculated from flow through the AV, the PV, the LVOT, the pulmonary artery (PA) or the MV, provided the structure is functionally normal. Tricuspid regurgitation is found in 90% of normal individuals (p.207), so the TV is unsuitable for this purpose. In the absence of regurgitation cardiac output (CO) is the product of SV and heart rate (HR):

$$CO = SV \times HR \qquad \text{(Equation 16.4)}$$

Cardiac index (CI) is obtained by dividing CO by body surface area (BSA):

$$CI = \frac{CO}{BSA} \qquad \text{(Equation 16.5)}$$

**Example 16.1:** cardiac output
Diameter of LVOT = 2.4 cm from the mid oesophageal AV long axis view (see Figure 10.1) in early systole; $VTI_{LVOT}$ = 20 cm from the transgastric long-axis view or the deep transgastric long axis view, using PW Doppler just proximal to the AV; heart rate = 70 beats per minute.
    Calculate cardiac output:

| | |
|---|---|
| $CSA_{LVOT} = \pi r^2 = 4.5\ cm^2$ | (see Table 16.1); |
| SV = 4.5 cm² × 20 cm = 90 cm³ | (= 90 ml: by Equation 16.3); |
| CO = 90 ml × 70 beats/min = 6300 ml/min or 6.3 l/min | (by Equation 16.4). |

Cardiac output measurement with TOE has been validated as a clinical alternative to thermodilution for the evaluation of the systolic function of the heart. Reasonable agreement between the two techniques has been shown using CW Doppler across the AV and PW Doppler positioned in the LVOT,[2,3] and using PW Doppler across a competent MV.[4] Experimental techniques have been developed to take into account the complexity of mitral flow geometry and dynamic changes in flow profile through the MV[5] but in practice the MV annulus is usually treated as an ellipse (see Table 16.1), or (more simply) as a circle.[1] The PA can also be used for cardiac output determination with TOE, but adequate views may be difficult to obtain.[6]

Other methods of estimating cardiac output and of evaluating systolic and diastolic function of the LV are discussed in Chapters 7 and 8.

# THE PRINCIPLE OF CONTINUITY OF FLOW

By the principle of continuity of flow, on average, in the absence of shunts, and under conditions of cardiovascular stability, net forward SV at any one part of the circulation must equal net forward SV at any other part (provided blood is neither added to nor removed from the system).

## Using the continuity principle to calculate valve orifice area from flow

This principle can be used to calculate the orifice areas of stenotic or regurgitant valves (with certain caveats in relation to prosthetic valves; p.196) in three distinct settings.

### Adjacent structures during the same phase of the cardiac cycle (e.g. AV and LVOT)

The assumption that flow through a stenotic valve is equal to flow proximal to the valve holds for maximum flow or stroke volume (and in theory for mean flow as well). Thus, for systole:

$$CSA_{AV} \times V_{max\text{-}AV} = CSA_{LVOT} \times V_{max\text{-}LVOT}$$

or

$$CSA_{AV} = CSA_{LVOT} \times \frac{V_{max\text{-}LVOT}}{V_{max\text{-}AV}} \qquad \text{(Equation 16.6)}$$

Similarly

$$CSA_{AV} = CSA_{LVOT} \times \frac{VTI_{LVOT}}{VTI_{AV}} \qquad \text{(Equation 16.7)}$$

The ratio of the maximum velocity in the LVOT to that through the AV ($^{V_{max\text{-}LVOT}}/_{V_{max\text{-}AV}}$) is called the **Doppler Velocity Index,** and has been used on its own as a simple index of the severity of aortic stenosis (p.197).

In theory, equivalent equations apply to the RVOT and PV, but these are less often used with TOE because the required views are more difficult to obtain, and because pulmonary stenosis is rare in adults.

**Example 16.2:** orifice area in aortic stenosis by continuity equation using VTI

In Example 16.1, $CSA_{LVOT} = 4.5$ cm$^2$ and $VTI_{LVOT} = 20$ cm were obtained; $VTI_{AV} = 70$ cm is now obtained with CW Doppler using the transgastric long axis view or the deep transgastric long axis view.

Calculate the effective orifice area of the AV:

$$CSA_{AV} \text{ cm}^2 = 4.5 \text{ cm}^2 \times \frac{20 \text{ cm}}{70 \text{ cm}} \qquad \text{(by Equation 16.7).}$$

Therefore

$$CSA_{AV} = 1.3 \text{ cm}^2 \quad \text{(i.e. mild aortic stenosis).}$$

**Example 16.3:** orifice area in aortic stenosis by continuity equation using maximum flow

In the same patient, CW Doppler is now used to obtain $V_{max-LVOT} = 1.5$ m/s and $V_{max-AV} = 5.2$ m/s using the "double-envelope technique" (see Figure 10.7); recall that $CSA_{LVOT} = 4.5$ cm$^2$.

Calculate the effective orifice area of the AV:

$$CSA_{AV} \text{ cm}^2 = 4.5 \text{ cm}^2 \times \frac{1.5 \text{ m/s}}{5.2 \text{ m/s}} \qquad \text{(by Equation 16.6);}$$

therefore

$$CSA_{AV} = 1.3 \text{ cm}^2 \quad \text{(in agreement with Example 16.2).}$$

## Non-adjacent structures on the same side of the heart during different phases of the cycle (e.g. the MV in diastole and the AV in systole)

At steady state over a reasonable period of time, the same net amount of blood must enter a given cardiac chamber as leaves it. Thus, for the LV, inflow in diastole must equal outflow in systole. In this situation the assumption of flow equality applies only to net forward stroke volumes (calculated using VTI); the maximum and mean flows (calculated using $V_{max}$ or $V_{mean}$), and indeed the entire velocity profile, will be different. Thus, *assuming no shunts or valvular regurgitation:*

$$CSA_{MV} \times VTI_{MV} \text{ in diastole} = CSA_{LVOT} \times VTI_{LVOT} \text{ in systole} \qquad \text{(Equation 16.8)}$$

If one of the structures is normal, its CSA can be calculated from the 2-D echo; the VTI can then be obtained for both (using Doppler), and the area of the other (i.e. the stenotic) orifice can be calculated. This method can be used in the evaluation of mitral stenosis, but it is unreliable if either mitral or aortic regurgitation is present (which, in the context of mitral stenosis, is often the case). Equation 16.6 or 16.7 would usually be preferable for assessing the severity of aortic stenosis.

**Example 16.4:** orifice area in mitral stenosis by continuity equation

Diameter of LVOT = 2.0 cm from the mid oesophageal AV long axis view; $VTI_{LVOT} = 20$ cm (in systole) from the transgastric long axis view or the deep transgastric long axis view, using CW Doppler; $VTI_{MV}$ (in diastole) = 65 cm from the mid oesophageal four-chamber view.

Calculate the effective orifice area of the MV:

$$CSA_{LVOT} = \pi r^2 = 3.14 \text{ cm}^2 \qquad \text{(see Table 16.1);}$$

$$CSA_{MV} \text{ cm}^2 \times 65 \text{ cm} = 3.14 \text{ cm}^2 \times 20 \text{ cm} \qquad \text{(by Equation 16.8).}$$

Therefore

$$CSA_{MV} = 1 \text{ cm}^2 \text{ (approx)} \qquad \text{(i.e. severe MS).}$$

If the valves are both regurgitant, mitral inflow + aortic regurgitant flow in diastole must equal aortic outflow + mitral regurgitant flow in systole. It is not possible to solve this equation but if only one of these valves is incompetent, and there are no shunts, then an equation applies from which the area of the effective regurgitant orifice (ERO) can be obtained. Thus, for mitral regurgitation:

$$CSA_{MV} \times VTI_{MV} \text{ in diastole}$$
$$= CSA_{LVOT} \times VTI_{LVOT} + ERO_{MV} \times VTI_{MV\text{-}regurgitant} \text{ in systole.} \qquad \text{(Equation 16.9)}$$

For aortic regurgitation:

$$CSA_{MV} \times VTI_{MV} + ERO_{AV} \times VTI_{AV\text{-}regurgitant} \text{ in diastole}$$
$$= CSA_{LVOT} \times VTI_{LVOT} \text{ in systole.} \qquad \text{(Equation 16.10)}$$

The **regurgitant volume** in isolated mitral or aortic regurgitation is the difference between the aortic outflow and the mitral inflow. The **regurgitant fraction** is the regurgitant volume divided by the forward flow through the regurgitant valve. A fraction greater than one-half is usually a sign of severe regurgitation.

### Structures on opposite sides of the heart (e.g. PA and MV)

The continuity equation can be applied to structures on opposite sides of the heart. For example, the PA diameter and the VTI are sometimes used to estimate stroke volume in the evaluation of mitral stenosis with transthoracic echocardiography[7] and, in the presence of a left-to-right intracardiac shunt, the pulmonary to systemic flow ratio ($Q_P/Q_S$) can be quantified by measuring stroke volume separately for the PA and for the LVOT. However, the required views of the PA are often difficult to obtain with TOE, and it is necessary to take an average of 5–10 measurements of flow to allow for left-to-right respiratory variation in stroke volume.

## PROXIMAL ISOVELOCITY SURFACE AREA

As blood flow converges towards a narrow orifice it accelerates. At any distance ($r$) from the orifice, the velocity ($V$) will be constant. Imagine an infinite series of hemispheres, of radius $r$, centred on the orifice; the velocity at the surface of any one of these hemispheres will be constant. Each of these surfaces is called a proximal isovelocity surface area (PISA). A PISA becomes clearly visible with colour flow Doppler at every point where the velocity exceeds the Nyquist limit (NL) or a multiple thereof, and aliasing occurs, represented by a marked change in colour (see Figure 16.1).

### Calculating the surface area of a PISA

It is usually possible to adjust the NL so that a particular PISA assumes the contour of a hemisphere (see Table 16.1). Then:

$$CSA_{PISA} = 2\pi r^2 \qquad \text{(Equation 16.11)}$$

If adjustment of the NL produces a PISA whose contour is too flat, its area will be overestimated by Equation 16.11, and if its contour is too tall its area will be underestimated. The morphology of the valve on which the PISA is formed may also alter the shape of the PISA. For example, a regurgitant MV will be closed at the time of PISA formation, so the base of the PISA will (theoretically) be flat (see Figure 16.1), whereas a stenotic MV will be partially open, and the base of the PISA will be cone-shaped (Figure 16.3). In the latter situation, if the angle between the two cusps is $\alpha$ (in degrees), then, by proportions:

$$CSA_{PISA} = 2\pi r^2 \times \frac{\alpha}{180} \qquad \text{(Equation 16.12)}$$

Obviously there is potential for error in the assumption that measurement of the angle in one plane reflects the shape of a symmetrical cone, and also in the assumption that no correction is required in the case of mitral (or aortic) incompetence.

## Using a PISA to calculate valve orifice area from flow

The velocity at the outermost PISA associated with aliasing will be the NL, which is under the control of the operator, and therefore known. Flow through this PISA will equal its surface area multiplied by the NL. In effect, the PISA and the valve orifice are adjacent structures during the same phase of the cardiac cycle (p.233), so the CSA of the valve can be calculated using the continuity equation:

$$CSA_{valve} \times V_{max\text{-}valve} = CSA_{PISA} \times NL$$

or

$$CSA_{valve} = CSA_{PISA} \times \frac{NL}{V_{max-valve}} \qquad \text{(Equation 16.13)}$$

The continuity equation can be used with a PISA formed at a stenotic MV in diastole (p.153), a regurgitant MV or regurgitant TV in systole (pp.144 and 211) and a regurgitant AV during diastole (p.168). In mitral stenosis the method can be used even in the

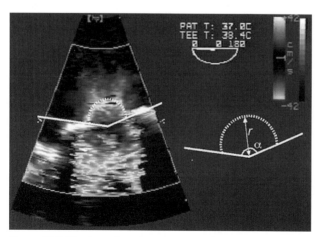

**Figure 16.3** The formation of more than one proximal isovelocity surface area (PISA) at a stenotic MV orifice: because the stenosis restricts the opening of the MV, the base of the PISA becomes cone-shaped, and a correction is necessary for the angle $\alpha$ between the valve leaflets.

presence of mitral regurgitation because the increased flow through the valve will apply equally to the PISA and the orifice.

**Example 16.5:** orifice area in mitral stenosis by PISA
From the mid oesophageal four-chamber view: PISA radius = 1.4 cm; MV angle = 120°; NL = 30 cm/s; $V_{\text{max-MV}}$ = 240 cm/s.
  Calculate the effective orifice area of the MV:

$$\text{CSA of PISA} = 2\pi r^2 \times \frac{120}{180} = 8.2 \text{ cm}^2 \qquad \text{(approx., by Equation 16.12)};$$

$$\text{CSA}_{\text{MV}} = 8.2 \text{ cm}^2 \times \frac{30 \text{ cm/s}}{240 \text{ cm/s}} \qquad \text{(by Equation 16.13)}.$$

Therefore

$$\text{CSA}_{\text{MV}} = 1 \text{ cm}^2 \qquad \text{(i.e. severe mitral stenosis)}.$$

## A simplified method for calculating the effective orifice area by PISA in mitral regurgitation

If the maximum regurgitant jet velocity is approximately 5 m/s (which is fairly typical of mitral regurgitation), a gradient from LV to LA of 100 mmHg can be assumed (by the simplified Bernoulli equation; see below). If the NL is set to 40 cm/s, then:

$$\text{CSA}_{\text{MV}} \text{ cm}^2 = \frac{(2\pi r^2 \text{ cm}^2 \times 40 \text{ cm/s})}{500 \text{ cm/s}} \qquad \text{(by Equation 16.13)}$$

Therefore

$$\text{CSA}_{\text{MV}} = 0.5 r^2 \text{ cm}^2 \qquad \text{(Equation 16.14)}$$

Since an effective regurgitant orifice >0.5 cm² implies severe regurgitation, it is possible to state the following simple rule of thumb:[8]

**If the NL is set to 40 cm/s, a PISA radius of ≥ 1 cm implies severe mitral regurgitation.**

# USING VELOCITY TO ESTIMATE PRESSURE GRADIENTS AND PRESSURES

## Pressure, flow and resistance

Flow ($Q$), assumed to be laminar, is a function of the pressure gradient ($P_1-P_2$) and the resistance ($R$):

$$P_1-P_2 = QR \qquad \text{(Equation 16.15)}$$

so that, if resistance is (effectively) zero (e.g. across an open normal valve), $P_1 = P_2$. This is true for widely open heart valves. Thus, in the absence of stenosis, pressures in the LV and aorta will be equal during systole, and pressures in the LA and LV will be equal during diastole (with similar equalities on the right side of the heart). Pressure gradients are often used to quantify the severity of valvular stenosis, but it is obvious from Equation 16.15 that, for any given resistance, the gradient will vary directly with flow, and may therefore be an unreliable index of the severity of valvular stenosis when a patient's haemodynamic state is unstable.

## The Bernoulli equation

The Bernoulli equation is based on the principle of conservation of energy. For a given volume, the work done by pressure (which is force per unit volume) in moving an incompressible fluid from one point to another along a rigid pipe is related to the gain in kinetic energy, the change in potential energy (a function of the difference in height between the two points) and work done overcoming viscous resistance. The kinetic energy at each of the two points is a function of the mass and the velocity squared. Mass per unit volume is density ($\rho$). Thus, where $P_1$ and $P_2$ are the proximal and distal pressures respectively, and where $V_1$ and $V_2$ are the proximal and distal velocities: $P_1 - P_2 \propto \frac{1}{2}\rho\,(V_2^2 - V_1^2)$. In the full form of the equation terms are added to allow for acceleration, viscous resistance and potential energy. For short orifices, viscous resistance is negligible and so is the change in potential energy across the orifice. Also, at the point of maximum velocity in systole or diastole, acceleration becomes zero as it changes from positive to negative. The density of blood can be taken as 1. Hence for maximum velocities, if $P_1 - P_2$ is expressed as $\Delta P$, and if a conversion factor is added for measuring velocity in m/s and pressure in mmHg, the Bernoulli equation can be reduced to:

$$\Delta P = 4(V_2^2 - V_1^2) \qquad \text{(Equation 16.16)}$$

If the proximal velocity is small compared with the distal velocity it can be ignored. For most purposes this provides the simplified Bernoulli equation:

$$\Delta P = 4V^2 \qquad \text{(Equation 16.17)}$$

### Important points about the simplified Bernoulli equation

Strictly speaking, the Bernoulli equation may not be applicable to pulsatile blood flow through compliant vessels and chambers, but in practice it has been found to give very accurate estimations of pressure gradients in various clinical situations. However, the Bernoulli equation does not apply to normal valves (where resistance is effectively zero), or to long tubular stenoses and extreme pinpoint stenoses (because viscous friction loss becomes significant). In severe anaemia, reduced blood viscosity may result in the overestimation of pressure gradients. With prosthetic valves, there may be some resistance to valve opening, and acceleration may be significant. With two stenoses in series (e.g. a valvular and a subvalvular stenosis), and with certain prosthetic valves, **distal pressure recovery** may occur (p.197). Changes in cardiac output will have a significant effect on the gradient across a stenotic valve (by Equation 16.15). The calculation of orifice area by the continuity equation is independent of flow, and should therefore be preferable for the evaluation of the severity of a stenotic lesion, but it involves several measurements and tends to be more demanding technically. If valvular regurgitation is present, total forward flow through a valve will be increased, and this will increase the pressure gradient for any given degree of stenosis; under these circumstances the continuity equation will also be unreliable for quantifying a stenotic orifice, except in relation to a PISA (pp.236–237).

The simplified Bernoulli equation has been found to apply to mean velocities as well as maximum velocities, but the mean pressure gradient should be obtained from the mean of the squared velocities (i.e. $\Delta P_{mean} = (4V_1^2 + 4V_2^2 + \ldots + 4V_n^2)/n$), not the square of the mean velocity.

Note carefully that units are embedded in the constant of the simplified Bernoulli equation. Therefore velocity must be in m/s if pressure is to be in mmHg. Note also that it is safe to use Equation 16.17 when the proximal velocity ($V_1$ in Equation 16.16) is <1 m/s (because squaring a number less than 1 reduces it), and reasonable accuracy can be expected provided $V_1$ < 1.5 m/s but if $V_1$ > 1.5 m/s Equation 16.16 should be used. The transvalvular velocity ($V_2$) is sometimes used directly as an index of the severity of valvular stenosis, or as evidence of an elevated pressure gradient (see, for example, pp.163 and 196). This may be misleading if $V_1$ > 1.5 m/s.

## The Venturi effect

It follows from Bernoulli's equation that high kinetic energy will be associated with low pressure. Thus the fast-moving air over an aerofoil is associated with low pressure, which creates lift, and the passage of fluid through a Venturi will generate suction. This is the mechanism of systolic anterior motion of the anterior leaflet of the MV in hypertrophic obstructive cardiomyopathy. When blood passes through a stenotic valve, the kinetic energy is highest and the pressure lowest at the narrowest part of the stenosis.

# ESTIMATING THE PRESSURE GRADIENT ACROSS A STENOTIC VALVE

## Aortic stenosis

In aortic stenosis, maximum and mean gradients derived echocardiographically correlate well with the same gradients measured during cardiac catheterisation. However, the difference between the maximum LV and maximum aortic pressures reported by catheter laboratories (often called the "peak to peak" gradient) is slightly smaller than the maximum gradient calculated from the echo-derived maximum velocity. In fact, the peak-to-peak gradient, measured at catheterisation, does not exist in real time, because pressure in the aorta peaks after pressure in the LV. The difference is of no significance, provided the type of gradient is specified precisely.

In the case of native AV stenosis, $\Delta P_{mean}$ is linearly correlated with $\Delta P_{max}$.[7] One expression of this relationship is:

$$\Delta P_{mean} = 2.4 \times (V_{max})^2 \qquad \text{(Equation 16.18)}$$

**Example 16.6:** aortic stenosis
$V_{max-AV}$ = 3 m/s and $V_{max-LVOT}$ = 1 m/s in the deep transgastric long axis view (see Figure 10.7).
Calculate maximum gradient:

$$\Delta P_{max} = 4 \times 3^2 = 36 \text{ mmHg} \qquad \text{(by Equation 16.17).}$$

It is usually reasonable to assume that $V_1$ (the proximal velocity, which in this case is the velocity in the LVOT) is < 1 m/s (approximately), but it is important always to check that this is the case; if $V_1$ >1.5 m/s (e.g. because of LVOT narrowing) it is safer to use Equation 16.16.

**Example 16.7:** aortic stenosis with proximal velocity >1 m/s
As in Example 16.6, but $V_{max-LVOT}$ = 1.5 m/s from PW Doppler in the deep transgastric long axis view:

$$\Delta P_{max} = 4 \times (3^2 - 1.5^2) = 27 \text{ mmHg} \qquad \text{(by Equation 16.16).}$$

## Mitral stenosis

It is usually straightforward to calculate the mean and maximum pressure gradients with TOE in mitral stenosis (p.152), but the effects of cardiac output (p.238) should be kept in mind.

## Pulmonary stenosis and tricuspid stenosis

The pressure gradient across a stenotic TV or PV (p.213) can be estimated in the same way as the gradient across a stenotic MV or AV, using the simplified Bernoulli equation.

# ESTIMATING UNKNOWN PRESSURES FROM KNOWN PRESSURES

## Right heart pressures

In *systole*, the gradient across a *regurgitant* TV can be used to calculate RV systolic pressure assuming RA pressure is known:

$$\Delta P_{\text{RV-RA}} = 4(V_{\text{TV-regurg}})^2 \qquad \text{(by Equation 16.17)}$$

$$P_{\text{RV-systolic}} = P_{\text{RA}} + \Delta P_{\text{RV-RA}} \qquad \text{(Equation 16.19)}$$

If the PV is normal, the resistance across it will be negligible and PA pressure will equal RV pressure (by Equation 16.15). If pulmonary stenosis were present (an unlikely scenario), then the calculation of PA systolic pressure would need to take this into account:

$$\Delta P_{\text{PA-RV}} = 4(V_{\text{PV}})^2 \qquad \text{(by Equation 16.17)}$$

$$P_{\text{PA-systolic}} = P_{\text{RV-systolic}} - \Delta P_{\text{PA-RV}} \qquad \text{(Equation 16.20)}$$

Similarly, in *diastole*, RV pressure will equal RA pressure if the TV is normal. On a CW Doppler recording of regurgitant velocity through the PV, a shoulder can be identified late in diastole (the waveform is similar to that seen in aortic regurgitation – see Figure 16.5); this can be used to estimate end diastolic PA pressure (p.208):

$$\Delta P_{\text{PA-RV}} = 4(V_{\text{PV}})^2 \qquad \text{(by Equation 16.17)}$$

$$P_{\text{PA-end diastolic}} = P_{\text{RA}} + \Delta P_{\text{PA-RV(end diastolic)}} \qquad \text{(Equation 16.21)}$$

**Example 16.8:** RV and PA pressures in systole from central venous pressure with normal PV
RA pressure = 5 mmHg from central venous pressure (CVP) line; maximum transtricuspid regurgitant velocity = 2 m/s from mid oesophageal RV inflow–outflow view (see Figure 13.2).
Calculate the RV systolic pressure and PA systolic pressure:

$$\Delta P_{\text{RV-RA}} = 16 \text{ mmHg} \qquad \text{(by Equation 16.17);}$$

$$P_{\text{RV-systolic}} = 21 \text{ mmHg} \qquad \text{(by Equation 16.19).}$$

During systole, RV pressure = PA pressure (if the PV is normal); therefore

$$P_{\text{PA-systolic}} = 21 \text{ mmHg}$$

## Left heart pressures

Equations equivalent to those described above may be applied to the left side of the heart. In particular, LA pressure may be estimated in the presence of a mitral regurgitant jet on the basis that LV systolic pressure is equal to arterial systolic pressure:

$$\Delta P_{\text{LV-LA}} = 4(V_{\text{MV-regurg}})^2 \qquad \text{(by Equation 16.17)}$$

$$P_{\text{LA}} = P_{\text{LV-systolic}} - \Delta P_{\text{LV-LA}} \qquad \text{(Equation 16.22)}$$

LV end diastolic pressure may be estimated from the jet of aortic regurgitation using an equation equivalent to Equation 16.21. However, results using transthoracic echocardiography have correlated relatively poorly with catheterisation values,[9] in part because peripheral arterial pressure may not equal central aortic pressure in the presence of aortic regurgitation. Other methods of estimating LA pressure with TOE are described in Chapter 8 (p.126).

**Example 16.9:** LV end diastolic pressure from diastolic blood pressure in the presence of aortic regurgitation
End diastolic AV regurgitant velocity = 4 m/s in the deep transgastric long axis view (see Figure 16.5); diastolic blood pressure = 75 mmHg from an arterial line.
  Calculate LV end diastolic pressure:

$$\Delta P_{\text{Aorta-LV}} = 64 \text{ mmHg} \qquad \text{(by Equation 16.17)};$$

$$P_{\text{LVED}} = 11 \text{ mmHg} \qquad (75 - 64 \text{ mmHg}).$$

## Ventricular septal defects

The simplified Bernoulli equation can be used to calculate the pressure gradient across a ventricular septal defect, and thereby to estimate RV pressure (and hence PA pressure) from LV systolic pressure (which equals aortic systolic pressure). However, depending on the location of the defect, it may be difficult to get a view with TOE in which the Doppler beam can be aligned adequately with flow. To some extent the presence of a high velocity across a VSD suggests that the orifice is restrictive, and that elevated right heart pressures are therefore unlikely (p.226).

# USING PRESSURE DECELERATION TO ESTIMATE VALVE AREAS

Pressure *acceleration* is used in the evaluation of systolic function ($^{dP}/_{dt}$; p.107) and can be used to estimate mean PA pressure (the pulmonary acceleration time: p.208). Pressure *deceleration* is the basis of the pressure half-time method of estimating valve orifice area in mitral stenosis and aortic regurgitation.

## Pressure deceleration and the pressure half-time

During diastole the rate of decrease in the pressure gradient between the LA and the LV (in mitral stenosis), or between the aorta and the LV (in aortic regurgitation), is a function of the severity of the respective valve lesions and to a lesser extent the compliance of the LV. In each case, this deceleration in pressure can be obtained from the slope of the velocity–time curve (Figures 16.4 and 16.5). The time from maximum to zero velocity will be the same as the time from maximal to zero pressure gradient, and is the

**deceleration time** (DT). In aortic regurgitation, as the lesion becomes more severe and the effective regurgitant orifice increases in size, DT will decrease. In mitral stenosis, as the lesion becomes more severe, the effective valvular orifice will become smaller, and DT will increase. However the *deceleration* of the pressure gradient is less dependent than DT on flow[7] and is preferable as an index of lesion severity.

The deceleration of the pressure gradient has been quantified as the time in milliseconds (ms) for the gradient to fall from any particular value ($P$) to half that value ($P/2$). This period is called the **pressure half-time** ($Pt_{1/2}$). Any value of the pressure gradient (calculated from the corresponding transvalvular velocity) could be used in the calculation of $Pt_{1/2}$ but the maximum is convenient. Because pressure is related to the square of velocity, the velocity associated with $P/2$ is obtained by dividing the velocity associated with $P$ by $\sqrt{2}$ ($= 1.4$), or multiplying it by the reciprocal of $\sqrt{2}$ ($= 0.7$):

$$V_{P/2} = 0.7 \ V_P \qquad \text{(Equation 16.23)}$$

$Pt_{1/2}$ is therefore defined as the time between $V_{max}$ and $0.7 \ V_{max}$ (Figures 16.4 and 16.5).

Although it is derived from similar principles, the interpretation of $Pt_{1/2}$ differs considerably between mitral stenosis and aortic regurgitation.

Mitral stenosis

In mitral stenosis (Figure 16.4) $Pt_{1/2}$, lengthens as lesion severity increases, is relatively independent of flow in any individual patient,[7] and is clinically useful (p.152).

It has been shown experimentally that (with CSA in cm$^2$ and $Pt_{1/2}$ in m/s):

$$CSA_{MV} = \frac{220}{Pt_{1/2}} \qquad \text{(Equation 16.24)}$$

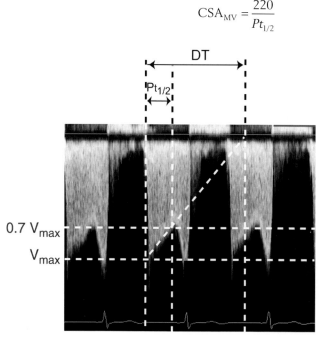

**Figure 16.4** Estimation of pressure half-time ($Pt_{1/2}$) in mitral stenosis (see text for details; DT = deceleration time; $V_{max}$ = maximum velocity).

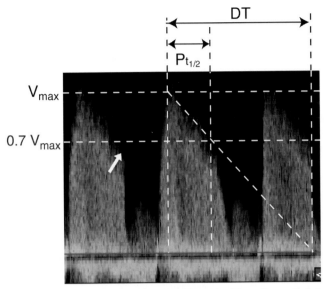

**Figure 16.5** Estimation of pressure half-time ($Pt_{1/2}$) in aortic regurgitation (DT = deceleration time; $V_{max}$ = maximum velocity). Note the shoulder late in diastole (arrow); this velocity can be used to estimate left ventricular end diastolic pressure (see text for details).

Furthermore, a MV orifice area $<1.0$ cm$^2$ is considered severely stenotic (see Table 9.6) and this result will be obtained if $Pt_{1/2} > 220$ ms. It has also been shown experimentally that $Pt_{1/2} = DT \times 0.29$; since $220/0.29 = 759$, it follows that orifice area $= 759/DT$, and stenosis is likely to be severe if DT $> 759$ ms (or 750 ms approximately). However, because DT is more dependent on flow than $Pt_{1/2}$, Equation 16.24 is preferable.

A number of factors may reduce the usefulness of the $Pt_{1/2}$ in the evaluation of the severity of mitral stenosis. In a normal MV, the $Pt_{1/2}$ is primarily a function of the compliance of the LV, and is not useful for estimation of orifice area. Although more robust than the transvalvular pressure gradient in relation to flow, $Pt_{1/2}$ is influenced by increased cardiac output (e.g. with inotropic support or volume loading), which tends to shorten it and therefore increase the estimated orifice area. Any cause of elevated LV end diastolic pressure (including mitral regurgitation) will also tend to shorten the $Pt_{1/2}$. More than mild aortic regurgitation may shorten the $Pt_{1/2}$, because the pressure in the LV will increase more quickly. Severe aortic regurgitation may impair the opening of the anterior leaflet of the MV, leading to a functional (i.e. misleading) increase in $Pt_{1/2}$ and therefore in the apparent severity of the stenosis. $Pt_{1/2}$ is shortened by tachycardia and restrictive filling, and lengthened by impaired relaxation. The compliances of the LV and LA change immediately after valvuloplasty, so $Pt_{1/2}$ should not be used to evaluate valvular function until several days after this operation. $Pt_{1/2}$ is unreliable as a measure of stenosis in mechanical valves (p.197). Atrioventricular block alters the profile of the mitral inflow E wave, making the $Pt_{1/2}$ method unreliable.

## Aortic regurgitation

In aortic regurgitation (Figure 16.5) $Pt_{1/2}$ shortens as lesion severity increases. The validation of the use of $Pt_{1/2}$ is less secure than in mitral stenosis (p.166). Nevertheless, severe aortic regurgitation is associated with DT $< 1000$ ms and $Pt_{1/2} < 300$ ms. $Pt_{1/2}$ is shortened by increased systemic vascular resistance and reduced LV compliance, either of which may lead to overestimation of the severity of the lesion. The $Pt_{1/2}$ is an unreliable index of aortic regurgitation in the presence of MV disease.

## TECHNICAL DETAILS IN THE MEASUREMENT OF VELOCITIES AND DIMENSIONS

For all measurements, data from three to five cardiac cycles (more in the presence of atrial fibrillation) and from more than one view should ideally be obtained. For a dimension the average should be taken. When measuring velocity with Doppler (whether for use in the continuity equation or for the calculation of a pressure gradient) the ultrasound beam should be parallel to the direction of blood flow in all planes, so more than one view should be examined, and the view providing the *highest* velocity used (p.35).

With 2-D imaging it is important that the ultrasound plane is orthogonal to the structure, and passes through its centre (Figure 16.6). Any error in the measurement of the dimensions of a structure will be magnified when squared during calculation of an area. In theory measurements are most accurately taken from leading edge to leading edge (see Figure 2.12), but in practice leading edges may be difficult to identify correctly on 2-D imaging, and structures are commonly measured from inner edge to inner edge.

With PW Doppler the outer edge of the most dense or brightest portion of the tracing (the modal velocity – the velocity of most of the red cells) should be used. With CW Doppler the outer edge of the envelope should be used.[1]

The dimensions of cardiac structures vary with the cardiac cycle, so the Doppler and 2-D measurements used in the continuity equation need to be made at the same time, as well as at the same place. The end of diastole should be timed from the R wave of the ECG, or from the moment of initial coaptation of the MV leaflets. The end of systole should be timed from the moment of initial closure of the AV, or from the smallest visible ventricular size. For determination of stroke volume the LVOT should be measured in early systole (in the mid oesophageal long axis view), and the MV annulus in mid-diastole (p.63). The measurements of velocity and VTI are described on pages 162 and 63–65.

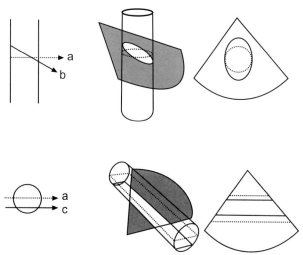

**Figure 16.6** Errors in the measurement of dimensions with TOE. Beam a is well placed in each case; beam b is not orthogonal to the structure; beam c does not pass through the centre of the structure.

# REFERENCES

1. Quinones MA, Otto CM, Stoddard M, et al. Recommendations for quantification of Doppler echocardiography: a report from the Doppler Quantification Task Force of the Nomenclature and Standards Committee of the American Society of Echocardiography. *Journal of the American Society of Echocardiography* 2002;15:167–183.
2. Royse CF, Royse AG, Blake DW, et al. Measurement of cardiac output by transesophageal echocardiography: a comparison of two Doppler methods with thermodilution. *Anaesthesia and Intensive Care* 1999;27:586–590.
3. Perrino AC Jr, Harris SN, Luther MA. Intraoperative determination of cardiac output using multiplane transesophageal echocardiography: a comparison to thermodilution. *Anesthesiology* 1998;89:350–357.
4. Ryan T, Page R, Bouchier-Hayes D, et al. Trans-oesophageal pulsed wave Doppler measurement of cardiac output during major vascular surgery: comparison with the thermodilution technique. *British Journal of Anaesthesia* 1992;69:101–104.
5. Rusk RA, Li X-N, Mori Y, et al. Direct quantification of transmitral flow volume with dynamic 3-dimensional digital color Doppler: a validation study in an animal model. *Journal of the American Society of Echocardiography* 2002;15:55–62.
6. Savino JS, Troianos CA, Aukburg S, et al. Measurement of pulmonary blood flow with transesophageal two-dimensional and Doppler echocardiography. *Anesthesiology* 1991;75:445–451.
7. Otto CM. *Textbook of Clinical Echocardiography*, 2nd ed. Philadelphia: WB Saunders Company, 2000.
8. Pu M, Prior DL, Fan X, et al. Calculation of mitral regurgitant orifice area with use of a simplified proximal convergence method: initial clinical application. *Journal of the American Society of Echocardiography* 2001;14:180–185.
9. Beyer RW, Ramirez M, Josephson MA, et al. Correlation of continuous-wave Doppler assessment of chronic aortic regurgitation with hemodynamics and angiography. *American Journal of Cardiology* 1987;60:852–856.

# Appendix 1.

# Cleaning and Care of the Probe

Appropriate care of TOE probes is essential to prolonging the life of the equipment and maintaining patient safety. For each type of probe the manufacturer's specific recommendations regarding cleaning, disinfection, storage and maintenance must be followed. However, the following comments are generally applicable.

Most TOE probes are designed for **high-level disinfection** (or occasionally sterilisation) in 2% or greater glutaraldehyde solutions, such as Metricide and Omnicide (devices that are used against intact skin require **low-level disinfection** and devices that are directly exposed to blood or compromised tissue require a sterile sheath or formal **sterilisation**). In some cases, non-glutaraldehyde-based solutions (e.g. Cidex OPA) may be used for high-level disinfection (but not sterilisation) on the manufacturer's specific recommendations.

Glutaraldehyde is used for the cold high-level disinfection or sterilisation of heat-sensitive equipment. It is toxic by direct contact and by inhalation. Symptoms of toxicity include throat and lung irritation, wheezing, headaches, nausea, burning eyes and rashes. Additional information is available from the Centers for Disease Control website (http://www.cdc.gov/niosh/2001-115.html) or product manufacturers.

Glutaraldehyde should be used only in a dedicated cleaning facility with appropriate ventilation and chemical storage and disposal capabilities. The glutaraldehyde bath should be kept in a sealed container under a fume hood at room temperature. Staff should be appropriately trained in the safe handling of glutaraldehyde (along with the principles of infection control and universal precautions), which should include the use of protective goggles, splash shields and gloves (nitrile or butyl rubber – not latex) during direct contact.

The probe should be cleaned and high-level disinfected (or sterilised) as follows:

- Wipe the acoustic coupling gel from the probe.
- Remove any organic matter from the shaft of the probe using soapy water or an approved enzymatic cleaner such as Metrizyme.
- Wipe down the handle of the probe and connector with a 70% alcohol solution. Avoid wetting or immersing these areas because, for most probes, the steering mechanism and connector are not sealed and can be damaged by water or cleaning fluids.
- Rinse the shaft of the probe in water.
- High-level disinfect the shaft of the probe by immersing in glutaraldehyde (or similar) for 45 minutes, or per instructions. For sterilisation, immerse for 10 hours or according to the manufacturer's instructions.
- Remove from the glutaraldehyde solution and thoroughly rinse the shaft of the probe in water, as per manufacturer's instructions.
- Allow to air dry in a hanging storage facility.
- Do not routinely soak the probes for extended periods (e.g. overnight) as this will, with time, weaken the outer sheath.

The following general precautions should also be observed to minimise injury to patients and prolong the life of the probe:

- Before use, inspect the probe for damage (particularly defects in the outer sheath) or inadequacy of cleaning (e.g. secretions or blood on the handle).
- Ensure that the probe is dry to prevent potential patient exposure to glutaraldehyde.
- When inserting, advancing or withdrawing the probe ensure the flexion lock is released and the probe is in a neutral position. The probe should also be stored with the tip in a neutral position.
- Do not bend or coil the shaft of the probe in a circle of less than 30 cm in diameter.
- Keep the probe straight and avoid movement during the synchronisation process with the ultrasound machine.
- A bite guard should always be used to prevent damage to the probe. In edentulous patients, it is prudent to use a bite guard to prevent pressure contact on the gums by the shaft of the probe.
- The probe should undergo regular current leakage testing (at least every 6 months). Failure in this test may be the first sign of a defect in the protective covering of the probe.
- Contact with certain antibacterial skin cleaning solutions that can damage the probe (e.g. phenol, benzoyl peroxide or benzothonium chloride) should be avoided. The acoustic coupling medium should be glycol, glycerol or water based; gels containing acetone, methanol or mineral oil can damage the probe.

In addition to the care of the probe, the echocardiography machine itself requires regular cleaning, disinfection, servicing and software updates according to the manufacturer's recommendations.

# Appendix 2.

## Normal Values

Values provided below are from a range of sources. Wherever possible 2-D TOE values are given. In situations where these values are not available, or are poorly documented, transthoracic echocardiography (TTE) or M-mode values are given.

| Normal 2-D dimensions | | |
|---|---|---|
| | Normal (± SD) (cm) | Range (cm) |
| **Aorta and aortic valve (end diastole)** | | |
| LVOT (TTE) | 1.9 (0.2) | 1.4–2.6 |
| Aortic valve annulus (TTE) | 1.9 (0.2) | 1.4–2.6 |
| Sinus of Valsalva (TTE) | 2.8 (0.3) | 2.1–3.5 |
| Sinotubular junction (TTE) | 2.4 (0.4) | 1.7–3.4 |
| Ascending aorta (TTE) | 2.6 (0.3) | 2.1–3.4 |
| Descending thoracic (proximal) | 2.1 (0.4) | 1.4–3.0 |
| **Pulmonary artery (end diastole)** | | |
| Pulmonary valve annulus (TTE) | 1.5 (0.3) | 1.0–2.2 |
| Main pulmonary artery (TTE) | 1.8 (0.3) | 0.9–2.9 |
| **Left atrium (MO four-chamber view)** | | |
| Length (apex to mitral annulus) | 3.8 (0.6) | 2.0–5.2 |
| Width (maximum dimension) | 3.9 (0.7) | 2.4–5.2 |
| **Right atrium (MO four-chamber view)** | | |
| Length (apex to tricuspid annulus) | 3.8 (0.5) | 2.8–5.2 |
| Width (maximum dimension) | 3.8 (0.6) | 2.9–5.3 |
| **Left ventricle (TG mid SAX view)** | | |
| End systolic dimension (A–P) | 2.8 (0.6) | 1.8–4.0 |
| End diastolic dimension (A–P) | 4.3 (0.7) | 2.3–5.4 |
| End diastolic area | | 10.6–17.8 cm$^2$ |
| Fractional area change | | 36–64% |
| Ejection fraction | | 55–75% |
| LV wall thickness (end diastole, M-mode, TTE) | | |
| Septum | <1.3 (male) | <1.2 (female) |
| Posterior wall | <1.2 (male) | <1.1 (female) |

| Normal 2-D dimensions (continued) | | |
|---|---|---|
| | **Normal (± SD) (cm)** | **Range (cm)** |
| **Mitral annulus (end systole)** | | |
| Anterior–posterior (MO LAX) | 3.02 | 2–3.6 |
| Intercommissural (MO commissural) | 3.72 | 7–4.6 |
| Tricuspid annulus (TTE) | | 1.3–2.8 |
| MO = mid oesophageal, TG = transgastric, SAX = short axis view, LAX = long axis view, A–P = anterior-to-posterior dimension. | | |

# REFERENCES INCLUDE:

Cohen GI et al. *Journal of the American Society of Echocardiography* 1995;8:221–230.

Triulzi M et al. *Echocardiography* 1984;1:403–426.

Devereux RB et al. *Journal of the American College of Cardiologists* 1984;4:1222–1230.

Malkowski MJ et al. *Journal of Heart Valve Disease* 1996;6:54–59.

Fyrenius A et al. *Journal of Heart Valve Disease* 2001;10:146–152.

Schiller NB et al. *Journal of the American Society of Echocardiography* 1989;2:358–367.

| NORMAL DOPPLER VELOCITIES | | |
|---|---|---|
| **Transmitral inflow** | | |
| $E_{max}$ (TTE) | $0.63 \pm 0.10$ m/s$_{(40–49 \, years)}$ | $0.55 \pm 0.11$ m/s$_{(60–69 \, years)}$ |
| $A_{max}$ (TTE) | $0.45 \pm 0.08$ m/s$_{(40–49 \, years)}$ | $0.55 \pm 0.10$ m/s$_{(60–69 \, years)}$ |
| $E/A$ ratio (TTE) | $1.44 \pm 0.26_{(40–49 \, years)}$ | $1.03 \pm 0.26_{(60–69 \, years)}$ |
| $E_{dec}$ (TTE) | $170 \pm 20$ ms$_{(<50 \, years)}$ | $210 \pm 36$ ms$_{(>50 \, years)}$ |
| **Pulmonary vein** | | |
| $S_{max}$ | $0.58 \pm 15$ m/s$_{(40–49 \, years)}$ | $0.64 \pm 19$ m/s$_{(>60 \, years)}$ |
| $D_{max}$ | $0.53 \pm 10$ m/s$_{(40–49 \, years)}$ | $0.44 \pm 13$ m/s$_{(>60 \, years)}$ |
| $S/D$ ratio | $1.13 \pm 0.4_{(40–49 \, years)}$ | $1.57 \pm 0.57_{(>60 \, years)}$ |
| $A_{max}$ | $0.24 \pm 0.09$ m/s$_{(40–49 \, years)}$ | $0.25 \pm 0.06$ m/s$_{(>60 \, years)}$ |
| **Transtricuspid inflow** | | |
| $E_{max}$ (TTE) | $0.41 \pm 0.08$ m/s$_{(>50 \, years)}$ | |
| $A_{max}$ (TTE) | $0.33 \pm 0.08$ m/s$_{(>50 \, years)}$ | |
| $E_{dec}$ (TTE) | $198 \pm 23$ ms$_{(>50 \, years)}$ | |
| $E/A$ ratio (TTE) | $1.34 \pm 0.4_{(>50 \, years)}$ | |

| NORMAL DOPPLER VELOCITIES (continued) | |
| --- | --- |
| **Superior vena cava** | |
| $S_{max}$ (TTE) | $0.41 \pm 0.012$ m/s$_{(>50 \text{ years})}$ |
| $D_{max}$ (TTE) | $0.22 \pm 0.05$ m/s$_{(>50 \text{ years})}$ |
| **Ascending aorta and left ventricular outflow tract** | |
| Peak velocity (ascending aorta) (TTE) | 1.0–1.7 m/s |
| Peak velocity (LVOT) (TTE) | $1.0 \pm 0.2$ m/s |

# REFERENCES INCLUDE:

Klein AL et al. *Journal of the American Society of Echocardiography* 1990;3:237.

De Marchi SF et al. *Heart* 2001;85:23–29.

Benjamin EJ et al. *American Journal of Cardiology* 1992;7: 508–515.

European Study Group on Diastolic Heart Failure. *European Heart Journal* 1998:19:990–1003.

Weymen AE. *Principles and Practice of Echocardiography*, 2nd ed. Philadelphia: Lea and Febiger, 1994.

# Interpretation of Echo Data

A full discussion of the statistical basis of clinical decision-making is beyond the scope of this book. However, the clinical use of TOE is underpinned by data from research that compares this modality with other methods of measurement, such as pulmonary artery catheterisation or cardiac catheterisation. It is therefore important to understand in principle how such comparative studies should be interpreted and how the information about a particular test (e.g. the use of TOE to determine the presence of severe aortic stenosis) should be applied in practice. The purpose of this appendix is to remind readers of some concepts important in the interpretation of echocardiographic data; for more detail, the text by Altman is strongly recommended.[1]

## THE INTERPRETATION OF DIAGNOSTIC TESTS

Assume $n$ patients are tested for a pathological condition, of which some have the condition and some do not. The test will be positive in some and negative in others. Unless the test is perfect, there will be some false positives and false negatives. This can be represented in a table in which $a + c$ patients have the disease, $b + d$ do not, $a + b$ test positive and $c + d$ test negative:

|  | Pathological condition | | |
|---|---|---|---|
|  | Present | Absent | Total |
| Test positive | $a$ | $b$ | $a+b$ |
| Test negative | $c$ | $d$ | $c+d$ |
| Total | $a+c$ | $b+d$ | $n$ |

**Sensitivity** $= a/(a+c)$ and is the proportion of patients with the condition who will be correctly identified by the test. **Specificity** $= d/(b+d)$ and is the proportion of patients without the condition who will be correctly identified by the test. **Positive predictive valve** $= a/(a+b)$ and is the proportion of patients in whom the test is positive who have the condition (i.e. the truly positive proportion of all positives). **Negative predictive valve** $= d/(c+d)$ and is the proportion of patients in whom the test is negative who do not have the condition (i.e. the truly negative proportion of all negatives). The **observed prevalence** of the condition in this tested group of patients is $(a+c)/n$. Prevalence is the proportion of patients in a population with a condition at a specified time. **Incidence** is the proportion who will develop the condition (or outcome) during a specified time.

In clinical practice we are generally in the position of knowing the result of a test (e.g. a particular measurement with TOE) and of wanting to understand the implications of this for the patient: in other words, we are primarily interested in the predictive values.

Unfortunately, these are a function of prevalence (or incidence, as the case may be). A positive test is more likely to be true in a group of patients with a high prevalence of the condition of interest than in a group with a low prevalence. In theory, Baye's theorem, and the concepts of **prior** and **posterior probability,** can be applied. However, in the context of practical perioperative TOE, the pragmatic approach is to recognise that the prevalence of a condition in a particular study may well be different from that in a clinician's own practice, and that this may make a substantial difference to the interpretation of a positive or negative finding. Therefore, in this book we have avoided undue emphasis on specific findings from individual studies and stressed the importance of integrating clinical information from many sources. It is much more likely that a particular inference from findings on TOE will be correct if other information has already placed the patient into a subgroup with a high prevalence of the condition of interest. Importantly, the converse is also true – unexpected findings in the absence of any other evidence of the suggested problem may well be misleading.

## AGREEMENT BETWEEN METHODS OF MEASUREMENT

We seldom know the absolute value of the variable we are trying to measure (cardiac output is a case in point), so a new method of measurement (such as TOE) is often assessed on the basis of whether it can be used interchangeably with an established method (e.g. thermodilution in the estimation of cardiac output). It is easy to forget that the reliability of the established method may be less than satisfactory. It is also possible to confuse *correlation* with *agreement*. **Correlation** simply measures the degree of association between two quantities. There may be a high degree of association in the presence of considerable **bias**. More problematically, a high degree of correlation may simply reflect a degree of variation in subjects that is substantial in comparison with the variation in test results. Studies comparing TOE with other methods of measurement should assess **agreement**. Differences between the results of two methods should ideally be distributed uniformly around zero; if they are not, then their mean is a measure of bias. The repeatability of any given method is also very important, and studies should include replicate measures to quantify this. The judgement of how well one test functions in comparison with another is not a matter of hypothesis testing, but rather one of quantifying variation and then making a clinical judgement about its acceptability. Furthermore, a test will often be much more accurate in skilled hands than in the hands of a beginner, so practitioners should validate their own skills against those of an expert before relying on any particular technique of measurement with TOE.

## REFERENCE

1. Altman DG. *Practical Statistics for Medical Research.* London: Chapman & Hall, 1991.

# Index

Page numbers followed by f indicate figures
Page numbers followed by t indicate tables